Statistics for Biology and Health

Series Editors:
Mitchell Gail
Jonathan M. Samet
Anastasios Tsiatis
Wing Wong

For further volumes:
http://www.springer.com/series/2848

Weili He • José Pinheiro • Olga M. Kuznetsova
Editors

Practical Considerations for Adaptive Trial Design and Implementation

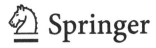 Springer

Editors
Weili He
Department of Clinical Biostatistics
Merck & Co., Inc.
Rahway, NJ, USA

José Pinheiro
Johnson & Johnson
Raritan, NJ, USA

Olga M. Kuznetsova
Department of Clinical Biostatistics
Merck & Co., Inc.
Rahway, NJ, USA

ISSN 1431-8776   ISSN 2197-5671(electronic)
ISBN 978-1-4939-1099-1   ISBN 978-1-4939-1100-4 (eBook)
DOI 10.1007/978-1-4939-1100-4
Springer New York Heidelberg Dordrecht London

Library of Congress Control Number: 2014949155

Printed on acid-free paper

Springer is part of Springer Science+Business Media (www.springer.com)

Preface

A great deal of progress has been made in the past couple of decades with regard to research and publications focused on technical and methodological aspects of planning and analyzing adaptive design. The major impetus behind the interest in the use of adaptive designs is the increased efficiency they offer, resulting in savings of cost and time, ultimately getting drugs to patients sooner. However, the adoption of adaptive designs in clinical development has been relatively low, approximately 20 % in recent years, according to a survey conducted by Tufts Center for the Study of Drug Development. One of the chief reasons for this has been the increased complexity of adaptive trials compared to traditional trials. Barriers, some perceived and some real, to the use of clinical trials with adaptive features still persist, and these may include, but are not limited to, the concerns about the integrity of study design and conduct, the risk of regulatory acceptance, the need for an advanced infrastructure for complex randomization and clinical supply scenarios, change management for process and behavior modifications, extensive resource requirements for the planning and design of adaptive trials, and the potential to relegate key decision makings to outside entities (such as Data Monitoring Committees). There have been limited publications on practical considerations and recommendations on adaptive trial designs and suggestions regarding best practices and solutions on implementation to address these real or perceived barriers.

This book aims to fill this publication void and serves as a resource for trialists who wish to consider adaptive trials in their clinical development programs, providing them with guidance on practical considerations for adaptive trial design and implementation. The target audience is anyone involved, or with an interest, in the planning and execution of clinical trials, in particular, statisticians, clinicians, pharmacometricians, clinical operation specialists, drug supply managers, infrastructure providers working in academic or contract research organizations, government, and industry. Our goal for this book is to provide, to the extent possible, a balanced and comprehensive coverage of practical considerations for adaptive trial design and implementation.

This book is comprised of three parts: Part I focuses on practical considerations from a design perspective, Part II delineates practical considerations related to the implementation of adaptive trials, and Part III presents a rich collection of practical case studies.

Part I includes a total of ten chapters. Chapter 1 discusses the need for and the future of adaptive designs in clinical development. Regulatory guidance documents on adaptive designs have been released by the European Medicines Agency (EMA) and US Food and Drug Administration (US FDA). Chapters 2 and 3 discuss key points in these two guidance documents from industry and regulatory perspectives, respectively. Improving clinical development efficiency starts at the program level. To provide trialists with the tools to strategically consider their clinical development plans, Chap. 4 describes adaptive program concepts and illustrates the efficiency of complex strategies for clinical program development through a case study, while Chap. 5 provides optimal Go/No Go decisions for clinical development. To provide guidance to practitioners on key issues associated with interim analyses, Chap. 6 presents a comprehensive and balanced discussion on optimal timing and frequency of interim analyses, including logistic and regulatory considerations. Adaptive design approaches provide greater efficiency, as compared to traditional design approaches, with regard to dose finding and optimal dose selection. The main statistical methods available for planning and analysis of adaptive designs in Phase I, II, and III are covered in Chap. 7. Chapter 8 provides a review of currently available simulation software tools, discussing detailing their specific features. Often evaluation of an adaptive design approach for a trial requires careful examination of randomization needs. Randomization challenges in adaptive design trials, and randomization techniques that help addressing these challenges, are described in Chap. 9. Chapter 10 discusses response-adaptive randomization, including regulatory concerns and recommendations for the path forward.

As reported in the DIA Adaptive Design Scientific Working Group (ADSWG) 2012 survey, the key barriers for the broader adoption of adaptive trials in clinical development include the lack of experience with and knowledge in the implementation of adaptive designs, along with a lack of appropriate processes and infrastructure to support efficient trial execution. Part II of the book deals with these issues in Chaps. 11 through 16. Chapter 11 highlights operational challenges that must be taken into consideration when conducting an adaptive trial and provides strategies for efficient execution of an adaptive design trial. Similarly, Chap. 12 illustrates various operational challenges via a case study, while Chap. 13 discusses logistic and operational challenges with a focus on IT and infrastructure improvement. A particularly critical issue for adaptive clinical trials, with potentially great impact on how large a role this type of studies will play in confirmatory stages of clinical development, involves the processes by which accruing data are collected and analyzed, and adaptation decisions are made and implemented. Chapter 14 discusses who should be involved in data review for adaptation decisions, how the data flow and access to results should be controlled, and the specific role that Data Monitoring Committees might play in this process. Drug supply and patient recruitment play critical roles in the ultimate success of adaptive trial execution. Chapters 14, 15, and 16 cover, respectively, the roles that modeling and simulation may play in successfully planning and carrying out clinical supply and patient recruitment strategies.

Putting it all together, Part III, featuring Chaps. 17 through 20, presents four illustrative case studies ranging from description and discussion of various specific adaptive trial design considerations to the logistic and regulatory issues faced in trial implementation. The solutions to practical challenges and recommended best practices, along with the rest of the chapters in the book, should equip clinical trialists with the much needed toolkit to embark on their journey to efficient adaptive trial design and implementation.

We would like to express our sincerest gratitude to all of the contributors who made this book possible. They are the leading experts in adaptive trial design and implementation from industry, regulatory and academia. Their in-depth discussions, thought-provoking considerations, and abundant advice based on a wealth of experience make this book unique and valuable for a wide range of audiences. We hope that you will find this book helpful as well. We would also like to thank Marc Strauss of Springer Science and Business Media for giving us the idea for this book and for providing us with the opportunity for publication. Thanks also go to Jonathan Gurstelle and Hannah Bracken, both of Springer Science and Business Media, for their patience and help in guiding us through the production phase of the book. Finally, our immense thanks go out to our families for their unfailing support.

Rahway, NJ, USA   Weili He
Raritan, NJ, USA   José Pinheiro
Rahway, NJ, USA   Olga M. Kuznetsova

Contents

Contributors

Keaven M. Anderson has worked in the pharmaceutical industry for over 20 years, most recently at Merck Research Laboratories. He has worked on drug development in many therapeutic areas. Previously, Dr. Anderson worked for the National Heart, Lung and Blood Institute at the Framingham Heart Study and received his Ph.D. in statistics from Stanford University. He has published frequently in the general area of adaptive design and specifically on group sequential design. He has designed and reviewed a large number of clinical trials throughout his career and has taught group sequential design at Joint Statistical Meetings for several years. Dr. Anderson has supported the gsDesign R package since 2006.

Suresh Ankolekar is Professor of e-Business at Maastricht School of Management (MSM, Netherlands) and consultant at Cytel Inc. (USA). He holds a Master of Technology from Indian Institute of Technology (IIT, Mumbai), and a PhD from Indian Institute of Management (IIM, Ahmedabad). At Cytel, he is involved in modeling of clinical trials, including randomization, patient recruitment, clinical supplies, and optimization of drug development portfolio. At MsM, he is involved in the executive education in IT management and business dynamics.

Zoran Antonijevic Senior Director, Strategic Consulting, Cytel, is responsible for strategic quantitative input at trial, program, or portfolio level. He also contributes to developing processes and tools for implementation of adaptive clinical trials. Research areas include: adaptive design, interim data monitoring, pharmaceutical portfolio optimization, and decision-making within clinical drug development process. Externally, Zoran is the chair of DIA Adaptive Design Scientific Working Group. Zoran's prior experience includes Quintiles Innovation, GlaxoSmithKline, and Harvard School of Public Health.

Robert A. Beckman an oncology clinical researcher and molecular biophysicist, has played leadership roles in developing new oncology clinical research groups at four pharmaceutical companies. He has coinvented novel clinical strategies for proof of concept studies and for biomarker driven clinical development. Educated at Harvard College and Harvard Medical School, Dr. Beckman has served on the

University of Michigan Biophysics faculty, as a Member in the Simons Center for Systems Biology, Institute for Advanced Study, Princeton, and in the Warner-Lambert Biomolecular Structure and Drug Design group. His versatile publication record, comprising greater than 135 articles and abstracts, ranges from computational chemistry to clinical oncology, emphasizing quantitative approaches. Dr. Beckman is currently Executive Director, Clinical Research Oncology, Daiichi-Sankyo Pharmaceutical Development and external faculty in the Center for Evolution and Cancer, University of California at San Francisco.

James A. Bolognese (BS math Bucknell, Masters Statistics, UF) joined Merck in 1976 and led clinical pharmacology projects, a pre-clinical statistics group, and late phase coxib projects, before forming and leading Merck's experimental medicine statistics group. He joined Cytel in 2008 to work on clinical project consulting, including adaptive trials, and software development. He has researched and published on dose-adaptive designs in early phase clinical development, and designed and served as blinded statistician on steering committees of large outcomes studies.

Dr. Frank Bretz joined Novartis in 2004, where he is currently Global Head of the Statistical Methodology group. He has supported the methodological development in various areas of drug development, including dose finding, multiple testing, and adaptive designs. He has authored or coauthored more than 90 articles in peer-reviewed journals and four books. He is an Adjunct Professor at the Hannover Medical School (Germany) and the Shanghai University of Finance and Economics (P.R. China).

Tomasz Burzykowski is Professor of Biostatistics at Hasselt University and Vice President of Research at the International Drug Development Institute (IDDI) in Louvain-la-Neuve (Belgium). He received an M.Sc. degree in applied mathematics (1990) from Warsaw University, and M.Sc. (1991) and Ph.D. (2001) degrees in biostatistics from Hasselt University. Tomasz published methodological work on, e.g., survival analysis, meta-analysis, and validation of surrogate endpoints. He is also a coauthor of numerous papers applying statistical methods to clinical data in different disease areas.

Marc Buyse holds a Sc.D. in biostatistics from the Harvard School of Public Health (Boston, MA). He worked at the EORTC in Brussels and at the Dana Farber Cancer Institute in Boston. He is the founder of the International Drug Development Institute (IDDI) and of CluePoints, Inc. He is Associate Professor of Biostatistics at Hasselt University, Belgium.

Xiting Cao is Associate Director in the department of Global Health Outcomes at Merck & Co. Inc. After completing her B.Sc. in Statistics from Peking University, in Beijing, China, she earned her M.Sc. and Ph.D. in Biostatistics from University of Minnesota. Dr. Cao's research interests encompass the areas of clinical trial design, statistical methods for network meta-analysis and outcomes research. She also conducts statistical analysis in the area of pharmacoeconomics and health policy.

Jerome Carlier is Associate Director, Randomization & Drug Supply Systems at the International Drug Development Institute (IDDI) in Louvain-la-Neuve, Belgium. He has over 15 years of experience in the implementation of computerized systems in clinical trials (such as IWRS, Drug Supply, EDC and CTMS).

Dr. Pravin A. Chaturvedi is the Chief Scientific Officer of Napo Pharmaceuticals and also Chief Executive and/or Board member of several enterprises. He has 25 years of experience in drug discovery and development. Prior to his senior roles at Napo, IndUS, Oceanyx and Scion, he headed Lead Evaluation at Vertex and served in the preclinical and product development groups at Alkermes and Parke-Davis/Warner-Lambert. Dr. Chaturvedi received his doctorate from West Virginia University and his undergraduate degree from the University of Bombay.

Dr. Cong Chen is Director of Oncology Biostatistics at Merck & Co., Inc. He joined Merck in 1999 shortly before he graduated from Iowa State University, Ames, USA, with a Ph.D. in statistics. At Merck, he has worked in oncology drug development and other therapeutic areas including infectious disease, diabetes, and cardiovascular disease. His publication record consists of over 50 papers on statistical design and analyses, and various clinical publications. He has coinvented new paradigms for biomarker directed clinical development, for proof-of-concept studies, and for studies using progression-free-survival as a surrogate endpoint for overall survival. He is a Board Member of International Chinese Statistical Association, a member of US-China Anti-Cancer Association, American Statistical Association, and International Society of Biopharmaceutical Statistics. He is also an Associate Editor of Statistics in Biopharmaceutical Research.

Christy Chuang-Stein joined the pharmaceutical industry in 1985. Currently, she is Head of the Statistical Research and Consulting Center at Pfizer. Christy is a Fellow of the American Statistical Association (ASA). She has authored or coauthored more than 140 papers including several book chapters and 2 books. Christy is a founding coeditor of the journal *Pharmaceutical Statistics* and has been active in several professional societies. She received ASA's Founders' Award in 2012.

Linda Danielson is Chief Operating Officer at the International Drug Development Institute (IDDI) in Louvain-la-Neuve, Belgium. She obtained her M.S. degree in 1990 from the University of Wisconsin, Madison. She has over 20 years of experience in the Pharmaceutical Industry and worked at UCB prior to IDDI. She has also been President of the Biostatistical Section of the Belgian Statistical Society and the Belgian representative to the European Federation of Statisticians in the Pharmaceutical Industry (EFSPI).

David DeMets, Ph.D. is currently the Max Halperin Professor of Biostatistics and former Chair of the Department of Biostatistics and Medical Informatics at the University of Wisconsin-Madison. He has coauthored numerous papers and four texts on clinical trials, two specifically on data monitoring. He has served on many NIH and industry-sponsored data monitoring committees for clinical trials in diverse disciplines. He also served as President of the Society for Clinical Trials in 1989–1990. In addition, he was Elected Fellow of the Society for Clinical Trials in 2006. In 2013, he was elected as a member of the Institute of Medicine.

Vladimir Dragalin, Ph.D. is a Vice President, Scientific Fellow in the Quantitative Sciences at Janssen. He is a well-known adaptive design expert with more than 25 years of experience in developing the statistical methodology of adaptive designs and with over 15 years of experience in pharmaceutical industry. His professional interests include model-based adaptive and Bayesian designs, response-adaptive dose escalations, simulation, monitoring and analysis of clinical trials, bioequivalence, multi center clinical trials, and adverse event monitoring in safety trials, with the major results published in more than 75 papers in peer-reviewed journals and books.

Paul Gallo is a Biometrical Fellow and a member of the Statistical Methodology Group at Novartis Pharmaceuticals in East Hanover, NJ. He received a Ph.D. in Statistics from the University of North Carolina in 1982. A main activity has involved support of Data Monitoring Committees; he has worked with DMCs in many key Novartis trials and authored company process documents and guidelines governing interim analysis procedures. He has been active in industry initiatives relating to adaptive trials, with particular focus on interim monitoring and DMC process issues. He was lead author of the PhRMA Adaptive Designs Working Group's Executive Summary in *Journal of Biopharmaceutical Statistics*, and coordinated the production and publication of the group's full White Paper. He has headed teams focusing on interim analysis process issues in adaptive trials for the PhRMA and DIA-sponsored working groups.

Christy Nolan, B.Sc., M.T.(A.S.C.P.) Vice President of Quintiles Innovation Business Unit. Christy Nolan has thirty years of health care industry experience to include clinical laboratory, pharmaceutical, diagnostics, and executive leadership in global clinical operations clinical research in clinical research organizations.

Lixin Han, Ph.D. is Director of Biostatistics at Infinity Pharmaceuticals. His previous positions included Director of Biostatistics at Pfizer, Senior Principal Biostatistician II at Wyeth, and Senior Statistician at Abbott Laboratories.

Weili He is a Director and Senior Principle Scientist of Clinical Biostatistics at Merck & Co., Inc. She has a Ph.D. degree in biostatistics. She has extensive experience in drug development, and has worked in many therapeutic areas over the years. Dr. He has been active both at Merck and in industry for initiatives relating to adaptive trials, with particular focus on adaptive trial design and implementation. She is a core member of the DIA Adaptive Design Scientific Working Group (ADSWG) and cochair of the DIA ADSWG KOL Lecture series. Her research and collaboration with colleagues in various disciplines has led to over 30 publications in statistical and medical journals.

Michael Krams, M.D. is the Global Head of Quantitative Sciences at Janssen Pharmaceutical. He is recognized as an expert in designing, implementing and executing adaptive designs, enabling real-time learning in Learn and Confirm studies. He has built an industry leading cross-functional team of drug developers, applying modeling and simulation techniques and integrating input from clinical, translational medicine, biostatistics, discovery and commercial. As cochair of PhRMA's working group on adaptive designs Mike has contributed to an ongoing debate with regulatory agencies, with a goal to establish a common position on "Good Adaptive Practices."

Olga M. Kuznetsova is a Senior Principal Scientist in the Late Development Statistics department of Merck & Co., Inc. She has a Ph.D. in probability theory and mathematical statistics and more than 15 years of experience in clinical trials. In the last decade, her research interests centered around randomization techniques in clinical trials, in particular, addressing the randomization needs of adaptive design trials. Her collaboration with colleagues on randomization issues resulted in more than 20 presentations and publications.

Lisa LaVange, Ph.D. is Director of the Office of Biostatistics in the Center for Drug Evaluation and Research at FDA. She is a former faculty member in the Department of Biostatistics at the University of North Carolina at Chapel Hill. Prior to that, she spent 10 years in the pharmaceutical industry and 16 years in nonprofit research. She is Fellow of the American Statistical Association and former President of the Eastern North American Region of the International Biometric Society.

David Lawrence Since completing a Ph.D. in epidemiology at the University of Edinburgh, UK, in 1999, David Lawrence has worked as a clinical trial statistician in both academia (Institute of Cancer Research and University College London) and the pharmaceutical industry. He has focused on phase II and III trials in the respiratory and oncology areas. He has been working at Novartis since 2008.

Olga Marchenko is Vice President and Head of Centre for Statistics in Drug Development at Quintiles. Prior to joining Quintiles, Dr. Marchenko' positions included Global Head of Data Services Therapeutic Consulting and Director of Biostatistics in Americas at i3Statprobe. She also worked at Pfizer, the Ohio State University, and the Belarusian State University. Olga received her PhD in Statistics from the University of Michigan, Ann Arbor. Dr. Marchenko' research interests include adaptive design methodology and implementation, and drug safety methods.

Cyrus Mehta is President and cofounder of Cytel Corporation and Adjunct Professor of Biostatistics, Harvard University. Dr. Mehta consults extensively with the biopharmaceutical industry. He has led the development of the StatXact, LogXact and East software packages, widely used in the biopharmaceutical industry. He is a Fellow of the American Statistical Association and an elected member of the International Statistical Institute. He is a past cowinner of the George W. Snedecor Award for the best paper in biometry, was named Mosteller Statistician of the Year by the Massachusetts Chapter of the American Statistical Association, and Outstanding Zoroastrian Entrepreneur by the World Zoroastrian Chamber of Commerce.

Nitin R. Patel has a Ph.D. in Operations Research from Massachusetts Institute of Technology and has been a visiting professor there for over a decade. He is currently a researcher at the MIT Center for Biomedical Innovation. He is a Fellow of the American Statistical Association and has served as vice president of the International Federation of Operations Research Societies. He has published over 70 papers in professional journals. He is a cofounder of Cytel Inc. where he is currently Chairman.

Inna Perevozskaya is Senior Director, Biometrics, Statistical Research and Consulting Center at Pfizer. She has 13 years of pharmaceutical industry experience, working at Pfizer, Wyeth, and Merck supporting various projects and also serving as an internal adaptive design expert and consultant. She received her Ph.D. in Statistics from University of Maryland where she specialized in novel dose-escalation designs for oncology. More recently, as a member of SRCC at Pfizer and DIA Working Group on Adaptive Designs, she continues to pursue her research interests while building expertise in other types of adaptive designs and their application.

Kristen Pierce, Ph.D. is currently an Associate Director of Biostatistics at Pfizer. Her focus while at Pfizer has been on early stage drug development for oncology clinical trials.

José Pinheiro has a Ph.D. in Statistics from the University of Wisconsin-Madison, having worked at Bell Labs and Novartis Pharmaceuticals, before his current position as Head of Statistical Modeling in the Model-Based Drug Development department at Janssen Research & Development. He has been involved in methodological development in various areas of statistics and drug development, including dose-finding, adaptive designs, and mixed-effects models. He is a Fellow of the American Statistical Association, former cochair of the PhRMA working group on Adaptive Dose-Ranging Studies, former core member of the PhRMA working group on Novel Adaptive Designs, and codeveloper of the nlme library/package in S-PLUS and R for linear and nonlinear mixed-effects models.

Judith Quinlan Following an initial career as a biometrician in agriculture in Western Australia, **Ms. Quinlan** later moved to the UK where she entered the pharmaceutical industry in 1996 as a statistician with SmithKline Beecham (later GSK). During her time at GSK she took on increasing roles of responsibility that included moving to the US to become Director of Statistics for Biopharmaceutical development. Ms. Quinlan has been a strong advocate for adaptive designs, and also played an active role as a member of industry's Adaptive Design Scientific Working Group (ADSWG). After leaving GSK, Ms. Quinlan spent 3 years as VP of Adaptive Trials Services at Cytel Inc., before joining Aptiv Solutions in 2011 as SVP Innovations Center, where her role has a strong focus on adaptive trial execution.

William F. Rosenberger is Professor and Chairman of Statistics at George Mason University. He received his Ph.D. in mathematical statistics from George Washington University in 1992 and since then has spent much of his career developing statistical methodology for randomized clinical trials. He has two books on the subject, *Randomization in Clinical Trials*: *Theory and Practice* (Wiley 2002), which won the Association of American Publishers Award for the best mathematics/statistics book published that year, and *The Theory of Response-Adaptive Randomization in Clinical Trials* (Wiley 2006). He is a Fellow of the American Statistical Association (2005) and of the Institute of Mathematical Statistics (2011). An author of more than 75 refereed papers, Prof. Rosenberger was named the 2012 Outstanding Research Faculty by the Volgenau School of Engineering, George Mason University.

Pralay Senchaudhuri has a Ph.D. in Biostatistics from Harvard University. He has published over 30 papers in professional journals and coauthored chapters of books on statistical methods. He is one of the main architects of several widely used statistical software products including East, StatXact, LogXact, and COMPASS. He has been a principal investigator on a number of SBIR grants from National Institutes of Health. Currently he is a Senior Vice President at Cytel Inc.

Dr. Linda Z. Sun is with Late Development Statistics at Merck & Co., Inc., focusing on oncology area. She received her Ph.D. in statistics from Northwestern University, Evanston, IL. Currently, Dr. Sun leads a team of statisticians in the Asia Pacific group of Merck, covering oncology, neuroscience, and respiratory and immunology areas. She published statistical papers about adaptive designs, early endpoint evaluation, cost effectiveness go-no-go decision, etc. She also has medical papers published in Journals like Lancet Oncology.

Yevgen Tymofyeyev is a Scientific Director in the Model-Based Drug Development department of Janssen Research & Development. He specializes in statistical modeling and simulation to support studies across multiple therapeutic areas including design and implementation of adaptive clinical trials. He has a Ph.D. in Statistics from the University of Maryland, Baltimore County. Over the last decade, he is actively involved in scientific collaborations in the field of randomization, adaptive design methodology, and software which led to an extensive list of publications.

Sue-Jane Wang received her Ph.D. in Biostatistics from the University of Southern California, having worked at Demographic Research Company and Cedars-Sinai Medical Genetics Institute, prior to her current position as Associate Director for Adaptive Design and Pharmacogenomics in the Office of Biostatistics, Office of Translational Sciences, Center for Drug Development and Research, U.S. Food and Drug Administration. Dr. Wang has received several awards at FDA including an FDA Scientific Achievement Award on Excellence in Analytical Science for a sustained record of published regulatory research in statistical design and methodology advancing complex and emerging clinical trial designs and analysis that support regulatory guidance, policies, and review. Dr. Wang is a Fellow of the American

Statistical Association, a DIA recipient of Thomas Teal Award for Excellence in Statistics Publishing. She has served Editor-in-Chief of Pharmaceutical Statistics, Guest (co)Editor-in-Chiefs for special issues: multi-regional clinical trials in Pharmaceutical Statistics, multiple comparison procedures in Biometrical Journal, subgroup analysis in Journal of Biopharmaceutical Statistics. She is an elected member of International Statistical Institute and is currently Guest Editor-in-Chief for the special issue on personalized medicine in Statistics in BioSciences.

Lanju Zhang is the Head of Nonclinical Statistics at Abbvie Inc. His research interests cover all areas of drug development process, including chemistry, manufacturing, and control (CMC). He has authored/coauthored more 30 publications in professional journals and books. He has performed editorial services for most major statistical journals.

Part I
Design Considerations

Chapter 1
The Need for and the Future of Adaptive Designs in Clinical Development

Christy Chuang-Stein and Frank Bretz

Abstract There has been much progress in the development and implementation of adaptive designs over the past 20 years. A major driver for this class of novel designs is to increase the information value of clinical trial data to enable better decisions, leading to more efficient drug development processes and improved late-stage success rates. In this chapter, we review common types of adaptive designs that have been developed and the frequently encountered challenges associated with their implementations. We discuss reasons why, in our opinion, the interest in adaptive designs will continue to rise. Furthermore, we describe what still needs to be done to move adaptive designs into our standard toolbox of design options. We emphasize the importance to implement adaptive designs with thorough upfront planning. The business case mandates that we treat the opportunities offered by adaptive designs carefully so that we can successfully foster a broad acceptance of properly designed and executed adaptive designs, when they represent the best design options based on their performance characteristics to address the need of a particular situation.

Keywords Adaptive randomization design • Adaptive dose–response design • Group sequential design • Sample size re-estimation • Software development • Treatment selection design

C. Chuang-Stein (✉)
Pfizer Inc, 5857 Stoney Brook Road, Kalamazoo, MI 49009, USA
e-mail: Christy.j.Chuang-Stein@pfizer.com

F. Bretz
Novartis Pharma AG, WSJ-27.1005, 4002 Basel, Switzerland
e-mail: Frank.Bretz@novartis.com

W. He et al. (eds.), *Practical Considerations for Adaptive Trial Design and Implementation*, Statistics for Biology and Health,
DOI 10.1007/978-1-4939-1100-4_1, © Springer Science+Business Media New York 2014

1.1 Introduction

The first decade of the twenty-first century saw a great interest in the research and implementation of adaptive designs in clinical trials to support product development. A major driver for this was the observation that the confirmatory trials were failing at an alarmingly high rate. The rate was allegedly to be between 50 % and 60 %. While safety issues contributed to the high failure rate, a majority of the failures occurred because of the inability to demonstrate the benefit of the new treatment over the comparator in a superiority trial setting (Milligan et al. 2013). The finding prompted many to conduct root cause analyses and look for solutions to reduce the failure rate. This effort led to the investigation of alternative designs that may allow trialists to critically examine the design features, especially the assumptions underlying a design, and modify certain aspects of the design in a prespecified manner while the trial is ongoing.

The desire for alternative designs led researchers to look beyond group sequential designs (GSD) which became popular for trials of mortality or major morbidity endpoints in the 1990s (Jennison and Turnbull 2000). A GSD allows a study to be stopped early for efficacy or lack thereof. A traditional GSD does not allow changing design features such as sample sizes or the primary study population once the study is started.

Other than GSDs, the most noted early research on adaptive designs focused on sample size re-estimation, both in a blinded (i.e., not using treatment assignment information) and an unblinded (i.e., using treatment assignment information) manner (Wittes and Brittain 1990; Cui et al. 1999; Gould 2001; Friede and Kieser 2001; Kieser and Friede 2003; Proschan 2005; Chuang-Stein et al. 2006). The former is a response to inaccurate assumptions on the variability associated with a continuous endpoint or an assumed event rate for a binary endpoint among those who received the control treatment in the enrolled population. By comparison, the unblinded sample size re-estimation is in response to an assumed treatment effect that is overly optimistic judged by the interim data collected in the study. As a result, the trial sponsor may wish to increase the sample size so that the study has a reasonable chance to detect a smaller, and still clinically meaningful, treatment effect. The resulting designs include proper statistical analysis that controls the overall type I error rate and addresses the estimation of the treatment effect.

Even early on, researchers of adaptive designs realized the importance of operational support needed to implement these designs. This is so because an adaptive trial requires (1) availability of fit-for-use interim data in a timely manner to enable adaptation decisions, (2) a committee to oversee the decision process for the proposed adaptations, and (3) a proper communication channel by which major decisions could be relayed back to the sponsor or the study team. The absence of a well laid-out process with tight control could introduce operational bias to an adaptive trial. These considerations have led many to propose procedures that focus on the execution of adaptive trials (Gallo 2006a, b; Quinlan and Krams 2006; Gaydos et al. 2009; Antonijevic et al. 2013).

The research on sample size re-estimation started the trend of using simulation to thoroughly evaluate study designs for their performance characteristics. As efforts to look for alternative designs gathered momentum, clinical trialists realized that another major factor contributing to the high failure rate is the suboptimal choice of dose(s) from the dose–response study in phase II (Antonijevic 2009). A traditional dose–response study typically includes three doses with a concurrent control. Patients are randomized to the four treatment groups in fixed ratios throughout the study. At the end of the study, each dose is compared with the control to decide if it is worthy of further testing in phase III trials. This practice depends critically on our ability to include relevant doses that are in the appropriate range of the dose–response curve in the phase II dose–response study. Experience has shown that this has not always been the case. In fact, many dose–response studies had to be repeated with lower doses, a higher dose or doses between two previously chosen doses. Realizing the value of a more quantitative product development process (Kowalski et al. 2007), researchers began to advocate including more doses in a dose–response study and conducting model-based analyses to identify the minimum effective dose (Milligan et al. 2013).

Because dose–response studies focus more on estimation than testing, their designs allow more flexibility in which methods to use and are less concerned with type I error rate control. In fact, dose–response studies have proven to be the most fertile ground for adaptive designs (Bornkamp et al. 2007; Pinheiro et al. 2010). Proposed adaptations for these studies include modifying randomization ratio of patients to doses based on interim results, introducing new doses or dropping existing doses. The analysis as well as the decision criteria for progressing the compound to phase III development could be based on either the Bayesian or the frequentist approaches.

The logical progression of innovation in study designs took another forward step when researchers advocated the need to consider studies in the exploratory phase together with those in the confirmatory phase in an integrated manner (Julious and Swank 2005; Bretz et al. 2009a). They argued that while each study has its unique role in supporting product development and approval, studies need to be planned together so that the information produced by distinct studies fits together to tell a complete story. This observation has motivated active research to assess adaptivity at the program level. Metrics used to compare phase II designs under this new paradigm include the probability of a successful phase III trial (Antonijevic et al. 2010) and the expected net present value of the product (Patel et al. 2012).

Common interests among statisticians supporting clinical trials in adaptive designs led to the formation of the Adaptive Designs Working Group (ADWG) in the spring of 2005 under the auspices of the Pharmaceutical Research and Manufactures of America (PhRMA). The initial objectives of the group were to foster and facilitate wider usage and regulatory acceptance of adaptive designs to enhance clinical development through fact-based evaluation of the benefits and challenges associated with these designs (Gallo et al. 2006). Since 2005, ADWG has sponsored workshops, presentations and publications. Members of the group have also reached out to regulators to discuss best adaptive design practice and share experience from implementing adaptive designs (Enas et al. 2008; Chuang-Stein et al. 2009). Early interactions with regulators for confirmatory trials were considered especially important because regulatory buy-in was essential for these trials. In addition, the increasing trend of conducting multiregional trials to satisfy marketing authorization requirements in multiple regions implied that we needed regulators to hold similar views on this new class of designs.

Since its inception, ADWG ran multiple workstreams concurrently. Some earlier workstreams such as regulatory interactions and desirable features of software to support modeling and simulation were sunset after the workstreams had completed the planned activities. Other workstreams have spanned over many years. The most noted long-running activity has been the monthly key opinion leader lecture series. Early lectures focused on theory behind adaptive designs. Over time, the lectures have moved to case studies of adaptive trials. The sponsorship of ADWG was officially transitioned from PhRMA to the Drug Information Association (DIA) in 2010. The name of the group was changed to Adaptive Design Scientific Working Group (ADSWG) after the transition. ADSWG remained active with additional new workstreams such as adaptive program, precision medicine and portfolio evaluation. A survey workstream repeated a survey (Jorgens-Coburger 2012) previously reported by Quinlan et al. (2010). The repeat survey showed the uptake in adaptive designs, not just by pharmaceutical sponsors, but also by academic institutions. The survey also showed a clear increase in the use of adaptive designs in all phases of drug development.

The interest in adaptive trials has led the European Medicines Agency to issue a reflection paper on adaptive designs in 2007 (CHMP 2007). In the US, the Food and Drug Administration issued a draft guidance in February 2010 (US FDA 2010) for the public to comment. EMA's reflection paper focuses primarily on confirmatory trials while FDA draft guidance covers trials in both the exploratory and the confirmatory space. At the time this chapter was finalized (February 2014), the FDA has yet to finalize its draft guidance on adaptive designs.

The advent of personalized medicine has offered another application of adaptive designs because changing the primary patient population is an adaptive feature. Research work supporting this aspect of adaptation has initially focused on oncology trials (Wang et al. 2007; Brannath et al. 2009). It will undoubtedly expand to other disorders where there are good clinical and biological rationales for choosing specific subgroups. We will describe the role that adaptive designs can play in helping deliver personalized medicine in Sect. 1.3.

In the next section, we will give a high-level overview of the advancements in adaptive designs. In Sect. 1.3, we will argue why interest in adaptive designs will continue to rise. While research on adaptive designs has made significant progress in recent years (Bretz et al. 2009a; Gaydos et al. 2009), there remains much work to do to turn theory into practice. We will describe such work in Sect. 1.4.

We have confidence that statisticians, with their expertise and collaborative spirit, will take a leadership role in making adaptive designs part of the design armamentarium for clinical trials in the twenty-first century.

1.2 Advancements in Adaptive Designs

In this section we describe major types of adaptive designs used at different phases of drug development and link them to topics covered in the various chapters of this book. A detailed taxonomy of adaptive designs in the context of clinical development is given in Dragalin (2006). An overview of applications of adaptive designs throughout drug discovery and development is given by Bretz et al. (2009b). We also discuss advancements in the implementation and tool development for adaptive trials. We offer two examples of confirmatory adaptive trials.

1.2.1 Types of Adaptive Designs

1.2.1.1 Adaptive Randomization Designs

One of the earliest types of adaptive designs described in the literature is adaptive randomization which allows changing the treatment randomization probabilities during an ongoing study. Adaptive randomization can be grouped into four categories (Hu and Rosenberger 2006): (1) Restricted randomization, where the allocation probability is conditional on past treatment assignments, such as the biased coin design from Efron (1971); (2) covariate-adaptive randomization, where the allocation probability is conditional on past treatment assignments, covariates and the covariate vector of the current patient, such as the minimization design from Pocock and Simon (1975); (3) response-adaptive randomization, where the allocation probability is conditional on past treatment assignments and responses, such as the randomized play-the-winner rule from Wei and Durham (1978); and (4) covariate-adjusted response-adaptive randomization that combines covariate-adaptive and response-adaptive randomization. For a recent overview of adaptive randomization we refer readers to Rosenberger et al. (2012).

To motivate the use of adaptive randomization techniques in clinical practice, consider, for example, a clinical study with four important covariates: study site (20 centers), gender (male or female), age (<65 or ≥65), and prognosis (good, poor). Applying stratified randomization one would have to balance treatment assignment in each of $20 \times 2 \times 2 \times 2 = 160$ strata, which is clearly infeasible in a study of moderate size. However, if marginal balance is sufficient (i.e., balanced on the four covariates individually), adaptive randomization techniques applied to the $20 + 2 + 2 + 2 = 26$ covariate levels are possible. Covariate-adaptive randomization approaches incorporate information on important patient baseline covariates into the randomization design in order to prospectively balance prognostic profiles of patients in different treatment groups while maintaining randomization. For a more general discussion of randomization challenges in adaptive design studies, we refer readers to Chap. 9. Chapter 10 focuses on response-adaptive randomization designs.

1.2.1.2 Adaptive Dose–Response Designs

Another important application of adaptive designs occurs in phase I and II studies to estimate dose–response and/or target doses of interest. This includes Bayesian adaptive dose-escalation designs, such as the continual reassessment method (CRM) proposed by O'Quigley et al. (1990) to estimate the maximum tolerable dose in phase I studies. The original CRM chooses the first dose level based on some assumed dose–response model. After each cohort of patients, the model is updated. The updated model is used to calculate the probability of dose-limiting toxicity (DLT) at each dose of interest. The statistical dose recommendation for the next patient cohort is communicated to the clinical team, who decides on the next dose based on the statistical input as well as other relevant information (e.g., toxicities that do not qualify for a DLT). The basic CRM has led to much research (Garrett-Mayer 2006) and numerous extensions (Neuenschwander et al. 2008; Cheung 2011).

A challenge in selecting the right dose is the trade-off between desired and unwanted effects. A prerequisite for informed decision and dose selection at the end of phase II is a solid characterization of the dose–response relationship. In the past, phase II dose finding studies were often designed using a small number of doses and a narrow dose-range, focusing on the upper end of the dose–response relationship. Only in recent years has there been a noticeable shift towards investigating the full dose–response range and estimating the minimum effective dose. This shift was partially driven by the PhRMA "Adaptive Dose-Ranging Studies" (ADRS) working group. The objectives of this group were to develop and evaluate novel adaptive and non-adaptive dose-ranging methods and to provide methodological recommendations for industry and regulatory agencies alike.

Extensive simulation work conducted by the ADRS working group showed that no single type of clinical trial design or analysis is universally best, though novel approaches outperform conventional designs in many plausible scenarios. Simulations also showed that with current phase II trial sizes, even novel dose-ranging approaches have non-negligible chance of making erroneous dose selection. It is clear that both the design and the amount of information to be generated need careful consideration. The working group also concluded that the probability of success was increased by including a wider range of doses in these trials. Despite these findings, adaptive designs are not always optimal, and are not always feasible. Trial sponsors should maximize their success rates by employing a "toolbox" approach, selecting different designs for different experimental situations. Details on adaptive dose-ranging designs can be found in the white papers from the ADRS working group (Bornkamp et al. 2007; Pinheiro et al. 2010).

1.2.1.3 Group Sequential Designs

Although there is a vast literature on sequential designs, with initial ideas dating back to the 1920s, for most clinical trials it is unrealistic to assess data after every observation. This restriction has led to group sequential designs (GSDs) that include only a small number of interim analyses as groups of observations become available. GSDs have been used for clinical trials since the 1970s (Pocock 1977; O'Brien and Fleming 1979) and are now standard for many long-term trials because these trials often include hundreds or thousands of patients and may last for several years. Ethical and economic reasons often mandate the conduct of interim analyses for these trials because: (1) patients should not be treated with a new therapy if the ongoing trial gives no indication of a potential benefit associated with the new therapy; (2) clinical trials should not be continued if a clear tendency favoring a particular treatment emerges. Thus, clinical trial designs that include the possibility for early decisions may help reduce the overall costs and timelines of the development while meeting the ethical obligation.

To properly control the type I error rate when interim analyses could result in early declaration of efficacy, researchers have developed a variety of stopping procedures for different types of data (e.g., continuous, binary, survival). The theory of GSDs is well described in, for example, the review paper by Emerson (2007) and the books by Whitehead (1997), Jennison and Turnbull (2000), and Proschan et al. (2006). GSDs have been implemented in software packages such as ADDPLAN, EAST, PEST and S+SeqTrial (Wassmer and Vandemeulebroecke 2006). Some of them are also described in Chap. 8.

Despite their popularity, GSDs have some limitations. For example, it is necessary to prespecify the required sample size for a GSD in the study protocol. While conceptually simple, choosing an appropriate sample size could be challenging due to uncertainties around nuisance parameters or the definition of a clinically meaningful treatment difference. GSDs address the latter issue by allowing the study to stop early if the observed effect is larger or smaller than the effect for which the study was powered to detect. However, modifying the sample size for future stages of the trial based on the interim efficacy information is not allowed under the traditional GSDs.

1.2.1.4 Sample Size Re-estimation

Sample size re-estimation (SSR) methods have been developed since the 1990s. SSR allows one to adjust the sample size of the trial based on emerging interim data of the ongoing trial. SSR methods fall into two main categories, depending on whether the treatment randomization information is used (unblinded SSR) or not (blinded SSR). In the latter case, an SSR approach adjusts sample size that were calculated using assumed nuisance parameters that are judged to be erroneous from blinded data at a prespecified interim look. Wittes and Brittain (1990) first introduced this concept and referred such designs as internal pilot study designs. They have found that such designs can be used in large randomized clinical trials to assess key nuisance parameters (e.g., the error variance for continuous data, the response rate with binary data in the control group, or the accrual rate with time-to-event data) and make appropriate modifications to the sample size with little impact on the type I error rate.

In contrast, unblinded SSR is based on a revised estimate of treatment effect using unblinded interim data. While using unblinded data could provide more accurate sample-size estimates, concerns exist over potential bias that may result from knowledge of observed treatment effect at interim. External data monitoring committees (i.e., external to the trial sponsor) are typically used to handle unblinded SSR for registration trials. As the type I error rate might be affected when using unblinded data to effectuate trial adaptations, care is necessary when conducting the final analysis. Chapters 11 through 14 discuss blinding and unblinding issue associated with adaptive trials.

A common approach to control the type I error rate is the combination test principle that combines stage-wise p-values using a prespecified combination function (Bauer and Köhne 1994). The key idea is to calculate separate test statistics from the samples at the different stages (e.g., before and after an interim analysis) and to combine them in a prespecified way for the final decision. Examples of such p-value combination functions include Fisher's product test and the inverse normal method (Lehmacher and Wassmer 1999; Cui et al. 1999). A closely related approach is based on the conditional error principle, which computes the conditional type I error rate based on the observed data at the interim analysis under the null hypothesis (Proschan and Hunsberger 1995; Müller and Schäfer 2004). Chapter 6 discusses at a strategic level the optimal timing of an interim analysis for futility and/or sample size re-estimation. Additional discussions on sample size re-estimation can be found in Chuang-Stein et al. (2006) and Friede and Kieser (2006).

1.2.1.5 Treatment Selection Designs

The p-value combination function approach and the conditional error rate principle can also be used for other types of adaptations such as changes in randomization ratio, study population, or number of treatment arms with a strict type I error rate control (Hommel 2001; Bretz et al. 2006). A particularly appealing application occurs in phase III studies with treatment selection at interim. Consider, for example, a phase III study that starts with several treatments and a control. At a prespecified interim analysis, one (or more) treatment(s) would be selected based on the available information, external information, and expert knowledge. Recruitment would continue, but now patients will only be randomized to the selected treatment(s) with a possibly reassessed sample size. The final analysis of the selected treatment(s) consists of patients in both stages and is performed in such a way that the overall type I error rate is controlled at a prespecified level, thus providing confirmatory evidence of efficacy that is of the registration quality. Chapter 7 includes a case study of a confirmatory treatment selection design.

1.2.2 Implementation of Adaptive Trials

The overall statistical methodology to implement confirmatory adaptive designs seems to be reasonably developed (Bretz et al. 2009a). Strict type I error rate control is mandatory for acceptable phase III adaptive designs. This implies that the experimental questions and hypotheses to be tested need to be clearly specified upfront in the study protocol. The number of possible adaptations should be kept to a minimum. Explorative, hypotheses-generating adaptive designs are not acceptable for confirmatory trials.

While adaptive designs often increase the information value given the same number of patients and lead to shorter overall development time and earlier access to effective treatments by patients, their implementations are subject to several factors such as time needed to assess treatment response, recruitment speed, procedures to protect trial integrity, and drug supply management. These factors may hinder the smooth implementation of an adaptive trial. For example, when a trial has the option to terminate treatment arms or change the allocation ratio of patients to a set of dose groups, drug supply personnel needs to be ready to make the necessary adjustments to study medications. Chapter 15 discusses drug supply issues associated with adaptive trials. Similarly, accurate prediction on patient enrollment is critical for a timely decision because too slow or too fast patient enrollment may put the planned adaptations at risk. Chapter 16 discusses different models to predict patient recruitment patterns.

Increasingly, sponsors use interactive voice randomization systems (IVRS) to manage treatment randomization. Prespecified algorithms could be built into the system to allow minimum sponsor intervention. Such a system requires careful upfront validation to ensure that the system is capable of handling the foreseeable scenarios. Interim results for adaptive trials are generally assessed by data monitoring committees that are independent of the study teams. For confirmatory trials, the data monitoring committees are typically external to the trial sponsors to avoid the possibilities that the sponsors might subtly affect the trials if they are aware of the comparative interim results. Chapter 14 discusses the planning, conduct and monitoring of interim results. Considerations on other key operational challenges, such as protecting trial integrity and minimizing operational bias, are further discussed in Chaps. 11–13.

1.2.3 Other Impact of Adaptive Designs

The endeavors of assessing adaptive designs over the last two decades have resulted in a number of positive by-products. For one, the efforts have led to better integration of clinical, statistical, operational, and regulatory perspectives when designing a trial. This is a topic of Chap. 4. Another important by-product is to expand the focus from the trial to the program level. Focusing the clinical development strategy at the program level means that an adaptive trial is of benefit only if it offers more evidence to the overall development program than a non-adaptive counterpart. Chapter 5 discusses making optimal Go/NoGo decisions that incorporate cost considerations at different stages of drug development.

A third positive impact from the adaptive design evolution is the heavy use of modeling and simulation techniques. In addition to adaptive designs, statisticians have begun to use modeling and simulations to assess a wide range of issues associated with trial designs such as missing data and multiple comparison procedures. The latter has started a shift towards model-based drug development and more quantitative decision making.

In our opinion, recent advancements in adaptive designs and their by-products have contributed substantially to the ultimate objective of employing more efficient designs and analyses in support of product development.

1.2.4   Two Examples of Confirmatory Adaptive Trials

Adaptive designs are increasingly being used in both the exploratory and the confirmatory settings. Bauer and Einfalt (2006) performed a literature review of clinical trials employing adaptive designs that employed methods like p-value combination functions or conditional error rate functions. Schmidli et al. (2006) provided applications and case studies of adaptive designs addressing more complex trial objectives (e.g., treatment selection, population enrichment) from their experience. Quinlan et al. (2010) and Jorgens-Coburger (2012) reported the results of cross-industry surveys, which showed a clear increase in the use of adaptive designs in all phases of clinical development during the time between the two surveys. In the following, we illustrate this trend with two examples where adaptive trials provided confirmatory evidence for product approval. Further case studies of adaptive trial designs are presented in Chaps. 17–20.

The first example is an adaptive trial that compared latanoprost in combination with timolol maleate against latanoprost alone in reducing intraocular pressure. An unblinded sample size reestimation was planned when approximately 50 % of patients were half-way through an 8-week treatment period. At this interim analysis, conditional power to detect a difference between the combination and latanoprost alone, based on the interim treatment effect estimate, will be calculated. If the conditional power is ≥90 %, there will be no change in the sample size. If the conditional power is ≥50 % but <90 %, the sample size will be increased to obtain a conditional power as close as possible to 90 %, but the increase will be no greater than 33 % of the originally targeted sample size. If the conditional power is <50 %, there will be no change in the sample size and the study will continue to the scheduled end. This approach is based on the method in Chen et al. (2004). As stated in Ando et al. (2011), sample size was not increased after the interim analysis in the actual trial. The study was found to be positive, leading to the approval of the combination of latanoprost and timolol for glaucoma and ocular hypertension.

The second example is a two-stage adaptive design with treatment selection at interim. This trial is one of two pivotal trials to support Indicaterol for marketing authorization for chronic obstructive pulmonary disease (COPD) (Barnes et al. 2011). The aim of the trial was to provide pivotal confirmation of efficacy, safety, and tolerability of the selected Indicaterol doses, where the dose selection is done at a prespecified interim analysis. In the first stage, patients were randomized to one of seven treatments arms (four different doses of Indicaterol, placebo and two active control groups). Based on the observed interim data, two Indicaterol doses were continued to the second stage, together with placebo and one of the two active controls. The final analysis compared the two selected dose groups with placebo and the continued active control on a prespecified sequence of primary and secondary endpoints. Evidence from both stages was combined in the final analysis, using a one-sided Bonferroni adjusted significance level of 0.025/4 for comparing each of the two Indicaterol doses with the placebo in the final analysis since the study started with four Indicaterol doses. More powerful approaches using, for example, p-value combination functions or conditional error rates, could have been applied, but were not chosen because of the complexity of the trial design and the desire to test for both primary and some key secondary endpoints.

For the COPD study, different dose selection rules were extensively simulated in order to understand the operating characteristics of the rules. It is worthwhile to note that Bayesian decision tools or modeling approaches could have been used to guide the interim decision without compromising the overall type I error rate. A set of dose selection guidelines for a variety of possible interim scenarios was compiled and included in the data monitoring committee charter. The charter, however, allowed the data monitoring committee to deviate from these guidelines, if necessary (mainly in case of unexpected results), and select doses on its own, possibly after consultation with senior representatives of the sponsor. In the actual trial, the intermediate two Indicaterol doses were selected for the second stage. Efficacy, safety, and tolerability of both doses were confirmed in the final analysis of this two-stage adaptive trial as well in the second parallel pivotal trial. This case study is presented in more detail in Chap. 7; see also Lawrence et al. (2014).

1.3   Why Will the Interest in Adaptive Designs Continue to Rise?

In this section, we will discuss reasons why, in our opinion, the interest in adaptive designs or in adaptations more generally will continue to rise.

1.3.1   Responding to Emerging Scientific Knowledge or Regulations

When developing products in diseases with emerging new knowledge or regulations, a sponsor needs to be able to adjust to knowledge from both within a trial and outside of the trial. While this flexibility may lead to a small reduction in trial design efficiency measured by the expected sample size needed for the study (Tsiatis and Mehta 2003), this trade-off is often considered worthwhile.

For example, in Nov 2010, the US FDA issued a draft guidance for hospital-acquired and ventilator-associated bacterial pneumonia (HABP and VABP). The draft guidance sets the 28-day mortality rate as the primary endpoint. The draft guidance targets a patient population with an approximately 20 % mortality rate and describes a 10 % non-inferiority margin for an active control trial. The draft guidance also states that if the 28-day all-cause mortality rate in the active-controlled group is lower than 20 %, a sponsor should consider using the odds ratio metric as the measure for assessing treatment efficacy. In the latter case, the non-inferiority margin expressed on the absolute difference scale will be a function of the mortality rate in the control group.

Many groups submitted comments to the agency including the Society of Critical Care Medicine whose comments were posted publicly on March 23rd 2011 (http://www.regulations.gov/#!documentDetail;D=FDA-2010-D-0589-0015). The society stated its ongoing efforts to reduce mortality in HABP/VABP patients and questioned the targeted 20 % mortality rate. They cited a study by Chastre et al. (2008) that reports 28-day mortality rate of 10.8 % and 9.5 % in the two treatment groups. The Society commented that this study was the largest clinical trial ever conducted of an investigational drug for ventilator-associated pneumonia (VAP). The mortality rate was much lower than that in prior studies, but the Society argued that it was representative of current VAP mortality rates in Intensive Care Units. They expressed a significant concern that should the enrollment be expanded to include more unstable patients to increase the mortality rate in a VABP trial, the mortality rate will reflect the clinical and critical care management and not the efficacy of the antimicrobial being studied. The concern and uncertainty around the mortality rate and study population expressed by the Society means that some form of adaptation is necessary for a modern-day trial in HABP or VABP.

The need to respond to emerging information is equally compelling in areas of unmet medical needs. Increasingly, efforts are directed towards disease-modifying products. For example, with an aging population, it is highly desirable to have products that could delay the structural progression in osteoarthritis measured by joint space narrowing (i.e., disease-modifying osteoarthritis drug, DMOAD). Despite the existence of a pathway for a DMOAD indication, no DMOADs are currently available commercially. Similarly, many sponsors are interested in a disease-modifying claim for the Alzheimer's Disease (AD) even though no guidance yet exists for such an indication path. In both cases, a sponsor needs to have information on the rate of disease progression in the placebo group (which may be enriched through inclusion criteria) since the treatment effect is likely measured in terms of % reduction in disease progression. For AD, the Alzheimer's Disease Neuroimaging Initiative (ADNI, http://adni.loni.ucla.edu/) and other groups have been collecting longitudinal biomarker and clinical data in elderly normal subjects and patients at various stages of AD. As the management of AD moves to possible interventions in populations with an early symptomatic stage of AD, but without dementia (Aisen et al. 2011), a sponsor will need data on the rate of disease progression in this new subpopulation using validated measurements judged to be sensitive to treatment effect by the medical community. The latter often needs to come from the ongoing trial or a recently completed trial. When facing with this type of challenge, a sponsor needs to stay agile in responding to emerging information, both from the internal and the external source. Adaptive designs offer an answer to this need.

1.3.2   Allocating Resources to Support Multiple Programs in a Portfolio

Some critics of adaptive designs have argued that trialists should design studies to detect a minimum clinically important difference (MCID) and rely on early stopping rules of a group sequential design to stop the study early if the treatment effect is substantially higher than the MCID. While this strategy is a good one from the expected sample size perspective, it also means that a large commitment is necessary upfront to support the trial. This could be a challenge for many resource-constrained enterprises where many trials are competing for the same funding pool. Other than a few programs that are adequately funded, several programs need to share the remaining budget. Since programs could be terminated early for either safety or efficacy, programs that are suboptimally funded initially could have a chance to receive additional funding later when resources allocated to terminated programs are redirected. In other words, development decisions are often based on efficiency together with other considerations. If one insists on efficiency and a large upfront commitment for each program, many programs will not have a chance to be initiated.

The need to optimize on resource allocation occurs at all levels of product development. For example, a company may have a large exploratory portfolio. Experience tells us that only a very small number of candidates would have an efficacy that achieves or exceeds a target value. Limited resources would preclude one from pursuing a large study for every candidate to determine Go versus No Go with high confidence. An alternative strategy is to utilize an early signal of efficacy design as a screening tool to identify most failures and some clear winners (Brown et al. 2012). The few candidates with a superior efficacy profile could be identified quickly because of the smaller sample size. This, in conjunction with some good development planning, could enable acceleration to market. The obvious downside is that compounds in the Go Slow category are likely to take longer to develop if they are proven successful in a subsequent trial.

1.3.3   The Journey to Targeted Therapies

On December 14 2012, US FDA issued a draft guidance on "Enrichment Strategies for Clinical Trials to Support Approval of Human Drugs and Biological Products". The draft guidance discusses a variety of strategies to select a subset of the general population in which the effect of a drug, if it exists, can be more readily demonstrated. The strategies include investigating a new treatment in patients who did not respond to another treatment, patients who could not tolerate another treatment or patients who have a positive (or negative) response to a biomarker assay at baseline. The selection of patients based on a pretreatment marker assay has become increasingly frequent in our search of targeted therapies, particularly for cancer patients where drugs block the growth and spread of cancer by interfering with specific molecules (targets) involved in tumor growth and progression.

When treatment effect is suspected to vary as a function of a marker status, the ideal situation is to have reasonable evidence for this association before conducting a late-stage study to confirm a treatment effect in a subgroup defined by the marker status. Unfortunately, this is not always possible for studies where assessing treatment effect on a clinical outcome such as survival may take a long time. The draft enrichment guidance acknowledges this challenge. It specifically states that entry criteria or sample sizes can be modified for later stages of a trial if factors can be identified that increase the event rate or treatment response (e.g., discovery that the enrichment factor has a greater impact on response than anticipated or that the patients without the enrichment factor have a very poor response).

One option to carry out mid-trial enrichment is to enroll all subjects regardless of their marker status but collect samples for marker assessment. If a preplanned interim analysis shows a strong treatment effect in marker-positive subjects and little effect in the marker-negative subjects, the study may enroll only marker-positive subjects for the rest of the trial and change the primary analysis population to marker-positive subjects. It goes without saying that under such a design, the study results need to be properly analyzed to control the type I error rate (Brannath et al. 2009).

It is possible that a trial does not restrict enrollment but specifies multiple primary analysis populations in the final analyses, one of which being a genomic subset. Research work in this scenario is reported in Wang et al. (2007, 2009). It is also possible to use the same study to identify and confirm treatment effect in a subgroup. Freidlin and Simon (2005) proposed an adaptive signature design that uses genomic data collected on all randomized subjects to identify the subgroup. They propose to divide the study into two parts. The primary final analyses consist of testing the treatment effect in the overall population and also testing it based on data collected in the second part of the study in a subgroup identified from data collected in the first part. The allowed two-sided type-I error rate 0.05 is split so that the overall population is tested at the two-sided 0.04 level while the effect in the subgroup is tested at the 0.01 level. Jiang et al. (2007) propose an extension where the subgroup is defined by a threshold value on the biomarker measurement.

The approvals of targeted therapies such as crizotinib for patients with ALK-positive advanced non-small-cell lung cancer and vemurafenib for late-stage (metastatic) or un-resectable melanoma with the BRAF V600E mutation in 2011 by the FDA in the US were examples of what are surely to come as we accelerate the journey to personalized medicine. Information of these approvals is available at FDA's Web site on approved drugs and in the labels for these two products.

1.3.4   Other Reasons

Identifying subgroups is important not only from the safety and efficacy perspective, but also from the cost-effectiveness perspective. In countries that practice social medicine, cost-effectiveness assessment often resulted in coverage decisions for subpopulations of the population for which the product is indicated. Therefore, a sponsor may want to conduct interim economics assessment during a phase III study and consider restricting patients to subgroups for the remainder of the trial based on cost-effectiveness considerations during the interim analysis.

For some confirmatory trials with a long-term clinical endpoints, dose selection is often based on a short-term endpoint in a phase II study. Depending on the association between the short-term and long-term endpoints, adjustment to the doses may be necessary in the confirmatory trial, based on early results on the long-term endpoint within the trial.

1.4   What Is Still Needed to Support the Adaptive Design Evolution?

There are many situations for which more efficient designs (compared to existing standards) are available but are not yet widely used. Many senior leaders in pharmaceutical companies hold the belief that simple, conventional and tested designs mean quicker development and regulatory approval. They fear that, if the proposed trial designs and/or development strategies deviate from the standard approaches or are perceived to be more complex, the proposals will face difficulty in receiving regulatory endorsement even if the basis for decision-making is more robust. Because of this fear, it is not unusual for senior leaders within these companies to ask "Wouldn't something simpler be better?" when presented with adaptive designs at internal review meetings.

We need to create a culture where clinical trial designs are selected based on well-informed comparisons of operating characteristics of the designs, and not on traditions. To effectuate this cultural change requires educating all parties involved in clinical trial planning on the benefits of novel approaches, including adaptive designs. Education helps increase awareness. In addition to the cultural hurdle, it helps solve logistical hurdles for implementation because all parties are working together towards a common goal. Furthermore, education stimulates the development of software tools. While there are opportunities for further methodological research for adaptive designs, the most pressing need currently is a greater awareness of available methods and an expanded pool of expertise and software to facilitate their use.

In most companies, the key drivers for selecting a trial design are time, cost and quality. Among these three, time and cost are often more influential than quality. The current drug development strategy is often determined by the "shortest path to market". Whilst this may generate the greatest financial returns for a successful development program, it also has a greater risk because of a higher failure rate in most cases. Decisions in companies are typically made by scientists and project/ business managers. The latter are often more focused on meeting targets and milestones measured in time and cost rather than quality. Balancing between minimizing time to market and maximizing the probability of success requires rethinking by clinical trial sponsors, in particular the pharmaceutical companies. As scientists, we need to find ways to more effectively quantify risks and communicate them to the senior leaders and non-statisticians in our respective organizations in languages they can understand.

Clearer thinking is required to identify and formulate key questions to be answered from a trial and then to select the trial design that is the most efficient in providing data to answer the questions with sufficient precision. Innovative designs and methods need "top-down" (key decision makers and budget holders) and "bottom-up" (clinical teams and regulatory affairs colleagues) buy-in within organizations for wide implementation. A culture operated in this fashion will promote better decisions and lead to a lower late-stage failure rate. Such a culture is crucial to a successful future for drug development.

At present, the capacity to efficiently assess trial designs is not widely available. Some of the commercial software contain proprietary information and are not freely available to the broader clinical trial community. Attempts have been made to initiate cross-company and foster joint industry/academic collaborations (in the pre-competitive space) to develop effective simulation tools to evaluate different clinical trial scenarios. Such tools can help compare and present the performance characteristics of different clinical trial design more effectively.

Clinical trial sponsors tend to use "standard" clinical trial designs when developing medicines. The number of designs that can be called "standard" is still arguably too few. While some advances have been made as outlined in Sect. 1.2, the set of commonly used designs need to be substantially expanded. To assist the latter, it would be beneficial if sponsors would require their clinical development teams to consider adaptive design as an option on a routine basis. Based on the authors' experience, even where not selected, considering how to plan an adaptive trial has led to more carefully developed plans being submitted for internal decisions. The introduction of a culture where multiple designs are considered regularly and selections made on their comparative operating characteristics could have a positive impact on the practice of using the most efficient designs.

It is generally agreed that improving the scope, conduct or efficiency of exploratory development trials can help us identify eventual "failures" earlier in the development process. Unfortunately, the more sophisticated novel designs are not without their challenges. Since these methods are not routinely used by sponsors, the number of sponsors (and their partners, consultants and contracted clinical research organizations) who have the necessary expertise to implement them is limited. Clinical key opinion leaders are often not in a good position to help either. This problem extends to investigators who may be discouraged from participating because the trial design seems complicated and unfamiliar. In recent years, there are workshops and short courses on adaptive designs. These venues help educate trialists and clinical scientists on how to select the most appropriate design or series of designs for trials, particularly those in the exploratory stage. Sharing and publishing case studies of novel approaches is another way to increase the collective experience of the clinical trial community and help establish good practice for adaptive designs.

One prevailing impression is that regulatory agencies are generally not receptive to novel designs and methods. Our experience suggests that adaptive designs that are well-justified, well-planned and well-executed have generally been accepted by regulators. Similarly, our interactions with regulators suggest that regulators welcome more and earlier discussions on scientific matters including adaptive designs together with regulatory standards and requirements. Novel designs should not be avoided for fear of regulatory rejections. All clinical trial designs should be judged by their properties and design characteristics, and not by whether or not they are novel. With proper planning and explanation a well formulated adaptive design that does not compromise standards for making decisions or protecting patient safety should not pose any particular difficulty to the regulators. We need to work with internal decision makers to dispel the "regulators do not like adaptive designs" myth.

Implementing adaptive designs for multi-regional clinical trials can be particularly challenging when different regulatory agencies make different requests. That is, a sponsor may receive conflicting scientific advice about a proposed adaptive global trial from different regulatory agencies. If one agency disagrees with the trial design, it may not be possible to rework the entire trial and resubmit to each of the agencies for approval. When this happens, there is a tendency for a sponsor to default to a standard design, hoping for a speedy acceptance by all regulatory agencies involved. Thus, global harmony between regulatory attitudes is important. The latter, in our experience, seems to be generally the case when it comes to the role, conduct and interpretation of adaptive trials (Chuang-Stein et al. 2009; Laurie et al. 2008). We would like to point out that when a multi-regional trial is planned, a sponsor should consider seeking parallel scientific advice between EMA and FDA, which may lead to greater collaborations between international regulatory authorities.

1.5   Final Remarks

Adaptive designs require careful planning to protect trial integrity and reduce possible operational bias. This applies to all designs with at least one interim analysis, including group sequential design. Consider a group sequential design with boundaries to allow for early stopping for efficacy or futility. If the decision from an interim analysis is to continue the trial, an astute individual familiar with the stopping rules will know the range where the interim comparative results fall. The concern for possible information breach led many pharmaceutical companies to develop internal operating procedures to detail how interim results should be obtained, shared and communicated.

While many adaptive designs have been proposed, some of them might be more of an intellectual interest with less appeal for practical applications. An elaborate adaptive design, although may appear statistically sound, could encounter real challenges in implementation. Thus, focusing on those adaptations that are practically feasible will result in the most successful implementation as the research enterprise is collectively gaining experience with this new class of designs.

Incremental improvement is how we advance the field of clinical trial designs. Research on adaptive designs and our collective experience from implementing them contributes to the incremental improvement. Instead of letting our fear of potential misuse prevent us from benefiting from adaptive designs, we should help promote good practices for adaptive designs so that the designs are implemented appropriately.

Even though we take much pride in the progress made on adaptive designs and believe in the business needs for this class of innovative designs for both the exploratory and confirmatory trials, we want to emphasize that a critical consideration in choosing the design for a trial is to choose the design that can best answer the research questions at hand. In some situations, a fixed design may be the most appropriate design to answer the research questions. In addition, we want to make it clear that while we believe that adaptive designs could help increase the success rate of our late stage trials, they are not the panacea to solve our late stage failure problem. The latter will require a holistic approach to product development, of which smart designs are an important part, but not all of it.

Adaptive designs open many opportunities to make preplanned mid-trial adjustments. We offer some examples on why we believe clinical trialists will continue to welcome these opportunities. We want to emphasize that these opportunities should be used with care. The last thing we want to do is to treat the opportunities offered by adaptive designs haphazardly, which could result in rejected trials and lead to the mistrust in these designs. The latter will delay broad acceptance of properly designed and properly executed adaptive designs.

References

Aisen PS, Andrieu S, Sampaio C et al (2011) Report of the task force on designing clinical trials in early (predementia) AD. Neurology 76:280–286

Ando Y, Hirakawa A, Uyama Y (2011) Adaptive clinical trials for new drug applications in Japan. Eur Neuropsychopharmacol 21:175–179

Antonijevic Z (2009) Impact of dose selection strategies on the success of drug development programs. Drug Inf J 43:104–106

Antonijevic Z, Pinheiro J, Fardipour P, Roger JL (2010) Impact of dose selection strategies used in phase II on the probability of success in phase III. Stat Biopharm Res 2(4):469–486

Antonijevic Z, Gallo P, Chuang-Stein C et al (2013) Views on emerging issues pertaining to data monitoring committees for adaptive trials. TIRS 47(4):495–502

Barnes PJ, Pocock SJ, Magnussen H et al (2011) Integrating indacaterol dose selection in a clinical study in COPD using an adaptive seamless design. Pulm Pharmacol Ther 23:165–171

Bauer P, Köhne K (1994) Evaluation of experiments with adaptive interim analyses. Biometrics 50:1029–1041

Bauer P, Einfalt J (2006) Application of adaptive designs—a review. Biom J 48:493–506

Bornkamp B, Bretz F, Dmitrienko A et al (2007) Innovative approaches for designing and analyzing adaptive dose-ranging trials (with discussion). J Biopharm Stat 17:965–995

Brannath W, Zuber E, Branson M et al (2009) Confirmatory adaptive designs with Bayesian decision tools for a targeted therapy in oncology. Stat Med 28(10):1445–1463

Bretz F, Schmidli H, Koenig F et al (2006) Confirmatory seamless phase II/III clinical trials with hypotheses selection at interim: general concepts. Biom J 48:623–634

Bretz F, Koenig F, Brannath W et al (2009a) Adaptive designs for confirmatory clinical trials. Stat Med 28:1181–1217

Bretz F, Branson M, Burman C-F et al (2009b) Adaptivity in drug discovery and development. Drug Dev Res 70:169–190

Brown M, Chuang-Stein C, Kirby S (2012) Designing studies to find early signals of efficacy. J Biopharm Stat 22(6):1097–1108

Chastre J, Wunderink R, Prokocimer P et al (2008) Efficacy and safety of intravenous infusion of doripenem versus imipenem in ventilator-associated pneumonia: a multicenter, randomized study. Crit Care Med 36(4):1089–1096

Chen YH, DeMets DL, Lan KK (2004) Increasing the sample size when the unblinded interim results is promising. Stat Med 23:1023–1038

Cheung YK (2011) Dose finding by the continual reassessment method. CRC Press, New York

(2007) CHMP reflection paper: methodological issues in confirmatory clinical trials planned with an adaptive design. www.emea.europa.eu/pdfs/human/ewp/245902enadopted.pdf

Chuang-Stein C, Anderson K, Gallo P, Collins S (2006) Sample size re-estimation: a review and recommendations. Drug Inf J 40(4):475–484

Chuang-Stein C, Bretz F, Komiyama O, Quinlan J (2009) Interactions with regulatory agencies to enhance the understanding and acceptance of adaptive designs. A report by members of the PhRMA Adaptive Design Working Group. Reg Focus 14(4):36–42

Cui L, Hung HMJ, Wang SJ (1999) Modification of sample size in group sequential clinical trials. Biometrics 55:853–857

Dragalin V (2006) Adaptive designs: terminology and classification. Drug Inform J 40:425–435

Efron B (1971) Forcing a sequential experiment to be balanced. Biometrika 58(3):403–417

Emerson S (2007) Frequentist evaluation of group sequential clinical trial designs. Stat Med 26:5047–5080

Enas G, Anderson K, Bedding A et al (2008) Global harmonization of standards for adaptive clinical trial designs. Regul Focus 13(8):8–17

Freidlin B, Simon R (2005) Adaptive signature design: an adaptive clinical trial design for generating and prospectively testing a gene expression signature for sensitive patients. Clin Cancer Res 11:7872–7878

Friede T, Kieser M (2001) A comparison of methods for adaptive sample size adjustment. Stat Med 20:3861–3873

Friede T, Kieser M (2006) Sample size recalculation in internal pilot study designs: a review. Biom J 48:537–555

Gallo P, Chuang-Stein C, Dragalin V et al (2006) Adaptive designs in clinical drug development—an executive summary of the PhRMA Working Group. J Biopharm Stat 16(3):275–283

Gallo P (2006a) Operational challenges in adaptive design implementation. Pharm Stat 5:119–124

Gallo P (2006b) Confidentiality and trial integrity issues for adaptive designs. Drug Inf J 40(4):445–450

Garrett-Mayer E (2006) The continual reassessment method for dose-finding studies: a tutorial. Clin Trials 3:57–71

Gaydos B, Anderson K, Berry D et al (2009) Good practices for adaptive clinical trials in pharmaceutical product development. Drug Inf J 43(5):539–556

Gould AL (2001) Sample size re-estimation: recent developments and practical considerations. Stat Med 20:2625–2643

Hommel G (2001) Adaptive modifications of hypotheses after an interim analysis. Biom J 43:581–589

Hu F, Rosenberger WF (2006) The theory of response-adaptive randomization in clinical trials. Wiley, New York

Jennison C, Turnbull BW (2000) Group sequential methods with applications to clinical trials. CRC Press, New York

Jiang W, Freidlin B, Simon R (2007) Biomarker-adaptive threshold design: a procedure for evaluating treatment with possible biomarker-defined subset effect. J Natl Cancer Inst 99(13): 1036–1043

Jorgens-Coburger S (2012) Perception and use of adaptive designs in the industry and academia: persistent barriers and recommendations to overcome challenges. Presented at DIA EuroMeeting, Copenhagen

Julious SA, Swank DJ (2005) Moving statistics beyond the individual clinical trial: applying decision science to optimize a clinical development plan. Pharm Stat 4:37–46

Kieser M, Friede T (2003) Simple procedures for blinded sample size adjustment that do not affect the type I error rate. Stat Med 22:3571–3581

Kowalski KG, Ewy W, Hutmacher MM et al (2007) Model-based drug development—a new paradigm for efficient drug development. Biopharm Rep 15(2):2–22

Laurie D, Branson M, Bretz F et al (2008) Designing and conducting confirmatory adaptive clinical trials. Regul Aff J Pharma 19:86–91

Lawrence D, Bretz F, Pocock S (2014) INHANCE: an adaptive confirmatory study with dose selection at interim. In: Trifilieff A (ed) Indacaterol—the first once-daily long-acting Beta2 agonist for COPD. Springer, Basel, pp 77–92

Lehmacher W, Wassmer G (1999) Adaptive sample size calculations in group sequential trials. Biometrics 55:1286–1290

Milligan PA, Brown MJ, Marchant B et al (2013) Model-based drug development: a rational approach to efficiently accelerate drug development. Clin Pharm Therapeut 93:502–514

Müller HH, Schäfer H (2004) A general statistical principle for changing a design any time during the course of a trial. Stat Med 23:2497–2508

Neuenschwander B, Branson M, Gsponer T (2008) Critical aspects to the Bayesian approach to phase I cancer trials. Stat Med 27:2420–2439

O'Brien PC, Fleming TR (1979) A multiple testing procedure for clinical trials. Biometrics 5:549–556

O'Quigley J, Pepe M, Fisher L (1990) Continual re-assessment method: a practical design for phase I clinical trials in cancer. Biometrics 46:33–48

Patel N, Bolognese J, Chuang-Stein C et al (2012) Designing phase 2 trials based on program-level considerations: a case study for neuropathic pain. Drug Inf J 46(4):439–454

Pinheiro J, Sax F, Antonijevic Z et al (2010) Adaptive and model-based dose-ranging trials: quantitative evaluation and recommendations (with discussion). Stat Biopharm Res 2:435–454

Pocock SJ, Simon R (1975) Sequential treatment assignment with balancing for prognostic factors in the controlled clinical trial. Biometrics 31(1):103–115

Pocock SJ (1977) Group sequential methods in the design and analysis of clinical trials. Biometrika 64:191–199

Proschan MA, Hunsberger SA (1995) Designed extension of studies based on conditional power. Biometrics 51:1315–1324

Proschan MA (2005) Two-stage sample size re-estimation based on a nuisance parameter: a review. J Biopharm Stat 15:559–574

Proschan MA, Lan KKG, Wittes JT (2006) Statistical monitoring of clinical trials, a unified approach. Springer, New York, USA

Quinlan JA, Krams M (2006) Implementing adaptive designs: logistical and operational considerations. Drug Inf J 40:437–444

Quinlan J, Gaydos B, Maca J, Krams M (2010) Barriers and opportunities for implementation of adaptive designs in pharmaceutical product development. Clin Trials 7(2):167–173

Rosenberger WF, Sverdlov O, Hu F (2012) Adaptive randomization for clinical trials. J Biopharm Stat 22(4):719–736

Schmidli H, Bretz F, Racine A, Maurer W (2006) Confirmatory seamless phase II/III clinical trials with hypotheses selection at interim: applications and practical considerations. Biom J 48: 634–643

Tsiatis AA, Mehta C (2003) On the inefficiency of the adaptive design for monitoring clinical trials. Biometrika 90:367–378

U.S. Food and Drug Administration (2010) Draft guidance for industry: adaptive design clinical trials for drugs and biologics. http://www.fda.gov/downloads/Drugs/GuidanceCompliance RegulatoryInformation/Guidances/UCM201790.pdf. Accessed 16 June 2013

US FDA Guidance for Industry (2010) Hospital-acquired bacterial pneumonia and ventilator associated bacterial pneumonia: developing drugs for treatment (draft). http://www.fda.gov/ downloads/Drugs/GuidanceComplianceRegulatoryInformation/Guidances/UCM234907.pdf. Nov 26, 2010. Accessed 6 April 2013

US FDA Guidance for Industry (2012) Enrichment strategies for clinical trials to support approval of human drugs and biological products (draft). http://www.regulations.gov/#!document Detail;D=FDA-2012-D-1145-0002. Dec 14, 2012. Accessed 7 April 2013

Wang SJ, O'Neill RT, Hung JHM (2007) Approaches to evaluation of treatment effect in randomized clinical trials with genomic subset. Pharm Stat 6:227–244

Wang SJ, Hung HMJ, O'Neill RT (2009) Adaptive patient enrichment designs in therapeutic trials. Biom J 51(2):358–374

Wassmer G, Vandemeulebroecke M (2006) A brief review on software developments for group sequential and adaptive designs. Biom J 48:732–737

Wei LJ, Durham S (1978) The randomized play-the-winner rule in medical trials. J Am Stat Assoc 73:840–843

Whitehead J (1997) The design and analysis of sequential clinical trials. Wiley, Chichester, UK

Wittes J, Brittain E (1990) The role of internal pilot studies in increasing the efficiency of clinical trials. Stat Med 9:65–72

Chapter 2
Regulatory Guidance Documents on Adaptive Designs: An Industry Perspective

José Pinheiro

Abstract Adaptive designs have the potential to be a transformative methodology in clinical drug development, but acceptance by regulatory agencies is a prerequisite for their broader adoption and success, especially in the context of confirmatory studies. Both FDA and EMA have published guidance documents focusing on adaptive designs, which have been neither discouraging nor clearly supportive of the approach in their assessments and recommendations. As a result, the interpretation of the *regulatory position* on adaptive designs also has been mixed, with some citing the guidance documents as evidence that health authorities do not accept adaptive designs, while others mentioning the same documents as indication that regulators support their use in drug development, when properly planned, conducted, and analyzed. This chapter reviews and discusses the two main regulatory documents on adaptive designs issued by the time this book was published: the reflection paper by EMA (Reflection paper on methodological issues in confirmatory clinical trials with flexible design and analysis plan (draft CHMP/EWP/2459/02, 23-Mar-2006), 2007) and the draft guidance by FDA (Adaptive design clinical trials for drug and biologics draft guidance, 2010). Reactions from the biopharmaceutical industry to both documents, collated by industry trade groups, are also presented and discussed.

Keywords FDA draft guidance • EMEA reflection paper • Well-understood and not well-understood adaptive designs • Operational bias • PhRMA Adaptive Designs Working Group

J. Pinheiro (✉)
Quantitative Sciences, Janssen Research & Development,
920 Rt 202, Raritan, NJ 08869, USA
e-mail: jpinhei1@its.jnj.com

W. He et al. (eds.), *Practical Considerations for Adaptive Trial Design and Implementation*, Statistics for Biology and Health,
DOI 10.1007/978-1-4939-1100-4_2, © Springer Science+Business Media New York 2014

2.1   Introduction

Adaptive designs (AD) have the potential to transform clinical drug development, as discussed and illustrated throughout this book. The very reason that makes AD attractive to drug developers, the opportunity to make pre-planned design and analysis modifications to an ongoing clinical trial, also raises understandable concerns from regulatory agencies (RA), especially when utilized in confirmatory studies. The ultimate success, or failure, of AD in the context of drug development hinges on their acceptance by RA around the world. This was recognized early on by industry groups advocating the broader use of AD in drug development, most notably the PhRMA Adaptive Designs Working Group (ADWG). Members of the ADWG engaged in early discussions on AD with RA in the USA (FDA), Europe (EMA), and Japan (PMDA), emphasizing the importance of guidance documents to provide a clear position with regard to regulatory acceptance, or not, of AD.

Two guidance documents focusing on AD were issued, at least in part, as a result of the advocacy efforts by industry groups: the EMEA reflection paper (EMEA/CHMP 2007) and the FDA draft guidance (FDA 2010). The former is a relatively short, high-level document, focusing almost entirely on confirmatory studies—neither encouraging, nor ruling out the use of AD, from a regulatory perspective. The FDA draft guidance is considerably more detailed, covering both exploratory and confirmatory studies (but with greater emphasis on the latter), and providing not only potential regulatory concerns about the use of AD but also recommendations on how to circumvent them in drug development practice. Although its overall tone is broadly supportive of adequately planned, executed, and analyzed AD, the FDA draft guidance has been interpreted by some in the biopharmaceutical industry as evidence that FDA does not favor the use of AD.

Both guidance documents elicited strong, mostly positive reactions from industry groups, who provided many comments and suggestions during the respective review periods. The EMA reflection paper incorporated some of the suggestions received during the consultation period (and provided responses to those which were not adopted) in the final version adopted by CHMP. The FDA draft guidance was yet to be revised and finalized at the time of publication of this book.

This chapter reviews both the EMA and FDA guidance documents on AD from an industry perspective. Section 2.2 describes the FDA draft guidance, discussing its impact on the biopharmaceutical industry. The EMA reflection paper is covered in Sect. 2.3, being contrasted to the FDA draft guidance. The industry perspective on both guidance documents and, more broadly, on the perceived regulatory position on AD are discussed in Sect. 2.4, with a focus on comments and recommendations issued over time by the ADWG.

2.2   US FDA Draft Guidance on Adaptive Designs

Even though the EMA reflection paper was issued prior to the FDA draft guidance, the latter is presented and discussed first in this chapter, as it has a considerably broader scope and has had more impact in industry than the former. The guidance document on AD was a PDUFA IV commitment of FDA, originally scheduled to be issued by October 2008 and finally published in March 2010. The inclusion of a guidance document on AD as part of the PDUFA IV negotiations was a clear indication of the importance that the biopharmaceutical industry placed on this methodology as a tool for modernizing and improving the efficiency of drug development, as a well as a recognition that regulatory guidance was a critical prerequisite for its successful utilization. The formation of the PhRMA ADWG in early 2005 also provided clear indication of the industry support for and interest in AD. The ADWG played a critical catalyzing role with regard to broad awareness, early adoption, and regulatory engagement on AD. The ADWG went on to publish a series of highly impactful white papers (Gallo et al. 2006; PhRMA 2006; Bornkamp et al. 2007; Antonijevic et al. 2010; Gallo et al. 2010; Pinheiro et al. 2010), to engage in productive discussions on AD with RA around the world (FDA, in particular), and to disseminate AD at scientific conferences. A good number of issues advocated by the ADWG made their way into the FDA draft guidance, but many were left out.

The overall tone of the FDA draft guidance is *encouraging of AD, but with caution*: the document states that FDA recognizes AD as having the potential to improve the efficiency and success rate of drug development, but raises some concerns about their use, mostly in the context of pivotal studies. It also acknowledges that the main appeal of AD is to allow pre-planned midway corrections to ongoing trials, revising design assumptions and research goals in light of observed data. Two main regulatory concerns are expressed early on and throughout the guidance: the potential for *Type I error rate inflation* and *operational bias* that could compromise study integrity and the validity/interpretability of the final results. The cautionary tone is pretty much consistent with regulatory guidance documents issued on other topics, but it was perceived by some in industry as an indication that FDA would be reluctant to accept AD, especially for confirmatory studies.

2.2.1   Description and Motivation for Adaptive Designs

The guidance defines AD as a clinical study that includes a prospectively planned opportunity for modification of one or more aspects of its design and hypotheses, based on analysis of data (usually interim data) from subjects in the study. This is consistent with other references on AD, including the ADWG Executive Summary (Gallo et al. 2006), which defines AD as *a clinical study design that uses accumulating data to decide how to modify aspects of the study as it continues, without undermining the validity and integrity of the trial*. By *prospectively* the guidance means before any unblinded data analysis is performed, but the recommendation put forward in the guidance is that any adaptation be planned, described, and evaluated before the study protocol is finalized. In addition, the timing of any adaptations should be pre-specified. The adaptations can be based on blinded or unblinded data, and may or may not include statistical hypothesis testing. A number of potential study design modifications that can be implemented in an AD are listed in the guidance, including

- Study eligibility criteria
- Randomization procedure
- Treatment allocation (e.g., dose, schedule)
- Total sample size and/or study duration
- Concomitant medication
- Planned patient evaluation schedule
- Primary endpoint (e.g., single vs. composite)
- Secondary endpoints (selection and testing order)
- Analysis methods to evaluate endpoints

The two main types of adaptations discussed in the guidance are *treatment allocation* and *total sample size/study duration*. Some of those potential adaptations, like the *primary analysis method*, appear to be included in the guidance just for completeness as they are declared as *unlikely to be acceptable* from a regulatory perspective right after being listed.

FDA acknowledges the motivation for AD in the guidance, naming, in particular the improvement in knowledge efficiency compared to conventional (i.e., nonadaptive) study designs (same information faster and/or cheaper; or more information for the same investment and time). Additional potential advantages of AD also mentioned are the increased likelihood of success (via midtrial corrections), the reliable early termination via futility rules, and the improved understanding of treatment effects (e.g., better evaluation of dose–response profile or subgroup effects).

2.2.2 Study Types

The guidance differentiates between two types of studies for which AD can be considered: adequate and well-controlled (A&WC) effectiveness studies intended to support drug marketing and exploratory studies, which can be considered as the complement of A&WC studies. From the point of view of AD, the main difference between the two types of study is that for an A&WC study strict control of Type I error rate is paramount, while for exploratory studies it is less critical. The focus of the guidance is on AD in the context of A&WC, but AD in the context of exploratory studies are also discussed in the document.

From a methodological perspective, the main concern expressed in the guidance about the utilization of AD with an A&WC study is the potential inflation of Type I error rate, with possible bias in the estimation of treatment effects also being mentioned, but somewhat downplayed. It is acknowledged that statistical methods have been developed to adequately control Type I error for a wide range of AD based on unblinded data (there is less of a concern about Type I error inflation when adaptations are based on blinded data), but it is emphasized that it is incumbent upon sponsors to demonstrate, preferably analytically, that the proposed statistical analysis methods will indeed control Type I error under the planned AD.

The other main concern related to AD in A&WC studies expressed in the guidance is harder to pin down and ensure control over: potential for operational bias due to leaking of unblinded results as the study is ongoing. If present, it could jeopardize the scientific validity of study, making results difficult to interpret and accept. Changes in patient population after an unblinded adaptation are cited as an example of operational bias associated with AD. Of course, changes in patient population during a clinical trial can, and do, also occur when no adaptations are used in the study. They may be the result, for example, of different regions/sites starting recruitment later in the trial. The recommendation, implicit in the guidance and expressed by FDA representatives at conferences and public meetings following the publication of the draft guidance, is that sponsors should ensure, and document, "squeaky clean" execution of AD to avoid any potential indication, real or perceived, that access to unblinded data during the study led to operational bias. Since the publication of the draft guidance, different vendors have developed commercial software to support the execution of AD that can be used to document the data access operational integrity of AD (see Chap. 8, on available software for AD).

The draft guidance explicitly encourages the use of AD in the context of exploratory studies, stating that they provide a natural framework for learning about dose–response, subgroup effects, etc. and have the potential to lead to substantial gains in knowledge efficiency. It is also mentioned that exploratory studies provide a natural framework for implementing and getting familiarity with unblinded adaptations currently included in the less well-understood category. That is, the guidance suggests that utilization of (currently) less well-understood adaptive methods in exploratory studies may pave the way for their future acceptance as well-understood AD. One potential practical difficulty for the implementation of this recommendation is that sponsors often design exploratory studies, especially in Phase 2, as mini A&WC studies, in the hope that if great results are observed, the study may be accepted by RA as one of the required pivotal studies. The guidance specifically discourages this type of practice.

2.2.3 Well-Understood vs. Less Well-Understood Adaptive Designs

Within the class of A&WC studies, the guidance introduces a classification of *well-understood* and *less well-understood* types of adaptive designs. This has been mistakenly interpreted by many in industry, most notably by some in regulatory affairs groups, to mean that only AD of the well-understood type would be acceptable to FDA. Even though it has been clarified by FDA representatives (involved in the writing of the draft guidance) at public meetings and conferences that the categorization only referred to the state of regulatory knowledge of and familiarity with different types of AD at the time the draft guidance was published, the misunderstanding persists till the time of publishing of this book. There is an expectation that this issue will be addressed in the final version of guidance, when it is published.

The set of well-understood AD identified in the draft guidance is composed broadly of group sequential designs (with early termination for either demonstrated efficacy or futility) and adaptations that do not involve post-baseline unblinded data. Examples include adaption of study eligibility criteria based on baseline data, blinded sample size or study duration re-estimation, and adaptations based on outcome unrelated to efficacy (though the guidance warns that this may be difficult to ascertain). In general, adaptations based on blinded and/or baseline data (carried out by personnel without access to unblinded results) do not raise any regulatory concerns.

The fact that group sequential designs, though involving adaptations based on unblinded data, are included in the well-understood category gives further indication that the classification is more based on regulatory familiarity than acceptance. It also suggests that, as FDA is exposed to more AD trials involving unblinded adaptations, some of the methods currently in the less well-understood category may find their way into the well-understood group.

All designs involving adaptations based on unblinded post-baseline data, with the exception of group sequential designs, fall into the less well-understood category. Examples include unblinded sample size/study duration re-estimation, response-adaptive randomization, adaptive subgroup and/or endpoint selection-based observed treatment effects, and adaptive dose selection. With regard to the latter, the guidance recognizes its potential value in the context of A&WC studies (to allow some limited exploration of dose–response), provided strict control of Type I error rate can be demonstrated. Within the category of less well-understood AD, the guidance highlights designs with multiple types of adaptations and adaptations in non-inferiority studies. With regard to the first, the guidance expresses concerns related to the increasing complexity that results from combining different types of adaptations in the same study, which could lead to difficulties in interpreting the final results. The value of adaptations in the context of non-inferiority studies is acknowledged, but the guidance points out that some of the design elements in non-inferiority trials are not suitable for adaptation, most notably the non-inferiority margin.

Besides the usual concerns about potential Type I error rate inflation, bias in treatment effect estimates, and operational bias in trial conduct, the guidance also indicates the potential for Type II error rate increase in the context of less well-understood AD, citing too liberal futility rules and suboptimal dose selection as examples. Of course these are concerns that typically resonate and concern more sponsors than regulators, so it is refreshing to see them mentioned in the guidance. The discussion around less well-understood AD ends on a positive note, with the guidance stating that *cautious use of adaptive designs can advance overall development programs*. This is likely to be as supportive as one could expect to read in a guidance document.

2.2.4   Role of Trial Simulations

As well known among practitioners who have designed and/or implemented adaptive designs, modeling and trial simulations play a central role in their evaluation and the understanding of their operating characteristics. Even relatively simple AD, such as blinded sample size re-estimation, require simulations to properly characterize its performance under alternative scenarios (e.g., underlying effect and variability) and design choices (e.g., when to conduct the interim analyses). Modeling plays a central role in the characterization of alternative scenarios, such as the recruitment and dropout processes, dose–response profiles, and correlation between endpoints. The combination of modeling and trial simulation provides the backbone for the evaluation and comparison of alternative designs, including adaptive ones, and the planning of a specific adaptive design (e.g., number and timing of adaptations, impact on Type I error rate and power).

The guidance acknowledges the importance of trial simulations for the determination of operating characteristics of AD, the comparison of alternative designs to justify the selection of a particular AD, and the understanding of inferential properties of an AD. In fact, the guidance states that the reporting of trial simulations should be an important component of the documentation to be submitted to FDA when a sponsor proposes the use of an AD in the development program. The guidance goes further and indicates that the models, programs, and flow charts for possible adaptive pathways used in the simulations should also be included as part of the submitted documentation. Among the inferential characteristics of the design that can be investigated via simulation, the guidance names the impact on Type I error rate, power, and bias in the estimation of treatment effects. The document goes into some detail on the types of models that could be considered in the simulation-based evaluation of AD, including withdrawal and dropout models, models for selecting among multiple endpoints, and models characterizing the study endpoints (e.g., longitudinal models). It also includes a list of which elements should be included when reporting simulations used for AD evaluation, such as a listing of all possible adaptation branches, the design features and assumptions, and calculation of Type I error rate and power.

While discussing the importance and usefulness of trial simulations, the guidance goes on a short detour to discuss how Bayesian methods can play a relevant role in the context of AD. It indicates that Bayesian approaches provide a useful framework for describing the various choices and decisions available in an AD, placing them in a probabilistic context that is naturally handled under the Bayesian paradigm. The guidance even goes as far as to state that Bayesian decision rules can be used to guide adaptations while preserving the Type I error rate in a frequentist sense. It is unclear, though, if such framework would be accepted by regulators in the context of an A&WC study, or if it should have its use limited to exploratory studies.

On a side note that was disappointing to some, the guidance states that, though trial simulations are acknowledged as useful, or even essential, for the understanding of operating characteristics of an AD, their use to establish strict control of Type I error rate in an AD is *controversial and not fully understood*. Because many AD are complex enough not to allow the analytical derivation of its Type I error rate, this remark in the guidance has led to lively reactions from industry. In general, the available analytical solutions rely on rather inefficient upper bounds for the Type I error rate, in the sense that the true significance level is considerably smaller than the upper bound, under a wide range of realistic scenarios. This leads to loss in power, or increases in sample size to avert it (both of which, of course, are evaluated via trial simulations).

2.2.5   Protocol and SAP for an Adaptive Design

Because of the heightened concerns about operational bias and trial integrity surrounding AD, the prospective specification of all aspects of the study design and planned analyses is of paramount importance. As frequently mentioned in the ADWG publications and also highlighted in the draft guidance, to ensure the scientific validity of an AD, any potential adaptations need to be pre-specified: *adaptive by design*, as aptly stated in Gallo et al. (2006).

The protocol of an A&WC AD study, according to the draft guidance, typically needs to be more detailed than for a conventional design. The protocol and its supportive documentation (such as the simulation report) need to contain all critical information to allow FDA to evaluate the AD. These should include

- Study rationale
- Justification of design features, including any proposed adaptations
- Operating characteristics of proposed design, such as Type I error rate and power
- Plans to ensure study integrity when unblinded interim analyses are planned
- Role of AD in overall clinical development strategy
- Objectives and design features of the AD, all possible adaptations envisioned, assumptions, analysis methods, and quantitative justification for design choices at planning stage (typically via simulations)
- Impact of adaptations on frequentist operating characteristics (e.g., Type I error rate)
- Summary of models used in planning (e.g., disease progression, dropout, dose–response)
- Analytical derivations to demonstrate strict control of Type I error rate, if appropriate (e.g., A&WC studies)
- Charter of personnel involved in carrying out adaptations and study monitoring

It is acknowledged that data monitoring committee (DMC) charters will generally need to be more detailed for an AD compared to a more conventional design involving interim analyses (e.g., group sequential design).

The extensive list of protocol elements for an AD mentioned in the draft guidance has raised some concerns about the greater scrutiny that this type of design may receive at FDA. In reality, most of the items in the guidance list apply equally to nonadaptive designs and should be part of the checklist of good design practice. Adaptive designs have created greater awareness about the importance of proper scenario evaluation via modeling and trial simulations, which should lead to better design planning and justification across drug development, and not just for AD.

With regard to statistical analysis plans (SAP) for AD, the key message in the guidance is *prospective specification*. The guidance encourages sponsors to have the SAP finalized by the time of protocol finalization, a practice already adopted by some, but certainly not the majority of biopharmaceutical companies. Specific elements that should be included in an AD SAP listed in the guidance are the following:

- All prospectively planned adaptations
- Statistical methods to be used to implement adaptations (e.g., how to calculate a potential increase in sample size or trial duration, rule used to select a dose)
- Justification of Type I error control
- Statistical approach to be used for appropriately estimating treatment effects

The overarching message in the guidance with regard to regulating AD is that FDA understands that this type of design requires more in-depth regulatory review and evaluations. Accordingly, it is expected that sponsors will provide documentation, such as protocols and SAP, with the level of detail necessary to allow the proper regulatory oversight.

2.2.6 Interactions with FDA on Adaptive Designs

According to the guidance, it is anticipated that sponsors will need earlier and more intense interactions with FDA to discuss and reach agreement on planned AD. This will, of course, vary with the type of AD and the phase of development, being more critical for less well-understood A&WC trials. The guidance is not entirely clear on the type of meeting request that should be made for the discussion of AD. For exploratory studies, it is recommended that either a Type C or an end of Phase 2 (EOP2) meeting request be used. For an A&WC study, the guidance indicates that, when appropriate, an EOP2 meeting request should be used, but acknowledges that there will be instances in which this will not be adequate. The guidance states that a special protocol assessment (SPA) meeting would *not* be appropriate to discuss AD and discourages sponsors from submitting SPA requests for that purpose. Further clarity on the type of meeting request that would be most appropriate for engaging FDA in discussions on proposed AD would be useful to sponsors. Perhaps a new type of meeting, or the extension of existing meeting types, should be considered for AD.

The protection of study blind among trial personnel non-authorized to have access to treatment assignment during the trial is a recurrent theme in the draft guidance, identified as a critical issue to ensure the integrity and validity of an AD. The guidance indicates that SOPs specific to AD should be put in place by sponsors, clearly indicating who will implement adaptations and how access to unblinded data during the study will be controlled (in particular, when study personnel and investigators may have access to unblinded results). The guidance highlights that an independent group from the study personnel should be responsible for unblinded interim analyses and adaptive decision making. The role can be assigned to an independent DMC (IDMC) or some other group. There is still no consensus across the biopharmaceutical industry, or among regulators on whether conventional IDMC should have their role extended to also handle AD monitoring and decision making, or if a new type of independent group should be formed for this type of study (see Chap. 14, on DMC).

2.2.7   Final Remarks

The draft guidance concludes with some specific recommendations regarding the report of the final results of an AD. There should be strict compliance with the prospectively planned adaptation process and with the procedures for ensuring study integrity, such as the preservation of treatment blinding. The final documentation submitted to FDA should include a description of the processes and procedures actually carried out in the trial, any records from deliberations of the IDMC and any other groups involved in carrying out adaptations, interim results used for adaptations, and an assessment of the adequacy of firewalls to prevent access to unblinded results by unauthorized personnel. All analyses included in the final report should strictly adhere to the SAP. Because of concerns about shifts in patient population during the study, possibly induced by adaptations, the guidance recommends that the consistency of estimated treatment effects across study stages (i.e., before and after adaptations) should be explored and reported with the final results. If potential shifts are observed, they are likely to become a review issue.

The overall message of the guidance is positive on AD while being cautious about their proper planning, implementation, and reporting. The guidance recommends that sponsors keep AD simple, avoiding too many or too complex adaptations in the same trial. It encourages increased planning and early interactions with FDA, especially for more complex A&WC studies. Assurance that treatment blinding is preserved and adequately documented is paramount to regulatory acceptance of the results from an AD.

2.3   EMEA Reflection Paper on Adaptive Designs

The EMEA reflection paper played a pioneering role with regard to regulatory guidance on adaptive designs, being published at a time of active discussion on different aspects of adaptive designs, such as methodology, implementation, and regulatory acceptance. The EMEA document shed some critical light into the discussions taken place then and, in many ways, paved the way for the FDA draft guidance published years later. The EMEA document is considerably narrower in scope and less detailed than the FDA draft guidance. On the other hand, it emphasizes some regulatory concerns about AD that are only tangentially discussed in the FDA document, making it a useful complement to the latter with regard to regulatory thinking on AD at the time this book was published. This section summarizes the key points in the reflection paper, contrasting them to the FDA draft guidance and considering them from an industry perspective.

The EMEA document focuses almost exclusively on confirmatory trials, or, in the notation of the FDA draft guidance, A&WC studies. The overall tone of the document is accepting of the potential utility of AD, but with clear concerns about their adequate implementation in clinical trial practice. By comparison, the reflection paper is less encouraging about AD than the FDA guidance, but it does not strike a negative tone with regard to their utilization, when properly planned, conducted, and analyzed. In its opening remarks, the EMEA reflection paper recognizes that AD have the potential to speed up drug development and more efficiently allocate resources, without compromising the scientific and regulatory standards, while high-lighting that the basis for regulatory decision making will need to be improved to allow AD to be fully embraced by regulators. A less encouraging comment in the opening section of the document is that AD in the context of confirmatory trials is a contradiction in terms, as one should not need to adapt what is to be just confirmed. Of course this is too narrow a view of the regulatory dichotomization between the exploratory and confirmatory phases of development, being toned down in later sections of the document. It is not the case in drug development practice that all is known about a compound before it is taken into Phase 3 studies—development programs would take substantially longer, and approved drugs would cost significantly more, if this narrow interpretation of the regulatory process were to be followed to the letter.

An important and interesting difference between the EMEA reflection paper and the FDA draft guidance is the focus of the former on the assessment of homogeneity between stages of an AD. The issue is certainly discussed in the FDA draft guidance, but with considerably less prominence than in the EMEA document, where it appears to be central to the regulatory acceptance of AD. There are, of course, more similarities than differences between the EMEA and FDA documents and certainly no disagreement between them with regard to recommendations and regulatory requirements.

The EMEA reflection paper is less didactic than the FDA draft guidance, with no attempts at classifying AD, like is done in the latter. A more formal definition of adaptive designs is only included in the last page of document and it illustrates the narrow view of the document: "a study design is called '*adaptive*' if statistical methodology allows the modification of a design element ... at an interim analysis with full control the type I error." It is clear from this definition that the main concern in the document about the validity of an AD is the preservation of strict control of Type I error rate in the presence of possible adaptations. The definition of AD presented in the FDA draft guidance is much broader in scope and more in line with mainstream publications in the field.

The concern about potential operational bias induced by an AD is shared between the EMEA and FDA documents, though in the former such concern is almost exclusively associated with the possible change in patient population during the study. The document states that if substantial differences are observed in patient composition (e.g., demographics, baseline characteristics) and/or in trial results before and after an adaptation then there would be serious regulatory concerns about the validity of the final conclusions and the integrity of the study as a whole. It is not clear, though, what would characterize a *substantial difference* in this context, or whether it should be formally tested via a hypothesis test, or just explored via summary statistics and estimated effects. There is a clear tone of discouragement of unblinded interim analyses in the reflection paper, because of the perceived risks of information leak resulting from them. The recommendation is that unblinded interim analyses only should be used when there is a clear, justifiable need, should be kept to a minimum number, and with the flow of unblinded information should be carefully documented and controlled. One is left to wonder if the regulators who produced the reflection paper would find the implementation of an AD as sufficient reason to justify the inclusion of interim analyses in the study.

It is possible (and, one would hope, likely) that regulatory thinking at EMA has evolved since the publication of the reflection paper and a more accepting view of the ability of sponsors to preserve the blind in an AD and avoid the leaking of unblinded results via appropriate processes and firewalls now prevails. If that is the case, one would expect a more positive view of unblinded interim analyses, not only in the context of AD, but in confirmatory trials, more broadly. Interestingly, the reflection paper seems to be supportive, or at least not discouraging, of group sequential designs, which, of course, require unblinded interim analyses.

A topic discussed in the EMA reflection paper but omitted from the FDA draft guidance is that of overrunning, i.e., observed data on certain patients only becoming available after a decision to stop the study at an interim analysis point was made. This may be because overrunning is a topic that has been extensively discussed and addressed in the context of group sequential designs, being less of an issue in AD that do not include an early efficacy stopping rule. Of course, it is a nonissue in the case of futility stopping.

Similarly to the FDA draft guidance, the EMEA reflection paper states that any adaptation under consideration should be pre-planned, be properly justified in the context of the development program, and have their number kept to the necessary minimum. Strict control of Type I error rate is indicated as a prerequisite for the regulatory acceptance of any AD, but appropriate statistical methods for treatment effect estimation (point-wise and confidence intervals) in the context of an AD are also necessary. The reflection paper stresses at various points that AD should not be used as a substitute for good planning and thorough exploration in early phases of clinical development.

The reflection paper names and discusses a number of specific types of adaptations, a subset of which are briefly summarized below.

- *Sample size re-estimation*: The blinded version should be used whenever possible, but the unblinded alternative can also be considered, when properly justified. In either case, there should be good justification of why the use of this type of adaptation is not an indication of just insufficient investigation in exploratory studies.

- *Change or modification of primary endpoint*: This would be very difficult to justify in practice and would likely lead to difficulties in statistical inference if one were to combine results from stages utilizing different endpoints (e.g., rejection of a global null hypothesis).
- *Discontinuing treatment arms*: Discontinuing the placebo arm after an interim analysis is discouraged, as it may result in changes in patient population and lead to inferential hurdles at the end of the study; unbalanced randomization favoring active treatment over placebo throughout the study should be considered as an alternative. Multiple comparison approaches are required to properly control the Type I error rate.
- *Phase 2/3 combinations*: The reflection paper suggests that Phase 2/3AD are in principle acceptable, but need to be properly justified (and with any AD mentioned in the document) and would not provide sufficient evidence of efficacy for regulatory approval if it were the single pivotal study conducted in the program. That would be the case even in indications in which a single Phase 3 study could be accepted for approval. The use of two Phase 2/3AD studies is mentioned as a possible path for approval, though it may be challenging to ensure that the same decisions are reached in both trials. One assumes that the combination of one Phase 2/3AD design with one conventional Phase 3 design would also provide sufficient evidence of efficacy for regulatory approval. Single Phase 2/3AD studies could be considered for orphan indications.

The FDA draft guidance does not contradict any of the recommendations included in the EMEA reflection paper, but it certainly strikes a more positive note on the regulatory acceptability of and support for adaptive designs. One of the possible reasons explaining this difference in tone between the two regulatory documents is that the FDA document was crafted following innumerous discussions with industry groups focused on AD at scientific meetings and through visitations to FDA, as well as several white papers published by those same industry groups. The EMEA reflection paper did not benefit from the same level of open dialog between industry representatives and regulators on methodological and operational issues related to AD, and may reflect a more one-sided view on AD.

2.4 Industry Reaction and Perspectives on Guidance Documents

The biopharmaceutical industry, by and large, regards adaptive designs as a useful tool for its ongoing effort to modernize and improve the efficiency of drug development. Clear regulatory guidance on the acceptability, or not, of different types of AD is a precondition for the effectiveness and viability of these methods in practice. Therefore, both the EMEA reflection paper and the FDA draft guidance on AD were well received by industry, despite the less than encouraging tone of the former and the ambiguity of some elements in the latter. They were perceived as an encouraging sign of regulatory agency acknowledgement of the potential benefits of AD while providing some level of guidance on how to possibly address regulatory concerns about their use in clinical development practice.

Following the release of the regulatory documents, industry groups were organized and collated their concerns and suggestions on the guidance documents, submitting them during the corresponding comment periods. Some of those suggestions have been implemented in the published version of the EMEA reflection paper. The final version of the FDA draft guidance had yet to be released at the time of publishing of this book, being unclear on which, if any, of the industry suggestions would be incorporated in the revised document. We review here the comments and suggestions collated for each of the documents by PhRMA industry groups, following the same order used previously in the paper, namely starting with the FDA draft guidance, followed by the EMEA reflection paper.

2.4.1 FDA Draft Guidance

By the time the draft guidance was released, the ADWG was no longer affiliated with PhRMA, so a new group needed to be formed to review and produce the PhRMA response to the document. However, the majority of the PhRMA review team was composed of former members of the ADWG, so a certain level of continuity was achieved in the response to the FDA draft guidance submitted by PhRMA.

The overall reaction of the PhRMA review team (and industry as a whole) to the draft guidance was positive, with the group acknowledging that the document was quite helpful in clarifying FDA's position on and concerns about AD, and with the expectation that the guidance would positively impact the broader acceptance and proper utilization of AD in clinical drug development. There were also a number of comments, concerns, and suggestions for improvement put forward by the PhRMA review team, summarized below.

The main concern was the categorization of adaptive designs for A&WC studies into well understood and less well understood. The team indicated the fear that less well understood would be misunderstood as not-to-be-used by many in industry, which unfortunately turned out to be the case. A suggestion was made for FDA to clarify in the final version of the guidance that, when properly planned, implemented and analyzed, less well-understood AD were also acceptable for A&WC studies. Furthermore, one would expect that as FDA became more familiar with the appropriate utilization of those AD, they would be moved to the well-understood category in possible future revisions of the guidance. One point raised by the review team was that many of the cautions indicated in the guidance for less well-understood AD (e.g., potential for operational bias after unblinded interim analyses) also apply to well-understood AD (e.g., group sequential designs) and even conventional, non-adaptive designs. Adaptive designs may have motivated greater awareness and discussion around such issues, but they are not exclusive, or even more prevalent in AD.

While the draft guidance is clearly encouraging of the use of AD in exploratory studies, the message is somewhat ambiguous with regard to A&WC studies.

The many references to bias in the context of AD for A&WC studies (operational, estimation, and in hypothesis testing) go beyond cautionary to strike a somewhat negative tone. The PhRMA review team suggested that the final guidance included a clear message of FDA's willingness to consider AD both for exploratory and A&WC studies.

The lack of clarity in the guidance about which type of meeting request would be appropriate for discussion and review of AD with FDA was another important point raised by the PhRMA review team. The group suggested that there should be greater clarity in the final version of the guidance on how sponsors should seek input from FDA on AD with different degrees of complexity and the circumstances under which an SPA would be the appropriate type of meeting for such interactions.

The Biotechnology Industry Organization (BIO) also formed a review team that produced an industry response to the FDA draft guidance. The comments and suggestions submitted by the BIO review team were broadly similar to those of the PhRMA group, with a few noteworthy additions. The BIO group made the recommendation that, to avoid potential confusion, methods and statistical and logistical consideration for AD be separately described in the guidance for exploratory and A&WC studies. In addition, the review team suggested that there should be better balance between exploratory and A&WC AD studies in the document—the draft guidance focuses mostly on the latter (which is understandable, from a regulatory perspective).

2.4.2 EMEA Reflection Paper

The PhRMA response to the reflection paper was mostly driven by the ADWG, which was still affiliated with the trade association at the time the document was released. The comments from the PhRMA team were more directly targeted at defending certain types of AD and related implementation practices, compared to what was included in the PhRMA response to the FDA draft guidance. This reflects the less positive tone of the reflection paper on adaptive designs and practices.

Adaptive seamless Phase 2/3 designs were prominently discussed in the PhRMA response, reflecting the industry mindset at that time. The naming of this type of design has changed since, to avoid the explicit reference to combining exploratory and confirmatory phases in one study (though the essence of the AD remains very much present in clinical development). Regulators expressed concern about having exploratory elements (i.e., Phase 2) in a study intended to be confirmatory. An example of new naming for this type of design is adaptive A&WC study with dose/subgroup selection. In their response, the PhRMA review team lists the benefits of this type of AD, including increased information on doses and efficacy prior to triggering the confirmatory stage, reduced development timelines and costs (compared to running separate Phase 2 and Phase 3 studies), more safety information, and increased chance of treating patients in the trial with efficacious and safe drugs (see Chap. 20 for an example of a successful seamless two-stage design). The response also included a discussion of possible regulatory strategies for including an adaptive seamless Phase 2/3 trial as one of the pivotal studies in a submission. Some of the suggestions were incorporated in the final version of the reflection paper published by CHMP.

The PhRMA review team defended the opportunity for limited sponsor involvement in interim decision making during an AD, pointing out that IDMC members may not be prepared, or willing, to make decisions that have important commercial implications to sponsors. Processes and safeguards that would allow this type of limited sponsor involvement to take place while protecting the integrity of the study are proposed in the team's response (and have been presented and discussed in white papers published by the ADWG, such as Gallo et al. 2010; see also Chap. 14 for more recent thinking on DMC for AD).

The potential for operational bias as a result of a poorly planned and/or implemented AD was acknowledged by the PhRMA review team, but they pointed out that this risk is also present with classic group sequential designs and has long been successfully addressed by sponsors. The team suggested that the potential for operational bias in an AD should be prospectively mitigated via design and implementation safeguards discussed and agreed upon with regulators prior to the start of the study, and not via post-trial assessment of changes in patient population during the study (which may occur irrespective of and unrelated to adaptations).

The response from the PhRMA review team included a suggestion to have AD for confirmatory studies classified into two categories of regulatory support: acceptable and possible. Blinded sample size re-estimation and subgroup selection were cited as examples of regulatory acceptable AD, while unblinded sample size re-estimation was mentioned in the possible category. The intention of the suggestion, at the time, was to request clear regulatory guidance on what types of AD were endorsed by EMA and which would require further justification and discussions with regulators. Even though this suggestion was not implemented in the final version of the reflection paper, it possibly provided the seed for the classification of AD A&WC studies into well understood and less well understood. In hindsight, the suggestion may not have the most beneficial for advancing the broader use of AD, from an industry perspective.

Additional comments and recommendations on the reflection paper put forward by the PhRMA review team were related to adaptive dose-finding designs (use of parsimonious modeling), unblinded sample size re-estimation (should not be ruled out as a valid AD), and Bayesian approaches (to be included in the reflection paper and have its potential use in AD discussed).

2.5 Concluding Remarks

The regulatory guidance documents on AD published to date have had a critical impact on the acceptance and utilization of AD by the biopharmaceutical industry. Both documents, in particular the FDA draft guidance, have helped clarify the regulatory position and concerns on AD, which by itself is quite useful. However, the cautionary tone of both documents and the classification of some AD for A&WC studies as less well understood in the FDA guidance have caused some negative reaction in industry with regard to regulatory acceptance of AD, more generally. As a result, the increased utilization of AD that was expected after the release of the FDA draft guidance never materialized.

One important change that has occurred from the time prior to the release of the FDA draft guidance is that the ADWG is no longer affiliated to PhRMA and, perhaps for this reason, no longer active with regard to scientific advocacy for adaptive designs. The publication of the final version of the FDA guidance which addressed the key industry concerns listed in Sect. 2.4.1 would go a long way toward increasing the acceptance and utilization of AD in industry. We hope that FDA will be able to provide industry advocates of AD with this valuable support soon.

References

Antonijevic Z, Pinheiro J, Fardipour P, Lewis R (2010) Impact of dose selection strategies used in phase ii on the probability of success in phase III. Stat Biopharm Res 2(4):469–486

Bornkamp B, Bretz F, Dmitrienko A, Enas G, Gaydos B, Hsu CH, Koenig F, Krams M, Liu Q, Neuenschwander B, Parke T, Pinheiro J, Roy A, Sax R, Shen F (2007) Innovative approaches for designing and analyzing adaptive dose-ranging trials (with discussion). J Biopharm Stat 17:965–995

EMEA/CHMP (2007) Reflection paper on methodological issues in confirmatory clinical trials with flexible design and analysis plan (draft CHMP/EWP/2459/02, 23-Mar-2006). www.ema. europa.eu/pdfs/human/ewp/245902en.pdf

FDA (2010) Adaptive design clinical trials for drug and biologics draft guidance. www.fda.gov/ downloads/Drugs/GuidanceComplianceRegulatoryInformation/Guidances/UCM201790.pdf

Gallo P, Chuang-Stein C, Dragalin V, Gaydos B, Krams M, Pinheiro J (2006) Executive summary of the PhRMA working group on adaptive designs in clinical drug development. J Biopharm Stat 16:275–283

Gallo P, Fardipour P, Dragalin V, Krams M, Litman GS, Bretz F (2010) Data monitoring in adaptive dose ranging trials. Stat Biopharm Res 2(4):513–521

PhRMA Working Group on Adaptive Designs (2006) Full white paper. Drug Inform J 40: 421–484

Pinheiro J, Sax R, Antonijevic Z, Bornkamp B, Bretz F, Chuang-Stein C, Dragalin V, Fardipour P, Gallo P, Gillespie W, Hsu CH, Miller F, Padmanabhan SK, Patel N, Perevozskaya I, Roy A, Sanil A, Smith JR (2010) Adaptive and model-based dose ranging trials: quantitative evaluation and recommendations (with discussion). Stat Biopharm Res 2(4):435–454

Chapter 3
A Commentary on the U.S. FDA Adaptive Design Draft Guidance and EMA Reflection Paper from a Regulatory Perspective and Regulatory Experiences

Sue-Jane Wang

Keywords Adequate and well controlled • Bias • Consistency • Difficult experimental situations • Exploratory adaptive design trial • Less well-understood • One trial one studywise type I error rate • Rare disease • Regulatory submission • Simulated type I error

3.1 Historical Landscape

Fixed design confirmatory trials rely on emerging and reliable prior data and knowledge to provide necessary assumptions about the key design parameters including nuisance parameters. Traditionally, a fixed design has been the gold standard for its simplicity, validity, and ability to provide an unbiased estimate of the treatment effect. To allow for pre-specified flexibility in an ongoing trial, a simple two-arm controlled trial with a single primary efficacy endpoint, the repeated significance testing involving multiplicity adjustment becomes more complex than a fixed design approach. The repeated significance testing recognized in group sequential design and analysis was proposed as early as the randomization ratio adaptation in late 1960s (Zelen 1969), e.g., Armitage et al. (1969).

In a broader sense, is a group sequential design controversial in the context of confirmatory trials? It may be possible to judge if a study design is controversial by examining the design features on whether the null hypothesis and the statistical information (i.e., sample size or number of clinical events initially planned for) remain unchanged. In group sequential designs, neither the initial null hypothesis nor

S.-J. Wang, Ph.D. (✉)
Office of Biostatistics, Office of Translational Sciences, Center for Drug Evaluation and Research, US Food and Drug Administration, 10903 New Hampshire Avenue, Building 21, Room 3526, HFD-700, Silver Spring, MD 20993-0002, USA
e-mail: suejane.wang@fda.hhs.gov

W. He et al. (eds.), *Practical Considerations for Adaptive Trial Design and Implementation*, Statistics for Biology and Health,
DOI 10.1007/978-1-4939-1100-4_3, © Springer Science+Business Media New York 2014

the maximum statistical information, e.g., the number of clinical events in an event-driven trial, is changed. Although the only and critical concern with group sequential design seems to be the potential maneuvers caused by unblinding that occurs in an interim analysis, we have gone a long way from adhering to fixed designs to adopting group sequential designs and such proposals have been considered by regulatory health authorities for medical product developments and licensures.

The conference on the practical issues with data monitoring of clinical trials held in 1992 (Ellenberg et al. 1993) signifies the milestones embracing group sequential designs in clinical trial practice following the public debates among experts involved in design and analysis of clinical trials, and the general recognition among clinical trialists, academia, and regulators. To maintain the integrity of a trial, the data monitoring committee (DMC) or data and safety monitoring committee (DSMC) previously known as the data and safety monitoring board (DSMB) was instituted to serve as an independent third party to communicate the only necessary information to drug sponsors.

Furthermore, the additional flexibility to modifying the multiple design aspects, e.g., adapting to some specific dose hypotheses with the potential to increase sample size in an interim analysis, has been proposed. The overwhelming interests in proposing adaptive designs in lieu of group sequential designs in regulatory submissions since mid-2000 allow the clinical trial community to experiment alternative trial designs beyond those fairly understood fixed designs and group sequential designs. In this chapter, regulatory guidance and reflection paper from health authorities on adaptive design will be briefly introduced. Their similarities and differences in emphasis will be highlighted. Key additions to the European Medicines Agency (EMA) reflection paper (European Medicines Agency 2007) described in United States Food and Drug Administration (US FDA) draft guidance (FDA 2010) will be bulleted. In addition, adaptive design proposals submitted to the US FDA both before and following publication of the draft guidance will be briefly summarized. Some of the challenges observed in implementing adaptive design confirmatory trials will be shared. Regulatory perspectives on statistical considerations for use of adaptive designs will be articulated based on current thinking, and a summary will follow.

3.2   Regulatory Guidance Documents

Shortly after Dr. Robert O'Neill, the former Director of Office of Biostatistics, Center for Drug Evaluation and Research, US Food and Drug Administration (FDA), instituted the regulatory roles in preparation of FDA regulatory review functions on adaptive design submissions, the EMA (the European counterpart) had drafted the reflection paper on methodological issues in confirmatory clinical trials planned with an adaptive design, agreed by the Efficacy Working Party (EWP) of Committee for Medical Products for Human use (CHMP) on January 11, 2006 (European Medicines Agency 2007). With oversights of regulatory submissions and their experience building since late 2005, the US FDA draft guidance for industry on adaptive design clinical trials for drugs and biologics was released for public comment on February 26, 2010 (FDA 2010).

The term "adaptive" and the rationales behind the regulatory guidance may not be quite the same between the two continents as the term "flexible" (e.g., Bauer et al. 2001; Hung et al. 2006) was also used until the term "adaptive" was eventually adopted in the two regulatory guidance documents (European Medicines Agency 2007; FDA 2010). Earlier, the greater interests in applying adaptive design beyond group sequential design were from Europe with its majority in Germany due to the fact that the broad early research on the newer adaptive design topics that combine stages from a single trial was performed in the Europe region, see (Bauer 1989; Bauer and Kohne 1994). Such interests gradually emerged and received enthusiastic attention in U.S. As a result, the development of the US FDA draft guidance for industry on adaptive design clinical trials for drugs and biologics (FDA 2010) was necessary to define the boundaries of adaptive designs regarding what are flexible, what are exploratory and what are adequate and well controlled (A&WC) (FDA 2002a) for clinical trials aiming for drug and biologics development.

3.2.1 EMA Reflection Paper on Methodological Issues in Confirmatory Clinical Trials Planned with an Adaptive Design

The EMA reflection paper on methodological issues in confirmatory clinical trials planned with an adaptive design (European Medicines Agency 2007) adopted by EMA/CHMP in October 2007 is a 10-page document. The EMA reflection paper is structured into four sections. The main body of the texts is in section 4, which outlines general considerations for studies incorporating interim analyses that are pre-planned (4.1), followed by a set of minimal requirements for interim analysis with design modifications that must be fulfilled whenever confirmatory clinical trials are planned with an adaptive design (4.2).

More specifically, in section 4.1, three topics on interim analyses for general considerations are discussed in details. They are (1) the importance of confidentiality of interim results, (2) considerations about stopping trials early for efficacy, and (3) overrunning. Specific design modifications that have been proposed in the relevant literature on (1) sample size reassessment, (2) change or modification of the primary end-point, (3) discontinuing treatment arms, (4) switching between superiority and noninferiority, (5) randomization ratio, (6) phase II/phase III combinations, applications with one pivotal trial and the independent replication of findings, (7) substantial changes of trial design, and (8) futility stopping in late phase II or phase III clinical trials are commented in section 4.2. See Appendix 1 for table of contents of the EMA reflection paper (European Medicines Agency 2007).

3.2.2 FDA Draft Guidance for Industry on Adaptive Design Clinical Trials for Drugs and Biologics

The US FDA draft guidance for industry on adaptive design clinical trials for drugs and biologics (FDA 2010) targets multidisciplinary readers directly or indirectly involved in designing, planning, performing, monitoring, and analyzing clinical trials for drug development including, e.g., external experts/consultants. This draft guidance is a 50-page document structured into 12 sections. The earlier sections of the document give (1) description of and motivation for adaptive designs, and (2) general concerns associated with use of adaptive design in drug development. The mid-sections of the document elaborate extensively on (1) generally well-understood adaptive designs with valid approaches to implementation, (2) adaptive study designs whose properties are less well understood, (3) statistical considerations for less well-understood adaptive design methods, and (4) safety consideration in adaptive design trials.

The later sections of the document provide details on the processes, procedures, and documentations needed to maintain the integrity of the trial and its results when planning and implementing an adaptive design clinical trial. Specifically, these sections discuss (1) contents of an adaptive design protocol, (2) interactions with US FDA when planning and conducting an adaptive design, (3) documentation and practices to protect study blinding and information sharing for adaptive designs, and (4) evaluating and reporting a completed study. See Appendix 2 for table of contents of the FDA draft guidance (FDA 2010).

3.3 Basic Premises/Definitions

In discussing the guidance document of FDA (FDA 2010) and the reflection paper of EMA (European Medicines Agency 2007), one should keep in mind that each document has its own objectives. I begin by extracting the basic premises and their definitions of adaptive designs in clinical trials.

3.3.1 Basic Premises

The word "should" in the FDA draft guidance means that something is suggested or recommended, but, not required. Such concept is specific to FDA guidances. This is because guidances describe the Agency's current thinking on a topic and should be viewed only as recommendations, unless specific regulatory or statutory requirements are cited. There are two such requirements cited in the FDA draft guidance on adaptive design clinical trials for drugs and biologics (FDA 2010). One is "The major focus of this guidance is adequate and well-controlled effectiveness (A&WC)

studies intended to provide substantial evidence of effectiveness required by law to support a conclusion that a drug is effective (see 21 CFR 314.126 (FDA 2002a))." The other is "In addition to the full documentation required for a study protocol (21 CFR 312.23(a) (FDA 2002b)), there should be comprehensive and prospective written standard operating procedures (SOPs) ..." In this spirit, when the FDA adaptive design draft guidance is finalized, a sponsor can use an alternative approach if the approach satisfies the requirement of the applicable statutes and regulations.

Instead of regulatory or statutory requirements cited in the FDA draft guidance (FDA 2010), the EMA reflection paper (European Medicines Agency 2007), focusing on the learning and thinking via reflection, gives a list of minimal requirements on adaptation of design specifications with interim analyses anticipated in a confirmatory clinical trial. They are highlighted below.

- It requires pre-planning and a clear justification
- The number of design modifications should be limited
- It requires the control of the pre-specified Type I error, pre-specification of the corresponding methods to estimate the size of the treatment effect and to provide confidence intervals with pre-specified coverage probability in addition to the presentation of the p-value
- A measure for the treatment effect that is readily interpretable for clinicians should be preferred when the effect can be measured on different scales
- From a regulatory point of view, whenever trials are planned to incorporate design modifications based on the results of an interim analysis, the applicant *must* pre-plan methods to ensure that results from different stages of the trial can be justifiably combined.
- Depending on the nature of the design modification, the simple rejection of a global null hypothesis across all stages of the trial may not be sufficient to establish a convincing treatment effect
- The involvement of sponsor personnel in interim decision making remain controversial, which introduces an additional risk when the credibility of the trial results is challenged, since it would be more difficult to argue that importantly different results from different stages are only due to chance.

The following key points are also emphasized in the EMA reflection paper (European Medicines Agency 2007).

- The body of evidence justifying the final treatment recommendation *must* be discussed.
- The EMA reflection paper focuses on the opportunities for interim trial design modifications, and the prerequisites, problems and pitfalls that *must* be considered as soon as any kind of flexibility is introduced into a confirmatory clinical trial intended to provide evidence of efficacy.
- A set of minimal requirements is outlined that *must* be fulfilled whenever confirmatory clinical trials are planned with an adaptive design.
- Analysis methods that control the Type I error *must* be pre-specified.
- Effects *must* always be attributable to specific endpoints to clarify the capabilities of the drug treatment in a confirmatory setting.

3.3.2 Definitions

The EMA reflection paper (European Medicines Agency 2007) defines 'A study design is called "adaptive" if statistical methodology allows the modification of a design element (e.g., sample-size, randomization ratio, number of treatment arms) at an interim analysis with full control of the Type I error.' In this definition, a clinical trial with "adaptive" design may not be a group sequential trial, although this document begins with general considerations for studies incorporating interim analyses.

In contrast, a more extensive definition can be found in the FDA draft guidance (FDA 2010), which contains three components. That is, "an *adaptive design clinical study* is (1) a study that includes a *prospectively planned opportunity* for modification of one or more specified aspects of the study design and hypotheses based on analysis of data (usually interim data) from subjects in the study. (2) Analyses of the accumulating study data are performed at *prospectively planned timepoints* within the study, (3) can be performed in a fully blinded manner or in an unblinded manner, and can occur with or without formal statistical hypothesis testing." FDA definition of adaptive design includes group sequential design. This distinction will be elaborated later in Sect. 3.5 of this chapter.

3.4 Similarities

There are several similar concepts and principles between the FDA regulatory guidance and the EMA reflection paper for adaptive studies designed as confirmatory trials. We highlight a few in this section.

• Prospectively planned adaptation and its justification

ICH E9 (ICH 1998) emphasizes the concept of prospective planning of a confirmatory clinical. This concept is repeatedly stated in the FDA definition of adaptive design shown as italic phrases in Sect. 3.3.2. Although the definition of adaptive in the EMA reflection paper did not mention the concept of pre-planning, it is the first bullet in the list of minimal requirements summarized in Sect. 3.3.1. In fact, the EMA reflection paper does not recommend unplanned changes to the design of an ongoing confirmatory trial, even though such changes could be introduced with full control of the Type I error (p. 5 of European Medicines Agency 2007).

As for the need of justification for why pursuing an adaptive design, it is stated in the EMA reflection paper that "In all instances the interim analysis and the type of the anticipated design modification (change of sample size, discontinuation of treatment arms, etc.) would need to be described and justified in the study protocol." (European Medicines Agency 2007) Similarly, the FDA draft guidance states that document should include the rationale for the design, justification of design features, evaluation of the performance characteristics of the selected design (particularly less well-understood features), and plans to assure study integrity when unblinded analyses are involved, see the subsection A on "A&WC Adaptive Design Studies" of Section IX of the FDA draft guidance (FDA 2010).

- Control of pre-specified type I error

Both documents stress the need to control the pre-specified Type I error in adaptive design confirmatory trials or A&WC trials. The term "Type I error" occurs 11 times in the EMA reflection paper (European Medicines Agency 2007) and 52 times in the FDA draft guidance (FDA 2010). From the EMA reflection paper (European Medicines Agency 2007), a minimal prerequisite for statistical methods to be accepted in the regulatory setting is the control of the pre-specified Type I error, which is used as an abbreviation for "the control of the family-wise Type I error in the strong sense, i.e., there is control on the probability to reject at least one true null hypothesis, regardless which subset of null hypotheses happens to be true", see page 2 of CHMP Point to Consider on multiplicity issues in clinical trials (European Medicines Agency 2002). The importance of "controlling study-wide Type I error rate" can be found in Section VII, which is elaborated under subsection "A" of the FDA draft guidance (FDA 2010). This draft guidance further states that using Bayesian predictive probability may aid in deciding which adaptation should be selected, while the study design is still able to maintain statistical control of the Type I error rate in the frequentist design. The Type I error rate control here refers to the hybrid setting where adaptive design relies on the frequentist analysis and incorporates Bayesian predictive probability tool for the purpose of adaptation decision.

- Sample size re-estimation

There has been a great interest to preplan the possibility of modifying the study sample size or statistical information based on interim unblinded treatment effect estimate, e.g., (Gao et al. 2008) on the methodological relationship of the many references cited therein. However, both guidance documents encourage blinded methods for sample size re-estimation. The EMA reflection paper (European Medicines Agency 2007) states that whenever possible, methods for blinded sample size reassessment that properly control the Type I error should be used, especially if the sole aim of the interim analysis is the re-calculation of sample size. In cases where sample size needs to be reassessed based on unblinded data, sufficient justification should be made.

The similar concepts flow in the FDA draft guidance (FDA 2010) as such "sample size adjustment using blinded methods to maintain desired study power should generally be considered for most studies." The FDA draft guidance elaborates on the blinded interim analyses used to make decisions to increase the sample size and discourages it to decrease the sample size "because of the chance of making a poor choice caused by the high variability of the effect size and event rate or variance estimates early in the study."

• Sponsor personnel involvement in interim adaptive process and decision making

The concerns with the involvement of sponsor-affiliated personnel in interim adaptive decision making have been articulated in detail in the FDA guidance for clinical trial sponsors on establishment and operation of clinical trial data monitoring committees released in 2006, see section 6.4 Statisticians conducting the interim analyses (FDA 2006). A key concern is the conflicting nature between the sponsor-affiliated statistician and the sponsor regarding the ability to ensure the sponsor is unaware of the interim comparative data. This can be seriously questioned when the primary trial statistician or sponsor affiliated statistician is (extremely) knowledgeable about the study or is involved in regard to making decisions about design modifications.

In a similar vein, the EMA reflection paper (European Medicines Agency 2007) acknowledges that decision in certain types of adaptive trials are more complicated to set into an algorithm for independent interpretation than, for example, a sample size re-estimation problem or group-sequential stopping guidelines. Nevertheless, sponsor involvement introduces an additional risk when the credibility of the trial results is challenged as such with sponsor involvement it would be more difficult to argue that importantly different results from different stages are only due to chance. Therefore, "it remains controversial if the sponsor-affiliated personnel is involved in interim adaptive decision making." (European Medicines Agency 2007)

• When a number of design aspects need modification

In the section describing the minimal requirements, the EMA reflection paper (European Medicines Agency 2007) notes that "the need to modify a number of design aspects, e.g., re-assess sample size, change inclusion or exclusion criteria, change dosing, treatment duration, model of application, allow for alternative co-medications, may change the emphasis from a confirmatory trial to a hypothesis generating, or exploratory trial."

To articulate, the FDA draft guidance (FDA 2010) devotes a subsection VI.F to addressing "adaptation of multiple-study design features in a single study." The concerns include that the study will become increasingly complex and difficult to plan and increased difficulty in interpreting the study result. In addition, if there are interactions between the changes in study features, multiple adaptations can be counterproductive and lead to failure of the study to meet its goals. Because of these concerns, the draft guidance highlights that "an A&WC study should limit the number of adaptations and recommends exploratory studies may be better suited to circumstances when multiple adaptations are warranted." (FDA 2010)

• Investigate more than one dose in confirmatory clinical trials

The EMA reflection paper (European Medicines Agency 2007) notes that even after a carefully conducted phase II program, in some instances, some doubts about the most preferable dose for phase III may still exist and recommends that "investigators may wish to further investigate more than one dose of the experimental treatment in phase III". Similarly, the FDA draft guidance (FDA 2010) states that "fully evaluating more than one dose in the larger A&WC studies is almost always advisable whenever feasible."

3.5 Differences in Emphasis

Some of the emphases differ between the FDA draft guidance (FDA 2010) and the EMA reflection paper (European Medicines Agency 2007). Below, I comment on a few key aspects.

- A&WC versus confirmatory

The EMA reflection paper (European Medicines Agency 2007) focuses on confirmatory trials citing ICH E9 (ICH 1998) that a confirmatory trial is an adequately controlled trial in which the hypotheses are stated in advance and evaluated. As a rule, confirmatory trials are necessary to provide firm evidence of efficacy or safety.

Instead of using "confirmatory trials", the FDA draft guidance (FDA 2010) distinguishes between A&WC studies (used here to refer only to effectiveness studies) and other studies, termed exploratory studies. In US, Section 314.126 in Code of Federal Regulations (CFR) defines in details on what are adequate and well-controlled (A&WC) studies (FDA 2002a). From CFR 314.126, the key characteristics of an A&WC study includes (1) a clear statement of the objectives of the investigation and a summary of the proposed or actual methods of analysis in the protocol for the study and in the report of its results, (2) uses a design that permits a valid comparison with a control to provide a quantitative assessment of drug effect, (3) the method of selection of subjects provides adequate assurance that they have the disease or condition being studied, or evidence of susceptibility and exposure to the condition against which prophylaxis is directed, (4) the method of assigning patients to treatment and control groups minimizes bias and is intended to assure comparability of the groups with respect to pertinent variables such as age, sex, severity of disease, duration of disease, and use of drugs or thereby other than the test drug, (5) adequate measures are taken to minimize bias on the part of the subjects, observers, and analysts of the data, (6) the methods of assessment of subjects' response are well defined and reliable, (7) an analysis of the results of the study adequate to assess the effects of the drug.

The distinction between A&WC and exploratory adaptive design clinical trials stated in the FDA draft guidance has major implications. The rationales of this distinction are summarized in the second bullet of section 6 on "Additions", as such an exploratory adaptive design trial as designed cannot be converted to an A&WC adaptive design trial. The regulatory and statistical requirements will be demanded for A&WC adaptive design trials, which may not be the case for exploratory adaptive design trials. To build on practical experiences with use of more complex adaptations, the FDA draft guidance encourages sponsors to gain experience with the less well-understood methods in the exploratory study setting (FDA 2010).

- Interim analysis

The term "interim analysis" is not further explained, other than to note that adaptive design involves design modifications based on the results of an interim analysis in the EMA reflection paper (European Medicines Agency 2007). Interim analysis is defined in the ICH E9 (ICH 1998) as "any analysis intended to compare treatment arms with respect to efficacy or safety at any time prior to the formal completion of a trial." However, the FDA draft guidance (FDA 2010) gives a footnote specifically to explain its broader meaning for interim analysis than those defined in ICH E9 (ICH 1998) to accommodate the broader range of analyses of accumulated data that can be used to determine study adaptations at an intermediate point in the study. For instance, an interim analysis in this broader definition may include a pre-planned analysis of accumulating data without performing a formal statistical hypothesis test, but may make the decision to increase statistical information, e.g., sample size, event count (or study duration in certain circumstances), in an ongoing trial.

- Blinded versus unblinded interim analysis

In addition to "Routinely breaking the blind should be avoided …", general statements on whether interim unblinded data can be protected or when blind cannot be maintained in an interim analysis and use of blinded sample size reassessment are mentioned using group sequential design as the backbone in the EMA reflection paper (European Medicines Agency 2007). In contrast, the FDA draft guidance (FDA 2010) devotes four subsections in the generally well-understood adaptive designs session. This includes (1) V.A. on adaptation of study eligibility criteria based on analysis of pretreatment (baseline) data, (2) V.B. on adaptations to maintain study power based on blinded interim analyses of aggregate data, (3) V.C. on adaptations based on interim results of an outcome unrelated to efficacy, and (4) V.E. on adaptations in the data analysis plan not dependent on within study, between-group outcome differences. Note on the unblinded interim analysis in FDA draft guidance (FDA 2010) can be found under the bullet "Well-understood versus less well-understood" below.

Those described in V.A. are relatively commonly known. For V.B., it may include, e.g., blinded enrichment modification, blinded interim analysis to upsizing for power improvement in a noninferiority trial. For V.C., it may be in a situation where if an unexpected serious toxicity is observed in safety monitoring, dropping the dose groups early with excessive toxicity would be an outcome unrelated to efficacy. Examples of where V.E. may be useful to include situations in which the observed data violate prospective assumptions regarding the distribution of the data or where data transformations or use of a covariate is called for in the analysis to achieve adequate conformity with the method's assumptions, e.g., (Wang and Hung 2005). These subsections involve interim analyses that are used in a broader sense than those defined in ICH E9 (ICH 1998), i.e., blinded interim analyses not for early efficacy or futility stopping.

• Phase II/III or phase 2/3 or seamless

In statistical literature, the term "seamless Phase II/III" was getting popular, e.g., (Schmidli et al. 2006; Friede et al. 2011), during and after the development of the EMA reflection paper (European Medicines Agency 2007). Section 4.2.7 of the EMA reflection paper (European Medicines Agency 2007) is devoted to "Phase II/ Phase III combinations, applications with one pivotal trial and the independent replication of findings". This section further elucidates what criteria should be considered as a basis for drug licensing in Europe.

Since "phase 2/3" or "seamless" used to describe an adaptive design confirmatory trial introduces confusion on whether a study is initially designed to be adequate and well-controlled, and ultimately demonstrate effectiveness, they also do not add to understanding of the design beyond the already inclusive term "adaptive". The FDA draft guidance (FDA 2010) therefore acknowledges these terms citing statistical literature, but, uses the terms exploratory study versus A&WC study (FDA 2002a), each can be an adaptive trial in itself.

• Well-understood versus less well-understood

In the EMA reflection paper (European Medicines Agency 2007), there is no distinction made on whether certain types of adaptive designs would be well or less well understood. Interestingly, specific adaptive designs sub-bulleted for special considerations listed in section 2.1 mostly involve unblinded interim analysis. In their discussion, the document distinguishes between group sequential trials and adaptive designs.

Whilst, group sequential trials is a type of A&WC adaptive design clinical trials described in the FDA draft guidance (FDA 2010) as whose properties are well understood. In addition, those A&WC adaptive design clinical trials adopting blinded approaches listed in section V also belong to the well-understood category. The blinded approaches in the comparative studies do not make use of the treatment codes in their pre-specified interim adaptation(s). As for A&WC adaptive design clinical trials whose properties are less well-understood, the adaptive design methods are all based on unblinded interim analyses that estimate the treatment effect(s).

• Consistency of and bias in treatment effect estimates

The EMA reflection paper (European Medicines Agency 2007) repeatedly reminds of the importance and the need to check for consistency of treatment effect estimates before and after the interim analysis in an adaptive design trial with a preplanned method, but only notes once about the bias as "assessment of results from clinical trials involves, amongst other issues, a full discussion of potential sources of bias."

In contrast, the FDA draft guidance (FDA 2010) repeatedly articulates and cautions regarding the bias issue induced by adoption of an adaptive design in lieu of a fixed design. Here, the biases include both the statistical bias embedded in the design, analysis, and interpretation of study finding and the operational bias caused by the conduct of an adaptive design trial mostly resulting from unblinded adaptation. The term "bias" occurs around 70 times but only twice regarding the consistency of treatment effect estimates.

- Situations or settings for encouraging adaptive design use

The ideal setting to utilize adaptive designs, explained by the EMA reflection paper (European Medicines Agency 2007), is using it as a tool for planning clinical trials in areas where it is necessary to cope with "difficult experimental situations" in confirmatory trials. It goes on to state "In all instances the interim analysis and the type of the anticipated design modification (change of sample size, discontinuation of treatment arms, etc.) would need to be described and justified in the study protocol. Adaptations to confirmatory trials introduced without proper planning will render the trial to be considered exploratory".

Here, "difficult experimental situations" refer to diseases, indications, or patient populations, where it is common knowledge that clinical trials will be difficult to perform (European Medicines Agency 2007). Three examples given as difficult experimental situations are (1) placebo response is difficult to predict, even in situations where criteria for inclusion and exclusion of patients to trials are well defined, (2) small populations or orphan diseases with constraints to the maximum amount of evidence that can be provided, and (3) ethical constraints to experimentation.

In contrast, the FDA draft guidance (FDA 2010) acknowledges the greatest interest in adaptive design clinical trials has been in the adequate and well-controlled study setting intended to support marketing a drug. Because these studies have the greatest regulatory impact, it is critical to avoid increased rates of false positive study results and to minimize introducing bias. The FDA draft guidance also notes that many adaptive methods are also applicable to exploratory studies and encourages sponsors to gain experience with the less well-understood methods in the exploratory study setting (FDA 2010).

3.6 Additions

It is noticeable that the FDA draft guidance (FDA 2010) is much more extensive than the EMA reflection paper (European Medicines Agency 2007). Instead of discussing specific statistical methods, the EMA reflection paper (European Medicines Agency 2007) focuses on the opportunities for interim trial design modifications, and the prerequisites, problems and pitfalls that must be considered as soon as any kind of flexibility is introduced into a confirmatory clinical trial intended to provide evidence of efficacy. A few key additions described or discussed in the FDA draft guidance (FDA 2010) are listed below.

- Comprehensively describing the rationales, motivations, and clinical contexts in drug development that should also be understandable to non-statisticians.
- Rationally articulating "adaptive design exploratory studies are usually different in multiple aspects of design rigor from A&WC studies so that design revisions while the study is underway will usually not be sufficient to convert the study into an A&WC study. As such studies that are intended to provide substantial evidence of effectiveness should not be designed as exploratory studies, but rather as A&WC studies at initial planning." With this theme, safety considerations in adaptive design trials are mostly exploratory studies.
- Extensively elaborating on the roles of clinical trial simulation in adaptive design planning and evaluation. This includes, but are not limited to, reliance on statistical models for the disease or the drug, use of modeling and simulation strategies with either a Bayesian or a frequentist approach, comparison of the design performance characteristics among competing designs under different scenarios mostly in situations where multiple factors will be simultaneously considered in the adaptive process, but, with little analytical solution on the strong control of study-wide Type I error.
- Mindfully recommending an elaborate standard operating procedure (SOP) for an adaptive design study in the less well-understood category, in addition to what has been in place for traditional group sequential trials, such as, how adaptation decision will be made, actual interim analysis results and a snapshot of the databases used for that interim analysis and adaptation decision should also be retained in a secure manner, acknowledging these SOPs will be related to the type of adaptation and the potential for impairing study integrity.
- Cautiously stipulating two types of trial logistics/adaptive monitoring models: one is the typical DMC model with procedures in place to ensure certain kinds of information with possibly unblinded analyses do not become available outside of the committee. Alternatively, a model with two separate committees with a DMC delegated only the more standard roles (e.g., ongoing assessment of critical safety information) and a separate adaptation committee used to examine the interim analysis and make adaptation recommendations. In either case, the specific duties and procedures of the committees should be fully and prospectively documented.
- Extensively detailing the content of an adaptive design protocol, processes in the interactions with FDA when planning and conducting an adaptive design clinical trial for a drug development or drug developments, documentation, and practices to protect study blinding and information sharing for adaptive designs, and evaluating and reporting a completed study

3.7 Regulatory Submissions and Statistical Considerations

The FDA draft guidance (FDA 2010) offers an opportunity to take a fresh look of fixed designs, group sequential designs, and a broader class of adaptive designs. While the draft guidance pinpoints important differences among these designs, adaptive designs may be considered with care for improving the efficiency of a clinical development program, but it is necessary, at the minimum, to distinguish if a trial is designed at the outset an exploratory trial or a confirmatory trial (Wang 2010a).

3.7.1 Regulatory Submissions

The overwhelming interests in pursuing an adaptive design clinical trial appears to be where it has most regulatory impacts for its potential in gaining regulatory licensure, namely, adaptive design confirmatory trials by the EMA reflection paper (European Medicines Agency 2007) or adaptive design A&WC trials by legal statutes and regulations stated in the FDA draft guidance (FDA 2010).

In 2005, the results of CDER's preliminary survey to capture any interest in adaptive/flexible design strategy up to September 2002 were published (Wang et al. 2005). Of the 46 study cases reported involving any flavor of adaptive/flexible designs irrespective of methodological validity, approximately 80 % were investigational new drugs (INDs) and 20 % were new drug applications (NDAs). In this preliminary survey, the most frequently considered adaptation was the sample size re-estimation (43 %) where blinded and unblinded approaches were proposed. Twenty-two percent of submissions considered dropping at least one treatment dose arm and 20 % considered study objective change from superiority to non-inferiority and vice versa. About 9 % involved adaptation on primary endpoint, 4 % on primary statistical analysis method and 2 % on multiplicity adjustment method.

The newer adaptive designs attempt to combine data in the first stage with data in the second stage for statistical inference in a two stage adaptive design trial. The germane question is what is the study-wise Type I error rate when data from both stages are combined. If the adaptive design trial as proposed is an exploratory trial, the study objectives aim at learning; therefore, study-wise Type I error rate control standard may not be the focus. In contrast, if the adaptive design trial is proposed as a confirmatory trial, the study-wise Type I error rate would be at issue.

Since 2005, a part of the newer topics for adaptive/flexible design consideration geared towards pharmacogenomics trials due to overwhelming interests in personalized medicine drug development (Wang 2006, 2007). Other newer topics attempted to pursue a learn-and-confirm approach (Wang 2010a), which prompted regulatory research to investigating the impact of family-wise Type I error rate in the context of learning-free in Stage 1 that combines data from both stages for statistical inference (Wang et al. 2010). Gradually, the learn-and-confirm approach was recognized for its suitability in exploratory trials to demonstrate preliminary early evidence, which can serve as a priori knowledge for planning confirmatory trials that can employ fixed design or adaptive design.

We have since received many two-stage adaptive design clinical trial submissions that are either exploratory (such as, proof of concept studies) or A&WC (FDA 2002a). Often, we see Bayesian approaches are proposed in exploratory adaptive design clinical trials including early dose escalation or tolerability studies. Interestingly, the majority of the adaptive design proposals are still in the domain of sample size or statistical information adaptive design that adapt either statistical information alone (Wang et al. 2012) or in conjunction with adaptive selection (Wang et al. 2013).

Traditionally, the proof of concept studies and dose-ranging studies are mostly fixed design trials. To enhance the flexibility and consistent with the recommendation from FDA draft guidance (FDA 2010), we are seeing an increase in two-stage adaptive design proof of concept trial proposals seeking preliminary data information prior to launching A&WC clinical trials. We have also received submissions proposing a two-stage adaptive design dose ranging exploratory trial based on short-term endpoints.

Recent regulatory experiences on adaptive design A&WC trials leading to eventual drug approval identified a number of challenges, though efficacy evidence supported by statistical significance may not be critically challenged. In a few incidences, the treatment effect estimates before and after adaptation can easily be argued to be inconsistent but with unclear causes or may be speculated to be due to patient heterogeneity or baseline imbalance between stages (Wang et al. 2013). Fast accrual results in a haphazard adaptation on statistical information (Wang and Hung 2013a), interim selection of treatment arm may have been impacted by market competition on efficacy benefit when safety risks are not well understood (Wang 2009).

It can be questioned that interim data used for interim adaptation can be suboptimal if data quality at interim time can be of concern possibly due to timing for data cleaning versus for interim analysis to make adaptation recommendation and adaptation decision. We believe regulatory learning curve will continue, especially on challenges that may evolve from more regulatory reviews of the less well-understood completed adaptive design confirmatory trials. The accumulating experiences from overseeing the range of trial logistics models for interim analysis, recommendation, and decision to adapt may facilitate future development of good adaptive design implementation practices in those less well-understood adaptive design trials aiming for A&WC investigation.

3.7.2 Statistical Considerations

In discussing the evidential standards for a confirmatory or A&WC clinical trial, the term "family-wise" in (European Medicines Agency 2002) is referenced in the EMA reflection paper (European Medicines Agency 2007) and the term "study-wide" is used in the FDA draft guidance (FDA 2010). For commentary, I will use the term "study-wise" to refer to the various terms: "family-wise", "experiment-wise", "study-wise", "overall" seen in the statistical literature regarding multiplicity in a study, a family, or an experiment.

- One trial one study-wise Type I error rate

Multiplicity issues may arise in a single hypothesis adaptive design clinical trial if (1) there is adaptation of a design feature, e.g., sample size reassessment based on the interim observed treatment effect estimate, or (2) there is adaptation of an analysis feature, e.g., repeated significance testing using independent incremental data information for potential early rejection of the same null hypothesis at an interim analysis, or (3) both (Bauer and Kieser 1999). For the newer adaptive designs intended to perform unblinded interim evaluations for adapting statistical information or adaptive selection, either the initial null hypothesis and/or the initial alternative hypothesis may have been modified (Wang et al. 2011a).

A minimum requirement for a statistically valid A&WC trial is the strong control of the study-wise (family-wise) Type I error rate (European Medicines Agency 2002). An adaptive design clinical trial to be considered A&WC should be subjected to the same requirement in addition to prospective specification of the adaptation criteria. In this spirit, the study-wise error rate control of an adaptive design clinical trial can be achieved, for example, using p-value combination tests or weighted Z-tests; see the literature such as (Bauer and Kohne 1994; Bauer and Kieser 1999; Posch et al. 2005; Bretz et al. 2009; Wang et al. 2007, 2009) and some articles cited therein. The principle of strong control of the study-wise Type I error rate is also adopted in the EMA reflection paper (European Medicines Agency 2007).

However, methodologies that do not require pre-specification of what to adapt after an interim unblinded analysis exit, and yet these approaches can control the pre-specified overall Type I error by controlling the conditional Type I error, e.g., control of conditional Type I error (Proschan and Hunsberger 1995; Schäfer and Müller 2001), recursive combination tests (Brannath et al. 2002). With this flexibility feature, it is possible that at any (unscheduled) time the remainder of the pre-planned design, say, group sequential design, can be replaced by an "adaptive design which preserves the conditional type I error rate" (Müller and Schäfer 2004). As noted by Bauer (2006) "such designs can be looked at as perfect tool to deal with the unexpected. The price to be paid for such a wide field of flexibility is mainly known."

It should be obvious that such approaches to control the study-wise Type I error may be controversial in the context of an adaptive A&WC trial that has wide flexibility without the need for pre-specification (Wang 2010a; Wang et al. 2010, 2011a). Not only there is no pre-specified adaptation, the elements to adapt can also be wide and flexible. These features would be inconsistent with the principles laid out in both regulatory guidance documents. In fact, both Koch (2006) and Hung et al. (2006) hinted similar concerns and only commented directly on the logistical challenges cited by Bauer (2006). These three commentaries were published prior to the release of either regulatory document.

For a while, several regulatory submissions using an adaptive design clinical trial aiming for an A&WC consideration propose to adjust for multiplicity only on the selected hypotheses based on the stage 1 data when data from both stages are to be combined for final statistical inference, referred to as a learn-and-confirm adaptive design clinical trial (Wang et al. 2011a). The Type I error rate in a learn-and-confirm adaptive design trial has recently been coined as learning-free Type I error rate by Wang et al. (2010). In the learn-and-confirm framework without increasing the total sample size, the learning free Type I error rate in a confirmatory trial has been shown to be liberal. Depending on the particular adaptation scenarios, the Type I error rate inflation can increase substantially beyond the intended significance level, such as the conventional one-sided 0.025 or two-sided 0.05 level, see (Wang et al. 2010).

Wang et al. (2010) note that in the scenario of selecting the better dose regimen between two doses in stage 1, the simulation studies show that the learning-free Type I error rate control requires use of an extremely stringent criterion for an ad-hoc adaptive dose selection if necessary multiplicity adjustment is ignored. That is, the perceived minimum multiplicity adjustment due to only two hypotheses without adjusting for interim adaptation may not be as straightforward as one would expect. This is because the selection between one of the two dose regimens, if the criteria are not carefully considered, can lean toward random selection as such either dose regimen has equal probability of being chosen without adjusting for all sources of multiplicity.

- Simulated Type I error rate aiming at an A&WC investigation

An adaptive design clinical trial to be counted toward one of the registration trials but without an analytical solution to the study-wise Type I error rate control signals the complexity of the design and the complexity of the inter-relationship among the design elements desired for potential adaptation. Simulation tools have been highly recommended to consider aspects of modernizing drug development via clinical scenario planning and evaluation (Benda et al. 2009). Recently, the simulation studies with or without modeling have received wide acceptance to critically assess the utility of adaptive design in terms of the study power, bias, mean square error, and the sample size.

In simple setting, analytical solutions of Type I error probability are available, e.g., sample size reassessment. However, the assessment of study-wise Type I error rate via (modeling) simulations in the context of an adaptive design clinical trial where no analytical solution is available and the adaptive design trial is intended to be considered as A&WC has been debated; see, for example, (Posch et al. 2011) and views by Brannath in (Wang and Bretz 2010).

In principle, if the statistical behavior of the test statistic is mathematically tractable, using simulation to find the critical value or performing numerical integration can be well understood. In general, simulation studies should be routinely performed for power assessment when clinical scenarios are to be compared at the planning stage with adaptive design in mind. This will demand people who plan the trials to think about what are likely adaptive design clinical scenarios for power assessment. The drug sponsors are always encouraged to use simulation to assess the statistical efficiency of a trial design. However, it can be very risky if the study-wise Type I error in a complex adaptive design trial aimed for confirmatory evidences has to depend on the unknown mathematical models with no good pilot data.

• Bias

For all practical purposes, the bias associated with adaptations can come in several forms into a study. This includes study design, study conduct, analysis and interpretation of the study results, and can be grouped into statistical bias and operational bias, e.g., ICH E9 (ICH 1998; Wang and Nevius 2005). The statistical bias in the treatment effect estimate can be induced by design due to interim adaptive selection; see, for example, (Bauer et al. 2010; Bretz and Wang 2010; Hung et al. 2010). Statistical bias induced by design can be adjusted for, e.g., median unbiased estimates (Posch et al. 2005; Brannath et al. 2006), or mean unbiased estimates (Lawrence and Hung 2003) for sample size re-estimation, and (Bowden and Glimm 2008) for selected treatment means in two-stage adaptive design clinical trials.

The operational bias causing inaccurate treatment effect estimates can be the results of changes in trial conduct due to interim adaptive decision, in trial implementation due to adaptive monitoring by the unblinded parties who either have scientific interests or financial interests among other factors impacted by interim unblinding. To minimize the operational bias, it is often questioned to what degree a sponsor should be involved in making the adaptive decision based on interim unblinded data information (Benda et al. 2010; Wang et al. 2011b).

• Consistency of treatment effects before and after adaptation

In the section articulating the importance of confidentiality of interim results in the EMA reflection paper (European Medicines Agency 2007), checking for consistency of treatment effect estimates from the data collected before and after the interim analysis is highlighted for interpretable conclusions in studies planned with an adaptive design. The document notes its greater importance if treatments cannot be fully blinded, if it is suspected that the observed discrepancies are a consequence of (intentional or unintentional) dissemination of the interim results, or if the assessment of results incorporates some subjective elements.

Viewing it as an integral part of the adaptive design proposal for regulatory considerations, Koch (2006) notes that it is essential to pre-specify the approaches to evaluating consistency of treatment effects to avoid post-hoc discussions whenever observed data may only indicate that combination of results from different stages is questionable. Following this plea, some methods are proposed in statistical literature, e.g., (Wang et al. 2013; Friede and Herderson 2009; Wang and Hung 2013b).

3.8 Difficult Experimental Situations

Should an A&WC adaptive design clinical trial be best utilized as a tool for planning clinical trials in areas where it is necessary to cope with difficult experimental situations noted in EMA reflection paper (European Medicines Agency 2007) or experimentation in exploratory trials with the less well-understood methods encouraged by US FDA (FDA 2010) or both? In an editorial, Wang (2010b) commented that a well-understood experimental situation refers to a well-understood primary endpoint, patient population, likely range of treatment effect size based on a plausible dose regimen or regimens, etc. An A&WC adaptive design trial can then be used to design a study to deal with the remaining uncertainty, such as the variability of the effect size or limited uncertainty on the magnitude of effect size, and to avoid falling short of statistical significance, such as a p-value slightly greater than the pre-specified significance level when the completed trial is analyzed (Wang and Hung 2013b).

3.8.1 Some Philosophy in EMA Reflection Paper

Best use of adaptive design in difficult experimental situations appears to bear a different philosophy. Rather than dealing with the limited uncertainties, the common theme of those examples cited in the EMA reflection paper (European Medicines Agency 2007) is 'difficult'. In one situation, it is difficult to predict placebo response though inclusion and exclusion of patients are well defined, such as in pain medication development. In other situations, ethical constraints may make it difficult to experiment, e.g., not feasible to pursue a superiority trial in an active controlled trial but a statistical non-inferiority margin may not be readily available. Or, orphan or rare diseases may make it difficult to plan and conduct sufficiently powered trials due to limited number of patients and consequently poses constraints on the maximum amount of evidence that can be provided.

3.8.2 Types of Adaptive Design and Study Endpoint

Should different standards be considered in difficult experimental situations? For instance, should learn-and-confirm adaptive design (Wang 2010a) be an acceptable design choice for establishing regulatory evidence of efficacy in difficult experimental situations? It would be challenging if the only confirmatory trial for evidence setting relies only on a single learn-and-confirm adaptive design trial that does not have a clear intent of being adequate and well controlled. Such learn-and-confirm adaptive design does not consider strong control of the study-wise Type I error rate (Wang 2010a).

Should the less well-understood adaptive design approach proposed to be A&WC be viewed as A&WC? The less well-understood adaptive design trial would be scientifically sound if it follows an A&WC investigation (FDA 1998, 2002a). In the case that a second trial is not feasible, US FDA Moderization Act released in 1997 may consider data from one A&WC clinical investigation and confirmatory evidence of substantial evidence (FDA 1997). In such cases, one trial one study-wise Type I error rate (Wang et al. 2010) should ideally be the statistical criterion for the only feasible adaptive design clinical trial, in addition to meeting the criteria on the characteristics of an A&WC trial.

Can a shorter-term endpoint be acceptable in place of the long-term clinical benefit endpoint? The effect size of a shorter-term endpoint measuring biological activity, especially if the endpoint is a continuous measurement, is generally not small. In the spirit of adaptation acknowledging upfront the risks and uncertainties one has to bear, it may be pragmatically plausible to plan with an adaptive design clinical trial based on a shorter-term endpoint. Would it be public health sound for benefiting patients in a near term when there may not have sufficient plausible prior data to expect the shorter-term endpoint's likelihood of predicting a long-term clinical benefit/risk endpoint in difficult experimental situations?

For instance, can allowing pre-specified adaptation on statistical information and/or adaptive selection, early futility stopping, and possibly early efficacy stopping based on a shorter-term endpoint meet the challenges of ethical constraints given the limited patient population in orphan or rare diseases? Consequently, the ultimate clinical endpoint benefit risk assessment may take years to unravel the uncertainty. Learning will be a big part in such an adaptive design trial applied in difficult experimental situations.

3.9 Summary

In summary, based on my review of both regulatory guidance documents as well as my experience with US regulatory submissions, the criteria for an A&WC adaptive design clinical trial should possess, at a minimum, the following characteristics:

- Pre-specification of all hypotheses and adaptation elements at the planning stage based on clinical scenario planning with simulation studies to justify the 'adaptation' value
- Provision of the background information on what data information have been gathered thus far and where the particularly proposed adaptive design clinical trial is positioned within its own drug development program
- Use of a valid study-wise Type I error rate control method
- Utility of drawing strength from external trials, but, caution the credibility of external evidence when they are anecdotal, preliminary, or limited

- Careful use of "learning" for "confirming" in a single adaptive design trial by distinguishing whether the primary study objectives are confirmatory or exploratory at the planning stage
- Necessary interim communication firewalls on adaptive monitoring and for properly handling the adaptive design trial logistics via adequate standard operating procedures and charters
- Consideration of a valid point estimate and its corresponding interval estimates

The last bullet point may be subject to debate given that regulators have not required a properly adjusted point estimate and the corresponding interval estimates in a confirmatory or A&WC trial with a group sequential design. However, these estimates are critical for future study planning, especially for defining the non-inferiority margin in designing non-inferiority active-controlled clinical trials. Note that the inability to mask in open-label studies can confound many operational and logistic factors. In general, a double-blind adaptive design clinical study is preferred.

Traditionally, statistical efficiency discussed is at an individual trial level. But this consideration may not be sufficient in the context of adaptive design that aims to incorporate design efficiency considerations into the entire development program. Setting the efficiency debate aside, what could be the benefit of using an adaptive design in any disease indication, if the experimental treatment may not be effective or only minimally effective? Perhaps, the early futility stopping is a major advantage to minimize the loss in drug developments and would be ethical so as not to expose more patients than necessary to an experimental treatment, particularly when the experimental treatment is also toxic.

Acknowledgments The book chapter materials are based on the presentation "Adequate and well-controlled confirmatory clinical trials with adaptive design: reflections about similarities and options in two regulatory guidance documents" given at the 22nd Annual DIA Euro Meeting held in France on March 10, 2010, the webinar "U.S. FDA draft guidance adaptive design clinical trials for drugs and biologics: statistical/contents/documentation/trial integrity/interaction/reporting" given at DIA Webinar—FDA Discusses the draft guidance on May 05, 2010 and the collaborative regulatory science research conducted by the author and her collaborators. The author wishes to thank Professor Dr. sc. hum. Armin Koch, Director, Institute of Biometry, Hannover Medicine School, Hannover, Germany, the former Head of Biostatistics, Federal Institute for Drugs and Medical Devices (BfArM), one of the primary authors of the EMA reflection paper, for his extensive contribution to regulatory science. Thanks are due to Dr. Robert O'Neill's visionary leadership and Dr. H.M. James Hung's diligent input on the simulated Type I error rate and other aspects of adaptive design trials, and colleagues from Office of New Drugs, CDER, US FDA for their coordinated efforts with Office of Biostatistics on adaptive design regulatory submissions. The author would also like to thank the three book Editors for their kind invitation to contribute.

Appendix 1: Table of Contents of the EMA Reflection Paper on Adaptive Design

Executive summary

1. Introduction
2. Scope
3. Legal basis
4. Main reflection paper text

   4.1. Interim analyses—general considerations

      4.1.1. The importance of confidentiality of interim results
      4.1.2. Considerations about stopping trials early for efficacy
      4.1.3. Overrunning

   4.2. Interim analyses with design modifications

      4.2.1. Adaptation of design specifications: minimal requirements
      4.2.2. Sample size reassessment
      4.2.3. Change or modification of the primary end-point
      4.2.4. Discontinuing treatment arms
      4.2.5. Switching between superiority and noninferiority
      4.2.6. Randomization ratio
      4.2.7. Phase II/phase III combinations, applications with one pivotal trial and the independent replication of findings
      4.2.8. Substantial changes of trial design
      4.2.9. Futility stopping in late phase II or phase III clinical trials

   Definitions
   References

Appendix 2: Table of Contents of the FDA Adaptive Design Draft Guidance

   I. INTRODUCTION
   II. BACKGROUND
   III. DESCRIPTION OF AND MOTIVATION FOR ADAPTIVE DESIGNS

      A. Definition and Concept of an Adaptive Design Clinical Trial
      B. Other Concepts and Terminology
      C. Motivation for Using Adaptive Design in Drug Development

IV. GENERAL CONCERNS ASSOCIATED WITH USING ADAPTIVE DESIGN IN DRUG DEVELOPMENT

    A. Potential to Increase the Chance of Erroneous Positive Conclusions and of Positive Study Results That Are Difficult to Interpret

    B. Potential for Counterproductive Impacts of Adaptive Design

    C. Complex Adaptive Designs—Potential for Increased Planning and More Advanced Time Frame for Planning

    D. Adaptive Design in Exploratory Studies

    E. Study Design Changes That Are Not Considered Adaptive Design

V. GENERALLY WELL-UNDERSTOOD ADAPTIVE DESIGNS WITH VALID APPROACHES TO IMPLEMENTATION

    A. Adaptation of Study Eligibility Criteria Based on Analyses of Pretreatment (Baseline) Data

    B. Adaptations to Maintain Study Power Based on Blinded Interim Analyses of Aggregate Data

    C. Adaptations Based on Interim Results of an Outcome Unrelated to Efficacy

    D. Adaptations Using Group Sequential Methods and Unblinded Analyses for Early Study Termination Because of Either Lack of Benefit or Demonstrated Efficacy

    E. Adaptations in the Data Analysis Plan Not Dependent on Within Study, Between-Group Outcome Differences

VI. ADAPTIVE STUDY DESIGNS WHOSE PROPERTIES ARE LESS WELL UNDERSTOOD

    A. Adaptations for Dose Selection Studies

    B. Adaptive Randomization Based on Relative Treatment Group Responses

    C. Adaptation of Sample Size Based on Interim-Effect Size Estimates

    D. Adaptation of Patient Population Based on Treatment-Effect Estimates

    E. Adaptation for Endpoint Selection Based on Interim Estimate of Treatment Effect

    F. Adaptation of Multiple-Study Design Features in a Single Study

    G. Adaptations in Noninferiority Studies

VII. STATISTICAL CONSIDERATIONS FOR LESS-WELL UNDERSTOOD ADAPTIVE DESIGN METHODS

    A. Controlling Study-Wide Type I error Rate

    B. Statistical Bias in Estimates of Treatment Effect Associated with Study Design Adaptations

    C. Potential for Increased Type II Error Rate

    D. Role of Clinical Trial Simulation in Adaptive Design Planning and Evaluation

    E. Role of the Prospective Statistical Analysis Plan in Adaptive Design Studies

References

Armitage P, McPherson K, Rowe BC (1969) Repeated significance tests on accumulating data. J Roy Stat Soc A 132:235–244

Bauer P (1989) Multistage testing with adaptive designs (with discussion). Biometrie und Informatik in Medizin and Biologie 20:130–148

Bauer P (2006) Discussion: methodological developments vs. regulatory requirements. Biom J 48:609–612

Bauer P, Kieser M (1999) Combining different phases in the development of medical treatments within a single trial. Stat Med 18(14):1833–1848

Bauer P, Kohne K (1994) Evaluation of experiments with adaptive interim analysis. Biometrics 50:1029–1041

Bauer P, Brannath W, Posch M (2001) Flexible two-stage designs: an overview. Methods Inf Med 40(2):117–121

Bauer P, Koenig F, Brannath W, Posch M (2010) Selection and bias—two hostile brothers. Stat Med 29(1):1–13

Benda N, Branson M, Maurer W, Friede T (2009) A framework for the evaluation of competing development strategies. Drug Dev 4:84–88

Benda N, Brannath W, Bretz F, Burger HU, Friede T, Mauer W, Wang SJ (2010) Perspectives on the use of adaptive designs in clinical trials. Part II. Panel discussion. J Biopharm Stat 20: 1098–1112

Bowden J, Glimm E (2008) Unbiased estimation of selected treatment means in two-stage trials. Biom J 50(4):515–527

Brannath W, Posch M, Bauer P (2002) Recursive combination tests. J Am Stat Assoc 97: 236–244

Brannath W, Koenig F, Bauer P (2006) Estimation in flexible two stage designs. Stat Med 15: 3366–3381

Bretz F, Wang SJ (2010) From adaptive design to modern protocol design for drug development: part II. Success probabilities and effect estimates for phase III development programs. Drug Inform J 44(3):333–342

Bretz F, König F, Brannath W, Glimm E, Posch M (2009) Adaptive designs for confirmatory clinical trials. Stat Med 28(8):1181–1217

Ellenberg SS, Geller N, Simon R, Yusuf S (eds) (1993) Proceedings of 'practical issues in data monitoring of clinical trials', Bethesda, Maryland, USA, January 27–28, 1992. Stat Med 12: 415–646

(2007) Reflection paper on methodological issues in confirmatory clinical trials planned with an adaptive design. European Medicines Agency EMA CHMP/EWP/2459/02 October 2007. http://www.ema.europa.eu/docs/en_GB/document_library/Scientific_guideline/2009/09/WC500003616.pdf

Food and Drug Administration Moderation Act of 1997. http://www.fda.gov/RegulatoryInformation/Legislation/FederalFoodDrugandCosmeticActFDCAct/SignificantAmendmentstotheFDCAct/FDAMA/FullTextofFDAMAlaw/default.htm

(1998) FDA guidance for industry on providing clinical evidence of effectiveness for human drug and biological products. http://www.fda.gov/downloads/Drugs/.../Guidances/ucm078749.pdf

FDA (2002) Food and Drug Administration, Health Human Services, Code of Federal Regulation, 21CFR314.126. http://edocket.access.gpo.gov/cfr_2002/aprqtr/21cfr314.126.htm

FDA (2002) Food and Drug Administration, Health Human Services, Code of Federal Regulation, 21CFR312.23(a). http://www.accessdata.fda.gov/scripts/cdrh/cfdocs/cfcfr/cfrsearch.cfm?fr=312.23

(2006) Guidance for clinical trial sponsors: on the establishment and operation of clinical trial data monitoring committees. http://www.fda.gov/downloads/RegulatoryInformation/Guidances/UCM126578.pdf

U.S. Food and Drug Administration (2010) Draft guidance for industry on adaptive design clinical trials for drugs and biologics. Released on February 25, 2010 for public comments. www.fda.gov/downloads/Drugs/GuidanceComplianceRegulatoryInformation/Guidances/UCM201790.pdf

Friede T, Herderson R (2009) Exploring changes in treatment effects across design stages in adaptive trials. Pharmaceut Stat 8:62–72

Friede T, Parsons N, Stallard N, Todd S, Valdés-Márquez E, Chataway J, Nicholas R (2011) Designing a seamless phase II/III clinical trial using early outcomes for treatment selection: an application in multiple sclerosis. Stat Med 30:1528–1540

Gao P, Ware JH, Mehta C (2008) Sample size re-estimation for adaptive sequential design in clinical trials. J Biopharm Stat 18:1184–1196

Hung HMJ, O'Neill RT, Wang SJ, Lawrence J (2006) A regulatory view on adaptive/flexible clinical trial design. Biom J 48:565–573

Hung HMJ, Wang SJ, O'Neill RT (2010) Flexible design clinical trial methodology in regulatory applications. Stat Med. doi: 10.1002/sim.4021. www.interscience.wiley.com

ICH (1998) ICH topic E9: statistical principles for clinical trials. www.ich.org/LOB/media/MEDIA485.pdf

Koch A (2006) Confirmatory clinical trials with an adaptive design. Biom J 48:574–585

Lawrence J, Hung HMJ (2003) Estimation and confidence intervals after adjusting the maximum information. Biom J 45(2):143–152

Müller HH, Schäfer H (2004) A general statistical principle for changing a design any time during the course of a trial. Stat Med 23:2497–2508

Point to consider on multiplicity issues in clinical trials. European Medicines Agency EMA CHMP/EWP/908/99 September 2002. http://www.ema.europa.eu/docs/en_GB/document_library/Scientific_guideline/2009/09/WC500003640.pdf

Posch M, Koenig F, Branson M, Brannath W, Dunger-Baldauf C, Bauer P (2005) Testing and estimation in flexible group sequential designs with adaptive treatment selection. Stat Med 24: 3697–3714

Posch M, Maurer W, Bretz F (2011) Type I error rate control in adaptive designs for confirmatory clinical trials with treatment selection at interim. Pharmaceut Stat 10(2):96–104

Proschan MA, Hunsberger SA (1995) Designed extension of studies based on conditional power. Biometrics 51:1315–1324

Schäfer H, Müller HH (2001) Adaptive group sequential designs for clinical trials: combining the advantages of adaptive and of classical group sequential approaches. Biometrics 57:886–891

Schmidli H, Bretz F, Racine A, Maurer W (2006) Confirmatory seamless phase II/III clinical trials with hypotheses selection at interim: applications and practical considerations. Biom J 48(4):635–643

Wang SJ (2006) Regulatory update on pharmacogenomics: an FDA perspective. Special report in the first multi-track DIA workshop on DIA congress on the development and utilization of pharmaceuticals moving towards e-regulation/risk management—safety and efficacy/biostatistics in Japan. pp 16–20

Wang SJ (2007) Genomic biomarker derived therapeutic effect in pharmacogenomics clinical trials: a biostatistics view of personalized medicine. Taiwan Clin Trials 4:57–66

Wang SJ (2009) Discussant: adaptive dose-finding studies. Proceedings of the American Statistical Association, biopharmaceutical section [CD-ROM]. American Statistical Association, Alexandria, VA

Wang SJ (2010a) Perspectives on the use of adaptive designs in clinical trials: part I. Statistical considerations and issues. J Biopharm Stat 20(6):1090–1097

Wang SJ (2010b) Editorial: adaptive designs: appealing in development of therapeutics, and where do controversies lie? J Biopharm Stat 20(6):1083–1087

Wang SJ, Bretz F (2010) From adaptive design to modern protocol design for drug development: part I. Editorial and summary of adaptive designs session at the third FDA/DIA (Drug Information Association) statistics forum. Drug Inform J 44(3):325–331

Wang SJ, Hung HMJ (2005) Adaptive covariate adjustment in trial design. J Biopharm Stat 15:605–611

Wang SJ, Hung HMJ (2013a) Adaptive enrichment with subpopulation selection at interim: general concepts, applications and practical considerations. Contemp Clin Trials 36:673–681

Wang SJ, Hung HMJ (2013b) A conditional adaptive weighted test method for confirmatory trials. Ther Innov Reg Sci. doi:10.1177/2168479013513891

Wang SJ, Nevius SE (2005) On the commonly used design and statistical considerations in double blind, potentially unblind, and open-label clinical trials. Clin Res Regul Aff 21(4):213–229

Wang SJ, Hung HMJ, O'Neill RT (2005) Uncertainty of effect size and clinical (genomic) trial design flexibility/adaptivity. The Proceedings of American Statistical Association, biopharmaceutical section [CD-ROM]. American Statistical Association, Alexandria, VA

Wang SJ, O'Neill RT, Hung HMJ (2007) Approaches to evaluation of treatment effect in randomized clinical trials with genomic subset. Pharmaceut Stat 6:227–244

Wang SJ, Hung HMJ, O'Neill RT (2009) Adaptive patient enrichment designs in therapeutic trials. Biom J 51(2):358–374

Wang SJ, Hung HMJ, O'Neill RT (2010) Impacts of type I error rate with inappropriate use of learn for confirm in adaptive designs. Biom J 52(6):798–810. doi:10.1002/bimj.200900207

Wang SJ, Hung HMJ, O'Neill RT (2011a) Regulatory perspectives on multiplicity in adaptive design clinical trials throughout a drug development program. J Biopharm Stat 21:846–859

Wang SJ, Hung HMJ, O'Neill RT (2011b) Adaptive design clinical trials and logistics models in CNS drug development. Eur Neuropsychopharmacol J 21:159–166

Wang SJ, Hung HMJ, O'Neill RT (2012) Paradigms for adaptive statistical information designs: practical experiences and strategies. Stat Med 31:3011–3023

Wang SJ, Brannath W, Bruckner M, Hung HMJ, Koch A (2013) Unblinded adaptive statistical information design based on clinical endpoint or biomarker. Stat Biopharm Res 5(4):293–310. doi:10.1080/19466315.2013.791639, In honor of Dr. Robert T. O'Neill special issue

Zelen M (1969) Play the winner rule and the controlled clinical trials. J Am Stat Assoc 64:131–146

Chapter 4
Considerations and Optimization of Adaptive Trial Design in Clinical Development Programs

Michael Krams and Vladimir Dragalin

Abstract Although the efficiency of adaptive design on the trial level is well recognized, its impact is even greater when applied at the program or portfolio level. Besides its simplest form of sample size reestimation or early stopping in a given trial, the adaptive design achieves efficiency by combining in a single trial objectives that are usually addressed in two separate conventional studies. Another feature of adaptive design is population enrichment where drug response can be optimized to specific patient subpopulations that respond better to treatment. More complex adaptive strategies integrate the development of several compounds and/or indications into one process. We provide an overview of these types of adaptive designs and illustrate their value added in a case study of an adaptive "compound" finder that investigates several compounds in Alzheimer's disease area simultaneously approaching the proof-of-concept stage.

Keywords Adaptive compound finder • Adaptive compound/population finder • Adaptive design • Adaptive dose finder • Adaptive indication finder • Adaptive population finder • Allocation rule • Longitudinal modeling • Seamless design • Stopping rule

M. Krams (✉)
Janssen Pharmaceutical Research and Development,
1125 Trenton Harbourton Road, Titusville, NJ 08560, USA
e-mail: mkrams@its.jnj.com

V. Dragalin
Janssen Pharmaceutical Research and Development, 1400 McKean Rd, Spring House,
PA 19477, USA
e-mail: vdragali@its.jnj.com

W. He et al. (eds.), *Practical Considerations for Adaptive Trial Design and Implementation*, Statistics for Biology and Health,
DOI 10.1007/978-1-4939-1100-4_4, © Springer Science+Business Media New York 2014

4.1 Background

The adoption of an adaptive design strategy across the product development process brings a number of important benefits. These include increased R&D efficiency, increased R&D productivity, and importantly increased probability of success at phase III. We are all too familiar with the worrying industry statistic that 50 % of phase III studies fail and in some therapeutic areas such as oncology or Alzheimer's disease the failure rate is even higher. Innovative adaptive design trials offer the potential to change this industry statistic and dramatically increase the ability of pharmaceutical companies to successfully bring more effective treatments to the market.

Adaptive designs enhance development efficiency by mitigating the need to repeat trials that just miss their clinical endpoint or fail to identify the effective dose–response at the first attempt. By avoiding the need to run these trials again, significant cost and time savings are achieved. This is possible through use of adaptive designs that enable additional patients to be added to achieve statistical significance the first time around or by allowing a wider dose range to be studied and a better understanding of the dose–response relationship. In addition, early stopping of development programs because a product is ineffective enables scarce resources to be redeployed in additional trials which may show more promise. Early stopping of a trial for efficacy is also possible. All of these factors increase development efficiency.

Adaptive design increases development productivity by enabling more accurate definition of the effective dose in a phase II trial which enables better design of the pivotal phase III program, which in turn increases the probability of success of this trial. A number of phase III trials fail because the dose is either too high and causes unwanted safety issues or too low to show sufficient efficacy. Adaptive design enables optimized dose selection before the pivotal trial is initiated.

Another feature of adaptive design is population enrichment where drug response can be optimized to specific patient subpopulations that respond better to treatment. Many phase III studies fail because the overall efficacy of treatment is diluted as a consequence of the drug being evaluated in the full population rather than in the specific subset where the drug works best. Adaptive design enables early selection of the appropriate patient population and increases the probability of success.

Phases I and II are critical steps in the product development process as this is where important information about the product has to be generated and assessed, before the decision is taken to commit to expensive phase III pivotal studies. This early phase of development is known as the "learn phase" and the data that has to be generated relates to the effective dose–response, the safety profile and therapeutic index, appropriate endpoints, and the population of patients that will benefit best from the product under evaluation.

Choosing which development candidate to back when there is a large portfolio of products competing for a fixed level of investment can be a difficult and complex process. The adoption of an adaptive design strategy at the portfolio level can provide significant value to the critical decision making required to deliver an optimized pipeline of products.

Adaptive design can:

- Increase the value of the pipeline by maximizing the probability of success and reducing the cost of development
- Enable better management of resources across a pipeline of products
- Optimize investment decision making
- Increase portfolio value

In its simplest form adaptive design enables early termination of trials in which the product just does not work and as a consequence enables redeployment of funding and resources to more promising programs. Another type of adaptive design, applied on the program level of a compound, is achieving efficiency by combining in a single trial objectives that are usually addressed in two separate conventional studies. Such a strategy provides the obvious benefit of reducing the timeline by running the two studies seamlessly under a single protocol with the same clinical team and the same centers and achieves trial efficiency by combining the information from subjects in both studies in the final analysis. Examples are:

- Combining a conventional multiple ascending dose escalation in patients and proof of concept (POC) in a single trial
- Combining the proof of concept with the dose-ranging study, by starting the study with equal randomization of patients to the top dose and placebo and then opening enrollment to other doses of the compound only if a futility rule is overpassed
- Seamless phase II/III adaptive designs, by starting a confirmatory trial with couple of doses of the new compound with a pre-planned option of selecting the "best" dose for the second stage of the trial

Furthermore, such adaptive designs optimize the benefit/risk balance for participating subjects via improved efficiency of decision making in relation to the doses of the new drug studied. They minimize the number of subjects that are exposed to ineffective doses of the drug while simultaneously focusing subjects to doses that are most informative for accurate dose selection for subsequent stages of compound development.

More complex adaptive strategies integrate the development of several compounds and/or indications into one process. The principle is to keep one or more aspects of the trial fixed and pre-plan for several adaptation options that will be applied during the conduct of the study. Examples are:

- *Adaptive "population" finder*: The fixed aspect of the trial is the indication (e.g., breast cancer) and the treatment (e.g., epidermal growth factor receptor inhibitor). The design aims to establish which subset of the population benefits most.
- *Adaptive "compound" finder*: The fixed aspects of the trial are the indication (e.g., Alzheimer's disease), the patient population (e.g., mild to moderate), and the gold standard treatment we are comparing ourselves against (currently

available best standard of care). The competing options are three different compounds for the same indication. The adaptive design aims to identify the compound with the most impressive therapeutic index to pursue in the further development. See the case study in the next section.

- *Adaptive "indication" finder*: The fixed aspect of the trial is the compound (e.g., a cytostatic treatment). The competing options are different indications (e.g., different tumor histologies). The design aims to establish which of the indications show therapeutic benefit.
- *Adaptive "compound/population" finder*: The fixed aspect is the population, but its heterogeneity is recognized from the outset. Multiple development candidates are assessed in parallel and matched with biomarker signatures of different subpopulations. The design aims to dynamically change the allocation of new patients with a given signature to different compounds, graduating successful compound/biomarker pairs to small, focused, more successful confirmatory phase, as is the case with breast cancer in the well-publicized ISPY-2 trial (Barker et al. 2009); see also BATTLE trial in lung cancer (Zhou et al. 2008).

These approaches assist in and enhance the decision on which product to be developed. However, adaptive design offers much more than selecting the right candidate to develop. It enables more effective decision making throughout the whole development process by increasing the quality of information generated at each stage of a trial. This increases development efficiency, productivity, and the probability of success at phase III, and ultimately contributes to the success of the overall portfolio.

All these factors contribute to a decrease in the cost of the portfolio and an increase in portfolio success which culminates in increased portfolio value. Adopting an adaptive design strategy at the portfolio level will significantly increase the return on the investment in several areas including new product development, lifecycle decision making, and product repurposing.

In the next section, we illustrate the efficiency of such complex strategies in clinical development programs in a case study of an adaptive "compound" finder.

4.2 Case Study

The sponsor has up to three compounds simultaneously approaching the POC stage in the same therapeutic area—Alzheimer's disease (AD). A conventional development strategy is to investigate these three compounds in a sequential manner, one after another in separate trials. The conventional design of each of such study is a multicenter, randomized, double-blind, placebo-controlled trial with two active arms (low, high) and placebo in a 1:1:1 randomization, all as adjunctive to background therapy.

This conventional development strategy is compared and contrasted with an adaptive compound finder proof-of-concept study design that investigates several compounds in a single trial. The objective is to find with high probability the "best" compound using adaptive allocation of subjects to competing treatments. The primary endpoint for comparing the efficacy of the compounds is the change from baseline at 12 months in ADAS-Cog. A maximum sample size of 450 subjects is utilized to adaptively allocate to six active treatments (low and high doses for each compound), all as adjunctive to background therapy, and a placebo (standard of care). An early stopping for efficacy or futility is utilized.

The comparison of these two design strategies is done through intensive simulations. Response data is simulated under a dozen of possible scenarios and the two strategies are compared on different operating characteristics: the average number of subjects, the average study duration, and probability of correctly identifying the "best" compound.

4.2.1 Treatment Duration

To decide on the treatment duration of the trial, different time courses of the change from baseline in ADAS-Cog have been considered. In Pfizer's comprehensive meta-analysis (Ito et al. 2010) of public data sources from 1990 to 2008, as well as clinical studies that evaluated the rate of deterioration of AD patients, a model describing the time course of the change from baseline in ADAS-Cog for mild- to moderate-severity AD patients was developed. The model was used to investigate the required number of subjects per arm for a conventional parallel-group study design with a two-sample t-test at a two-sided significance level of 0.05. It is assumed that the standard deviation (SD) for the change from baseline in ADAS-Cog is 6 points for each treatment and at each time point. Treatment durations of 12, 26, 40, and 52 weeks are considered. Figure 4.1 plots the mean difference in change from baseline on ADAS-Cog between the active treatment and placebo, for the three drugs investigated in Ito et al. (2010): donepezil, galantamine, and rivastigmine. The dots show the mean difference used in the sample size calculation in Table 4.1.

It can be seen that the donepezil treatment effect is around −2 points and is almost constant starting at week 12. Therefore for drugs like donepezil the duration of treatment is not so important. However, the treatment effect of galantamine depends very much on treatment duration and changes from −2.3 at week 12 to −3.9 at week 52. For the rivastigmine, the treatment effect is small overall (only −1.36 at week 52), so the time course is also not very pronounced. As a result, the effect on the required sample size is different for different drugs. For donepezil, the range is 140–118 subjects per arm for 80 % power. In contrast, for the galantamine the range is from 105 to 39 for the same 80 % power. For the rivastigmine, because the treatment effect is so small the required number of subjects is more than doubled when considering 12-week treatment period versus 52-week period.

Because at this stage there is no information what might be the time course of treatment effect for these three drugs, the recommended treatment duration will be 52 weeks.

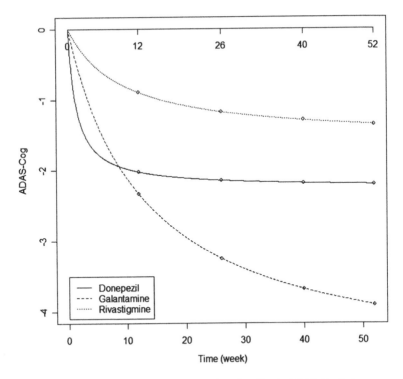

Fig. 4.1 Time course of mean difference in change from baseline in ADAS-Cog between an active drug and placebo

Table 4.1 Sample size per arm for a conventional parallel-group design with fixed sample size: Two-sample t-test at a two-sided significance level of 0.05, SD = 6 units

Time point	Donepezil Power 80 %	Power 90 %	Galantamine Power 80 %	Power 90 %	Rivastigmine Power 80 %	Power 90 %
12 weeks	140	187	105	140	702	940
26 weeks	124	165	52	70	395	528
40 weeks	120	160	43	57	338	452
52 weeks	118	158	39	51	309	413

4.2.2 Conventional Development Strategy

Each compound is investigated in a separate clinical trial. The primary endpoint is the change from baseline at 12 months in ADAS-Cog. A parallel-group design with two active treatment arms (low dose and high dose) and placebo is considered.

Literature review of studies with subjects treated with standard of care provides the following rates of decline over 12 months in the ADAS-Cog (Table 4.2):

Table 4.2 Rates of decline over 12 months in the ADAS-Cog in subjects treated with standard of care

Study	Sample size	Mean change in ADAS-Cog (SD)	Monthly decline
Reines et al. (2004)	327	5.4 (NA)	0.45
Thal et al. (1996)	211	7.0 (7.8)	0.58
Aisen et al. (2003)	111	5.7 (8.2)	0.48
Thal et al. (2000)	102	7.5 (8.0)	0.63
Aisen et al. (2000)	69	6.3 (6.4)	0.53

Table 4.3 Sample size per arm for a conventional parallel group design with fixed sample size: Two-sample t-test at a two-sided significance level of 0.05

	Difference in mean change from baseline/SD							
Power	−2/6	−2/7	−2.5/6	−2.5/7	−3/6	−3/7	−4/6	−4/7
80 %	143	194	92	125	64	87	37	50
90 %	191	259	123	166	86	116	49	66

A meta-analysis of 14 studies (Hansen et al. 2008) reported the mean change in ADAS-Cog from baseline to endpoint for active treatment (donepezil, galantamine, and rivastigmine) compared with placebo in subjects with mild-to-moderate dementia in a range of [−3.90, −1.60]. The pooled weighted mean difference in change between active treatment and placebo was −2.67 (95 % CI (−3.28,−2.06)) for donepezil, −2.76 (95 % CI (−3.17,−2.34)) for galantamine, and −3.01 (95 % CI (−3.80,−2.21)) for rivastigmine.

To calculate the required sample size for a given power, we use different standard deviations (SD) for the change from baseline in ADAS-Cog (6 and 7 points) and different treatment effects measured as the difference in mean change from baseline between active treatment and placebo (−2, −3, −4 points).

Table 4.3 provides the sample size per arm for a conventional trial assuming different treatment effects and required power. A two-sample t-test at a two-sided significance level 0.05 is assumed for comparing each dose with placebo with no adjustment for multiplicity.

The required number of subjects per group for 80 % power and a minimum treatment effect of −2 units is 143 (assuming SD=6). This might be too large for a proof-of-concept study; therefore we will assume that the expected treatment effect is −3 that results in 64 subjects per group for 80 % power. We will use this setup as the benchmark in our comparison with the adaptive design trial.

4.2.3 Adaptive Design Trial Structure

The structure of the adaptive trial is as follows.

Design: There is an initial burn-in period of 50 subjects equally allocated to each of the seven treatments. After this first look, additional interim analyses are conducted after every 50 subjects enrolled. If there are at least 100 subjects in the trial then the trial can stop for efficacy or futility. If the trial does not stop at an interim analysis then the trial continues with adaptive interim looks until 450 subjects have been randomized.

Allocation rule: Any active treatment with the posterior probability of being better than placebo Pr(T beats Plbo)<0.4 will be dropped for further allocations; that is, no new subjects will be allocated to this treatment. However, the subjects already allocated to this treatment will be followed up for their endpoint at 52 weeks. The new subjects will be equally allocated to the remaining active treatments and placebo.

Stopping rule: If there are at least 100 subjects in the trial, a decision is made at each interim analysis whether to stop the trial for success or futility.

- *Early success*: The trial is stopped for success if the active treatment group with the highest posterior probability of having the maximum effect has at least a 0.80 probability of achieving the clinical significant difference (CSD) of 3 points in ADAS-Cog change from baseline compared to placebo, Pr(CSD I T=Max)>0.80. If the condition is satisfied, the enrollment is stopped and the last subject is followed up for the endpoint at 52 weeks.
- *Early futility*: The trial is defined as futile if Pr(CSD I T=Max)<0.05. If the condition is satisfied, the enrollment is stopped and the last subject is followed up for the endpoint at 52 weeks.

Decisions at trial completion: At the conclusion of the trial, at full 52-week follow-up for the last subject enrolled, the trial is defined as follows:

- *Late success*: The trial is defined as a success if the active treatment group with the highest posterior probability of having the maximum effect has at least a 0.95 probability of being better than placebo, Pr(T beats Plbo I T=Max)>0.95 and has at least 0.25 probability of achieving the clinical significant difference, Pr(CSD I T=Max)>0.25.
- *Late futility*: Otherwise, the trial is defined as futile.

There is a possibility that the trial is stopped early (either for success or futility), but after the last subject is followed up for 52 weeks, the terminal decision is reversed. In the simulation study, this is counted as a "flip-flop" outcome.

Statistical hierarchical model: A Bayesian hierarchical model is used as the analysis working model. The change from baseline at 52 weeks in the ADAS-Cog score for each treatment $t=0,1,\ldots,6$ ($t=0$ means placebo arm) arm is modeled as normal distribution with mean μ_t and variance σ^2:

$$Y_t \sim N\left(\mu_t, \sigma^2\right).$$

The mean responses μ_t of the experimental treatments $(t=1,\ldots,6)$ are assumed to follow a normal distribution with a common mean μ ($\mu=-5$ is used) and variance τ^2:

$$\mu_t \sim N\left(\mu,\tau^2\right).$$

The prior distribution for the variance components is inverse-gamma:

$$\sigma^2 \sim IG\left(\frac{5}{2},\frac{2/5}{6^2}\right) \text{ and } \tau^2 \sim IG\left(\frac{5}{2},\frac{2/5}{6^2}\right),$$

that is equivalent to assuming 5 observations with differences between observations of 6.

Longitudinal modeling: The primary endpoint is the ADAS-Cog score. The change from baseline for the ADAS-Cog is observed at 12, 26, 40, and 52 weeks. These measurements will be used to inform the primary endpoint for subjects with partial information.

The early measurements of ADAS-Cog are modeled using a linear regression model:

$$Y_t \sim N\left(\alpha_k + \beta_k y_{t,k}, \lambda_k^2\right) \text{ for } k = 12, 26, 40 \text{ and } t = 0, 1, \ldots 6,$$

where $y_{t,k}$ is the ADAS-Cog change from baseline at week k and Y_t is the change from baseline at 52 weeks. Therefore, it is a piecewise linear model. Separate linear models are used for modeling the placebo $(t=0)$ and the other treatments $(t=1,\ldots,6)$.

The prior distributions are

$$\alpha_k \sim N\left(-5,1\right), \ \beta_k \sim N\left(-0.5,1\right), \ \lambda_k^2 \sim IG\left(\frac{12}{2},\frac{2/12}{5^2}\right).$$

The model helps guide the adaptive algorithm in allocating subjects and possibly stopping early for efficacy or futility. However, these longitudinal models do not affect the final conclusion when the final endpoint for a subject is known.

This piecewise linear longitudinal model is flexible enough to accommodate more complex ADAS-Cog time profiles investigated in the literature. For example, in a recent model-based analysis (Ito et al. 2010) of 52 literature sources consisting of 576 mean values of ADAS-Cog at each visit from approximately 20,000 subjects, the time profile models have been developed for both the placebo and active treatments (donepezil, galantamine, and rivastigmine). Figure 4.2 shows the time course of ADAS-Cog for these four treatments. It is easy to see that these nonlinear time courses can be well approximated by two or three piecewise linear segments. In our simulation study we will be generating the longitudinal time profile similar to the donepezil (the top-right panel), while the fitting longitudinal model will be the piecewise linear model described in this section.

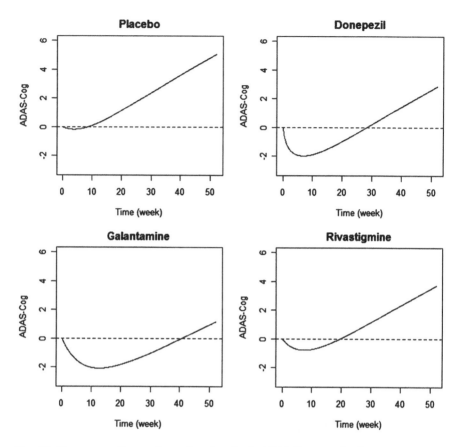

Fig. 4.2 Time course of mean change from baseline in ADAS-Cog on active drugs

4.3 Simulations

In order to evaluate the operating characteristics of the adaptive design, several simulation scenarios are created. In these simulations, virtual subjects with pre-specified distribution of the primary clinical endpoint (ADAS-Cog) are generated and their results simulated. These simulated subjects and the simulations have no bearing on the actual trial, but merely evaluate the characteristics of the described design.

In each simulation scenario presented in this section we assume that the standard deviation for the primary clinical endpoint ADAS-Cog is 6 points. The weekly accrual rate is assumed to be three subjects. Therefore, if the trial enrolls to the maximum number of subjects 450 without early stopping, the duration of the study will be 202 weeks (150-week accrual period plus 52-week follow-up).

The results of the simulations are described in the next section.

Table 4.4 Simulation scenarios: Assumed change from baseline in ADAS-Cog at week 52

| Scenario name | Assumed change from baseline in ADAS-Cog at week 52 | | | | | | |
	0	1	2	3	4	5	6
Flat	5	5	5	5	5	5	5
Equal 4pts	5	1	1	1	1	1	1
Nugget 4pts	5	4	4	4	1	4	4
2nuggets 4pts	5	4	4	4	1	4	1
2nuggets 3pts	5	4	4	4	2	4	2
Nugget 3pts	5	4	4	4	2	4	4

4.3.1   Operating Characteristics

This section presents the operating characteristics of the design under six different scenarios. For each scenario, assumptions about the change from baseline in ADAS-Cog at week 52 for each treatment, including placebo, are made. They are presented in Table 4.4. The treatments are numbered from 0 to 6, 0 being placebo, followed by low and high doses of each of the three active treatments.

The first scenario, called "flat," assumes that all treatments, including placebo, have the same change from baseline in ADAS-Cog of 5 points. The 5 points decline at week 52 in ADAS-Cog is consistent with the placebo effect derived by the modeling approach in Ito et al. (2010), and it is smaller than the annual rates of decline reported in Table 4.1, but close to the one (5.4 points) reported in the largest study (Reines et al. 2004).

The second scenario assumes that all active treatments are equally effective with the change from baseline in ADAS-Cog of 1 point compared to 5 points on placebo. Therefore, all treatments are very effective with a mean change difference of −4 points, a treatment effect that is greater than the 95 % CI reported in the meta-analysis by Hansen et al. (2008): (−3.28,−2.06) for donepezil, (−3.17,−2.34) for galantamine, and (−3.80,−2.21) for rivastigmine.

The third scenario, called "nugget 4pts," assumes that only one treatment (treatment 4) is highly effective (nugget effect); all the others have just 1 point mean difference from placebo.

The fourth scenario assumes that there are two nuggets, treatment 4 and 6. The fifth scenario assumes also that there are two nuggets, but the magnitude of the effect is only 3 points mean difference. The last scenario assumes the same magnitude but only for treatment 4.

For each scenario, 1,000 simulation runs have been conducted and the following operating characteristics are reported in Table 4.5:

- Average sample size
- Average study duration
- Probability of early stopping for success
- Probability of early stopping for futility

Table 4.5 Operating characteristics of the adaptive design

Scenario name	Mean number subjects	Mean trial duration	Prob. of early success	Prob. of early futility	Prob. of late success	Prob. of late futility	Prob. of flip-flop
Flat	370.75	176	0.021	0.499	0.045	0.425	0.010
Equal 4pts	257.40	138	0.915	0.000	0.084	0.000	0.001
Nugget 4pts	361.60	173	0.506	0.011	0.436	0.037	0.010
2nuggets 4pts	328.40	162	0.659	0.003	0.318	0.013	0.007
2nuggets 3pts	377.15	178	0.389	0.024	0.475	0.100	0.011
Nugget 3pts	400.80	186	0.238	0.050	0.501	0.198	0.013

Table 4.6 Average number of subjects allocated to each treatment

Scenario name	Treatment allocation						
	0	1	2	3	4	5	6
Flat	71.886	49.401	48.845	49.737	49.29	48.706	52.885
Equal 4pts	37.682	36.627	36.465	36.322	36.95	36.635	36.719
Nugget 4pts	62.716	47.711	47.294	47.801	59.833	48.410	47.835
2nuggets 4pts	52.949	42.633	42.427	43.722	51.902	43.488	51.279
2nuggets 3pts	62.207	49.296	49.479	49.486	58.325	49.049	59.308
Nugget 3pts	66.971	54.371	54.830	54.695	63.081	53.469	53.383

- Probability of late success
- Probability of late futility
- Probability of "flip-flop"

Across all six scenarios the mean number of subjects required by the adaptive design is smaller than 401. The smallest mean number of subjects (257.4) is required under scenario "equal 4pts" when all active treatments are very effective. The largest mean sample size (400.8) is required under scenario "nugget 3pts" when only one treatment achieves the mean change difference of 3 points.

The "flat" scenario is used here to quantify the false-positive rate of the adaptive design. It can be seen that the probability of wrongly claiming success under this scenario is only 0.045.

Probability of early futility is about 0.50, which means that in about 50 % of the simulations the trial did not enroll to the maximum of 450 subjects.

On the other hand, for "good" scenarios, the probability of early futility is well under 0.05. Under scenario "equal 4pts," the trial stops early for success in 91.5 % of cases. This is a good property of the design because in such situation it is good to find at least one good treatment as soon as possible to proceed to further development stage. In the case of only one treatment with effect of mean change difference of 3 points (scenario "nugget 3pts"), the trial requires about 400 subjects and the probability of early success is only 0.238. But overall, the probability of futility is only 0.25. As can be seen from Table 4.6, the average number of subjects allocated to

Table 4.7 Probability of being selected as treatment with the maximum effect

Scenario name	Probability of being selected as treatment with the maximum effect					
	1	2	3	4	5	6
Flat	0.155	0.163	0.171	0.188	0.149	0.174
Equal 4pts	**0.160**	**0.148**	**0.140**	**0.185**	**0.176**	**0.191**
Nugget 4pts	0.005	0.004	0.005	**0.974**	0.005	0.007
2nuggets 4pts	0.004	0.001	0.003	**0.488**	0.002	**0.502**
2nuggets 3pts	0.015	0.012	0.009	**0.452**	0.011	**0.501**
Nugget 3pts	0.032	0.029	0.030	**0.863**	0.029	0.017

placebo and the "nugget" treatment 4 is 67 and 63, respectively. This can be expected, because according to the sample size calculations in Table 4.3, 64 subjects per arm are required in such case for 80 % power.

In contrast, for the more effective scenario "nugget 4pts," the corresponding numbers of subjects on placebo and treatment 4 are only about 63 and 60, respectively, and the overall number of subjects is 361.6. Moreover, the probability of futility is reduced to 0.048. Therefore, in a situation of a single treatment effect with very effective mean difference of 4 units, the adaptive design reduces the false-negative rate by 20 % in comparison with the case of only 3 points difference, and achieves that also by reducing the overall number of subjects by about 40.

Under scenario "equal 4pts," the average number of subjects allocated to each dose is approximately 37, which is exactly the required number of subjects per arm for such situation (see Table 4.3, column 6). For scenario "nugget 4pts," most subjects are allocated to placebo and treatment 4. Similarly, for the other scenarios, the placebo and the treatments that have higher efficacy get more subjects allocated.

Another important operating characteristic is the probability of being selected as the treatment with the maximum effect that is presented in Table 4.7. The numbers in boldface correspond to treatments that are indeed the true treatments with the maximum treatment effect. For scenarios with a single nugget, the probability of correctly selecting it is very high, 0.974 and 0.863 for scenarios "nugget 4pts" and "nugget 3pts," respectively. For the scenarios with two nuggets, the probabilities of selecting them are split almost evenly, but overall the probabilities of correctly selecting either one are 0.99 and 0.95, respectively.

For each scenario two figures are presented to highlight specific operating characteristics; see Figs. 4.3, 4.4, 4.5, 4.6, 4.7, and 4.8. For each scenario, the top figure presents the box plots for the sample size per treatment. The bottom figure shows the probability each treatment is selected as the most likely treatment with the maximum effect (Max).

Table 4.8 presents the bias in estimating the primary endpoint at each treatment, including placebo. The bias is smallest at the treatments that are selected, which is very important, because the response at that treatment will be used for planning the future development.

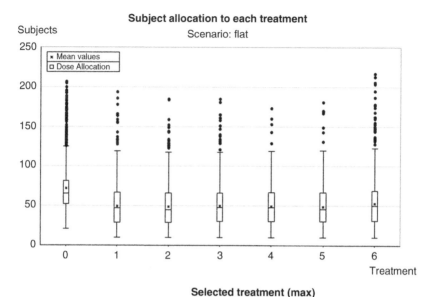

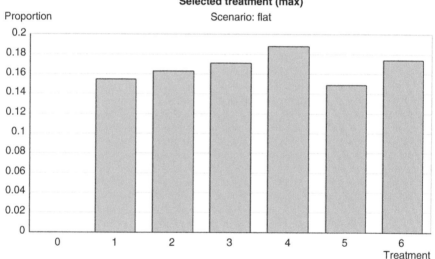

Fig. 4.3 Scenario "flat": Subject allocation to each treatment and selected treatment

4.3.2   Comparison to a Conventional Development Strategy

In this section the adaptive design is compared to a conventional development strategy, defined as follows. Each trial enrolls 192 subjects equally allocated (64 per group) to placebo, low, and high dose of the corresponding active treatment. From Table 4.3, this guarantees a power of 80 % to detect a mean difference of 3 points

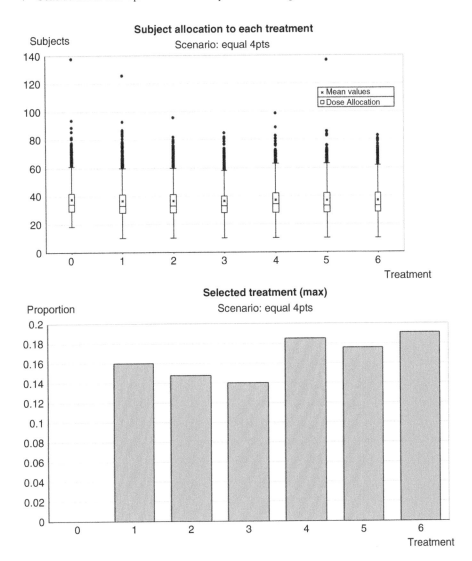

Fig. 4.4 Scenario "equal 4pts": Subject allocation to each treatment and selected treatment

with the assumed standard deviation of 6 points. Assuming the same accrual rate of 3 subjects per week, the trial duration is 116 weeks (64-week enrollment plus 52-week follow-up). Because the conventional strategy will run the three trials one after another, the total number of subjects will be 576 and the total duration of the program 348 weeks. These are both much larger than the maximum number of subjects required by the adaptive strategy: 450 subjects and 202 weeks. Therefore, the net benefit of the adaptive strategy versus the conventional one is total saving of 126 subjects and 146 weeks in POC study duration.

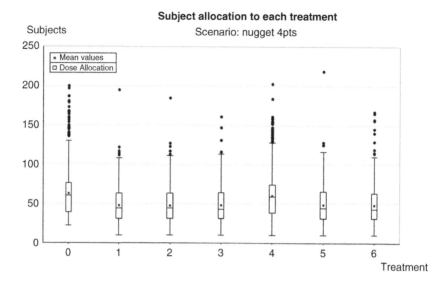

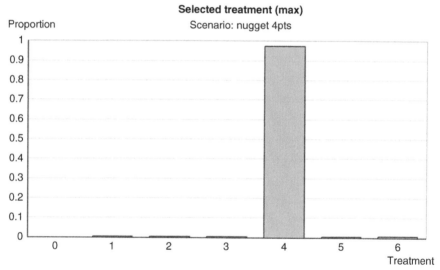

Fig. 4.5 Scenario "nugget 4pts": Subject allocation to each treatment and selected treatment

However, the adaptive design strategy provides additional efficiency by incorporating early stopping and dropping treatment arm options. On the other hand, the conventional strategy may also stop the program after finding an effective treatment. The comparison of this modified conventional strategy with the adaptive one is given in Table 4.9 that presents the mean number of subjects and average duration of the study for the two strategies under different scenarios. For the conventional strategy, three situations are considered for the order in which the trials will be run.

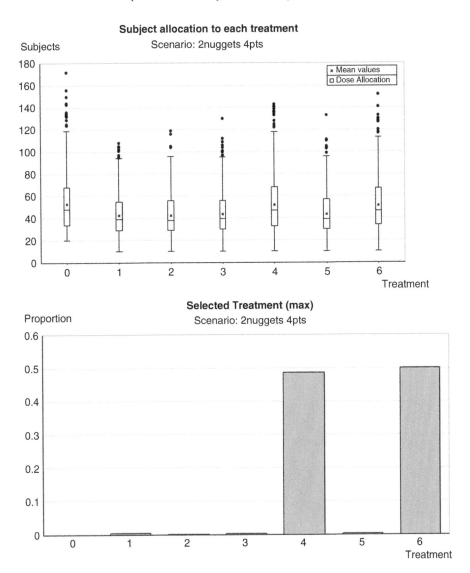

Fig. 4.6 Scenario "2nuggets 4pts": Subject allocation to each treatment and selected treatment

For example, "$12 \rightarrow 34 \rightarrow 56$" means that the low and high dose of the first active treatment will be run against placebo, followed if not successful by the low and high dose of the second active treatment against placebo, and then followed if not successful by the low and high dose of the third treatment against placebo.

Under "flat" scenario, the adaptive design is a clear winner, requiring on average 370.75 subjects and the average study duration of 176 weeks. The conventional strategy requires an additional 178 subjects and prolongs the study duration by

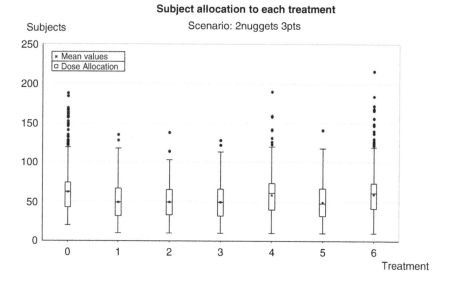

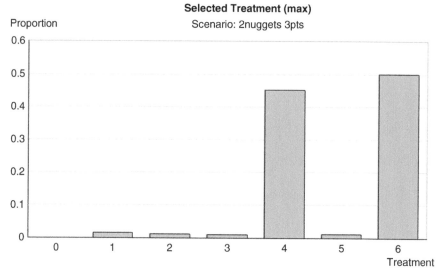

Fig. 4.7 Scenario "2nuggets 3pts": Subject allocation to each treatment and selected treatment

155 weeks. Under "equal 4pts" scenario, the situation is reversed because the conventional strategy stops with high probability (0.998) after the first trial.

The comparison results for the remaining scenarios depend on the order in which the conventional strategy will run the three trials. The situation "$34 \rightarrow 12 \rightarrow 56$" is the best, giving the treatment 4 the high chance of being selected after the first trial. The situation "$12 \rightarrow 56 \rightarrow 34$" is the worst, running the trial with the nugget treatment 4 only in the third trial. The situation "$12 \rightarrow 34 \rightarrow 56$" is in the middle, running the treatment 4 in the second trial.

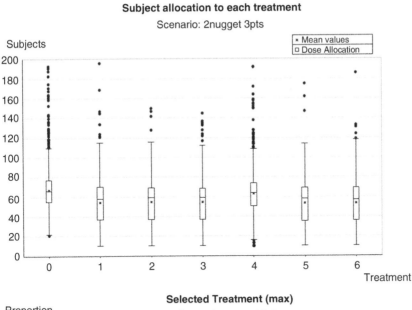

Fig. 4.8 Scenario "nugget 3pts": Subject allocation to each treatment and selected treatment

Although the conventional strategy may require smaller number of subjects (see, e.g., scenario "nugget 4pts" under first situation: 335.44 vs. 361.60), the duration of the study is greater than that of the adaptive strategy. Moreover, under the first and third situations, the study duration is greater than 202 weeks which is the maximum study duration for the adaptive strategy, irrespective of the scenario.

Notice that in the conventional strategy each patient has a 1/2 chance to be allocated to placebo, compared to 1/7 in the adaptive strategy trial.

Table 4.8 Bias in ADAS-Cog at week 52 estimate

Scenario name	Bias in ADAS-Cog at week 52 estimate						
	0	1	2	3	4	5	6
Flat	−0.0414	0.1889	0.1565	0.1543	0.0965	0.1810	0.1268
Equal 4pts	0.1114	0.1085	0.1546	0.1283	0.0735	0.1103	0.0657
Nugget 4pts	0.2020	0.1184	0.1686	0.1286	−0.0008	0.1153	0.1023
2nuggets 4pts	0.1605	0.1330	0.1087	0.0821	0.0404	0.1194	0.0602
2nuggets 3pts	0.1302	0.0854	0.1254	0.1577	0.0559	0.1327	−0.0083
Nugget 3pts	0.0780	0.1122	0.0538	0.0660	0.0312	0.1228	0.1240

Table 4.9 Comparison of adaptive and conventional strategies on the number of subjects (N Subj) and study duration (S Dur)

Scenario name	Adaptive strategy		Conventional strategy					
			$12 \rightarrow 34 \rightarrow 56$		$34 \rightarrow 12 \rightarrow 56$		$12 \rightarrow 56 \rightarrow 34$	
	N Subj	S Dur	N Subj	S Dur	N Subj	S Dur	N Subj	S Dur
Flat	370.75	176	548.03	331.1	548.03	331.1	548.03	331.1
Equal 4pts	257.40	138	192.31	116.2	192.31	116.2	192.31	116.2
Nugget 4pts	361.60	173	335.44	202.7	203.24	122.8	430.95	260.4
2nuggets 4pts	328.40	162	335.44	202.7	203.24	122.8	335.44	202.7
2nuggets 3pts	377.15	178	354.30	214.1	248.22	150.0	354.30	214.1
Nugget 3pts	400.80	186	354.30	214.1	248.22	150.0	430.95	260.4

Another important point to be made is the fact that the adaptive strategy gives each treatment a chance to be investigated and the treatment is dropped only if it shows a low chance of being effective, while the conventional strategy may very well never reach the point of investigating a given treatment.

The "white space" between closing a trial and starting another one was ignored in previous comparison, but this time may be considerable in practice.

4.4 Discussion

Although enormous progress has been made in recent years in understanding the pathophysiology of Alzheimer's disease, this progress has not yet translated into new treatments. The high cost and low success rate of drug development in Alzheimer's disease can be attributed, in large part, to late-stage clinical trial failures. Thus, identifying in "learn" phase drugs that are likely to fail could have a dramatic impact on the costs associated with developing new drugs.

In the case study, we illustrated the novel adaptive screening strategy of several compounds for treatment of mild-to-moderate Alzheimer's patients in the portfolio of a single company. However, the methodology can be applied in the setting of testing several candidate drugs from different sponsors simultaneously.

The Executive Director of the Innovative Medicines Initiative (IMI) Michel Goldman mentioned recently that "[T]he challenge of developing new treatments for Alzheimer's disease is too great for any single organisation, country or company to tackle alone. What is needed is an unprecedented, international, collaborative approach bringing together all stakeholders involved in the development of new treatments for Alzheimer's."

On December 11, 2013, the IMI launched a major new project that will pioneer a novel adaptive approach to clinical trials of drugs designed to prevent Alzheimer's disease, which is expected to affect 100 million people worldwide by 2050. The project will focus its efforts on speeding up drug development and patient access to the latest treatments by testing several candidate drugs from different sponsors simultaneously.

Furthermore, this novel "adaptive" trial design can allow researchers to consider patients with different stages of Alzheimer's disease and adapt the trial design in response to emerging results. For example, if a compound appears to be particularly effective in only early (the so-called prodromal) Alzheimer's disease patients, then assignment of that compound can be preferentially directed to those patients to confirm this finding and perhaps "promote" that compound to a confirmatory clinical trial. Similarly, new candidate drugs can be added to the trial and the ones that turn out to be ineffective can be dropped.

The strategy has already proved effective in the I-SPY 2 trial of new treatments for breast cancer. The adaptive trial design enabled two experimental breast-cancer drugs to deliver promising results after just 6 months of testing, far shorter than the typical length of a clinical trial. Researchers assessed the results while the trial was in process and found that cancer had been eradicated in more than half of one group of patients, a particularly favorable outcome.

References

Aisen PS, Davis KL, Berg JD, Schafer K, Campbell K, Thomas RG, Weiner MF, Farlow MR, Sano M, Grundman M, Thal LJ (2000) A randomized controlled trial of prednisone in Alzheimer's disease. Alzheimer's Disease Cooperative Study. Neurology 54(3):588–593

Aisen PS, Schafer KA, Grundman M, Pfeiffer E, Sano M, Davis KL, Farlow MR, Jin S, Thomas RG, Thal LJ, Alzheimer's Disease Cooperative Study (2003) Effects of rofecoxib or naproxen vs placebo on Alzheimer disease progression: a randomized controlled trial. JAMA 289(21): 2819–2826

Barker AD, Sigman CC, Kelloff GJ, Hylton NM, Berry DA, Esserman LJ (2009) I-SPY 2: an adaptive breast cancer trial design in the setting of neoadjuvant chemotherapy. Clin Pharmacol Ther 86:97–100

Hansen RA, Gartlehner G, Webb AP, Morgan LC, Moore CG, Jonas DE (2008) Efficacy and safety of donepezil, galantamine, and rivastigmine for the treatment of Alzheimer's disease": a systematic review and meta-analysis. Clin Interv Aging 3(2):211–225

Ito K, Ahadieh S, Corrigan B, French J, Fullerton T, Tensfeldt T, Alzheimer's Disease Working Group (2010) Disease progression meta-analysis model in Alzheimer's disease. Alzheimers Dement 6:39–53

Reines SA, Block GA, Morris JC, Liu G, Nessly ML, Lines CR, Norman BA, Baranak CC, Rofecoxib Protocol 091 Study Group (2004) Rofecoxib: no effect on Alzheimer's disease in a 1-year, randomized, blinded, controlled study. Neurology 62(1):66–71

Thal LJ, Carta A, Clarke WR, Ferris SH, Friedland RP, Petersen RC, Pettegrew JW, Pfeiffer E, Raskind MA, Sano M, Tuszynski MH, Woolson RF (1996) A 1-year multicenter placebo-controlled study of acetyl-L-carnitine in subjects with Alzheimer's disease. Neurology 47(3): 705–711

Thal LJ, Calvani M, Amato A, Carta A (2000) A 1-year controlled trial of acetyl-l-carnitine in early-onset AD. Neurology 55(6):805–810

Zhou X, Liu S, Kim ES, Herbst RS, Lee JJ (2008) Bayesian adaptive design for targeted therapy development in lung cancer—a step toward personalized medicine. Clin Trials 5:181–193

Chapter 5
Optimal Cost-Effective Go–No Go Decisions in Clinical Development

Cong Chen, Robert A. Beckman, and Linda Z. Sun

Abstract In late-stage drug development, drug developers have to make two critical Go–No Go decisions. The first one is whether to proceed to the definitive Phase III investigation after a Phase II proof-of-concept (POC) trial. The second one is whether to stop a Phase III confirmatory trial for futility after an interim analysis of the data. In practice, the two decisions are heuristically made with limited statistical input, usually amounting to statistical characterization of proposed options. We propose to find the optimal decisions by explicitly maximizing a benefit–cost ratio function, which is often the implicit objective in an otherwise qualitative decision-making process. The numerator of the function represents the benefit (proportional to the expected number of truly active drugs identified for Phase III development in the POC setting; proportional to the expected power for successful completion of Phase III in the interim analysis setting), and the denominator represents the expected total late-stage development cost. The method is easy to explain and simple to implement. The optimal design parameters provide a rational starting point for decision makers to consider. As an illustration, the method developed herein is applied to examples from the oncology therapeutic area including an adaptive seamless Phase II/III design. The same idea is applicable to any disease area where cost-effectiveness of a Go–No Go decision is a major concern.

C. Chen (✉) • L.Z. Sun
Biostatistics and Research Decision Sciences, Merck Research Laboratories (MRL),
UG1C-46, 375 Sumneytown Pike, Upper Gwynedd, PA 19454, USA
e-mail: cong_chen@merck.com; linda_sun@merck.com

R.A. Beckman
Oncology Clinical Research, Daiichi Sankyo Pharmaceutical Development,
Edison, NJ 08837, USA

Center for Evolution and Cancer, Helen Diller Family Cancer Center, University of California
at San Francisco, San Francisco, CA 94115, USA
e-mail: eniac1915@gmail.com

W. He et al. (eds.), *Practical Considerations for Adaptive Trial Design and Implementation*, Statistics for Biology and Health,
DOI 10.1007/978-1-4939-1100-4_5, © Springer Science+Business Media New York 2014

Keywords Adaptive design • Bayesian • Cost-effectiveness • Decision analysis • Futility analysis • Proof-of-concept • Seamless design • Surrogate • Type I/II error rates

5.1   Introduction

This chapter addresses two Go–No Go decision issues in late-stage drug develop-ment, followed by a real example of seamless Phase II/III design. As an illustration, the method developed herein is applied to examples from the oncology therapeutic area. The same idea is applicable to any disease area where cost-effectiveness of a Go–No Go decision is a major concern. The first issue comes from Phase II proof-of-concept (POC) trials. A POC trial is defined as a trial which provides the critical information about drug activity or lack thereof in a patient population for deciding whether to proceed to definitive Phase III investigation. The phenomenal expansion of our knowledge in the molecular biology in the last decade has led to an unprec-edented number of exciting new targets, which in turn lead to numerous opportuni-ties for POC. These opportunities are often of similar interest given the difficulty in picking the likely winners based on preclinical and early clinical data alone. Because the total resource budget is often capped, drug developers must decide how many POC trials to move forward, how large each trial should be and how to set the cor-responding Go–No Go decision criterion to Phase III. The second issue comes from the Phase III confirmation trial. Historically, the majority of Phase III oncology tri-als fail in spite of strong efficacy signals observed in POC trials. One way to reduce the consequences of failure in Phase III is to conduct an interim futility analysis of the data to reduce resource expenditure on therapies that appear unlikely to succeed. However, it remains a challenging issue when to perform the futility analysis and how to set the futility boundary.

At the center of each of these issues is how to appropriately balance benefit and cost. The balance of benefit and cost is particularly important when there is a fixed maximum resource budget (number of patients, or financial costs) which does not allow us to adequately investigate all possible drugs, schedules, and indications of interest. A fixed maximum total research budget is a common reality in both private and public sector drug development. In the face of a fixed maximum budget, maxi-mization of the benefit–cost ratio will maximize benefit.

In the literature, there are two quantitative approaches to finding the optimal bal-ance between benefit and cost. The first approach is to find optimal design parame-ters that minimize patient exposure (a surrogate to trial cost) at fixed type I/II error rates, e.g., under null as in Simon (1989) or under any prior distribution for treat-ment effect as in Anderson (2006). This approach (hereafter referred to as sample size minimization approach) is appealing to statisticians because it is parsimonious and avoids assumptions that could be controversial such as the overall benefit of the study drug. As a result, numerous publications have been generated in the statistical literature. However, this approach has limitations when the choice of type I/II error rates itself is an issue and when the benefit of the study drug has to be taken into account. The second approach is a decision-theoretic approach that applies Bayesian decision analysis techniques to find the optimal design parameters by directly maximizing the net return (i.e., benefit–cost). It is used for determination of optimal sample size for Phase III trials subject to budget constraints (Patel and Ankolekar 2007) as well as for determination of Phase II sample sizes (Stallard 1998 and Stallard 2003). Relevant work can also be found in Stallard et al. (2005) and O'Hagen et al. (2005). This approach is appropriate when benefit can be quantified upfront and the parameter space for decision-making is very well defined. When benefit is overestimated, which occurs often in practice, such analyses tend to recommend a low bar for a Go decision, making it hardly acceptable to stakeholders (Leung and Wang 2001).

We proposed a new simple-to-apply decision-theoretic approach with unique advantages (Chen and Beckman 2009a, b; Chen and Beckman 2014). The idea is to find optimal cost-effective parameters by maximizing a benefit–cost ratio function (a direct measure of expected benefit per expected resource unit expended). The numerator of the function is the probability-of-success (POS) and Type II error adjusted benefit, as given by the expected number of truly active drugs correctly identified for Phase III development (in the proof of concept application) or the expected power for successful completion of Phase III (Phase III interim analysis application), each multiplied by the benefit per drug if applicable, and the denominator is the expected total late-stage development cost, including that resulting from both Type I and Type II errors. From a high-level perspective, the sample size minimization approach is equivalent to the use of our denominator as a utility function while assuming a constant numerator. The decision-theoretic approach is equivalent to the use of the difference between our numerator and denominator as a utility function. One major difference among the three approaches resides on the way the intrinsic benefit of a study drug, denoted by B in Sects. 5.1–5.3 in this chapter, is handled. Our approach acknowledges the fact that variations in benefit, POS, and Type II error may be important, and therefore incorporates them into the utility function in contrast to the sample size minimization approach which simply attempts to minimize cost. However, in contrast to the decision-theoretic approach, our approach is less sensitive to small errors in estimation of benefit (and cost). When only one trial is considered, the optimal design is independent of the benefit; when more than one trial are considered, the optimal designs depend only on the relative benefit which is considerably easier to assess than the absolute benefits that the decision-theoretic approach relies on.

Our proposed approach is similar to the decision theoretic approach in its handling of POS (denoted by p in Sects. 5.1–5.3 in this chapter), the probability of the study drug being truly active in the study population. The probability of no treatment effect is then 1-POS (as can be seen in Sect. 5.2.3 in this chapter our proposed approach can accommodate a general distribution for treatment effect). For our illustrative purposes, the POS for an oncology study drug is assumed to be 0.1–0.3 before POC or is 0.3–0.7 after passing POC. The estimate seems reasonable or possibly generous from historical data. Prior information on POS as such, be it subjective or objective, is frequently cited by relevant decision makers in a drug development program. However, the information is rarely fully accounted for in the actual (mostly qualitative) decision-making process. It is not the focus of this chapter to estimate prior POS, or update posterior POS after data from the POC trial or the interim analysis becomes available. Our focus is how to properly use the same information for making quantitative decisions at the design stage, rather than as a data analysis tool. We assume data from the trial will be analyzed using a Frequentist approach.

To demonstrate the power and the flexibility of our proposed approach, we will address the two decision issues with several examples in the next two sections. We will further illustrate with a real example that shows how to apply the method to a complicated Phase II/III seamless design (Sun and Chen 2012). There are many ways to extend our proposed approach in both method and application. We briefly touch upon some of them without supplying full details.

5.2   Optimal Designs for POC Trials

Consider a typical POC trial with two arms (study drug or placebo, or more typically in oncology, standard of care plus study drug or standard of care plus placebo). Denote by Δ (>0) the standardized effect size (treatment effect divided by standard deviation) of clinical interest with respect to an endpoint, which is typically a surrogate marker to overall survival in oncology. Denote by (α, β) the doublet of one-sided Type I error rate and Type II error rate of the trial. The total sample size for the trial is approximately

$$N = 4\left(Z_{1-\alpha} + Z_{1-\beta}\right)^2 / \Delta^2 \qquad (5.1)$$

where $Z_{(\cdot)}$ denotes the respective quantile of the standard normal distribution. When a time-to-event variable is the primary endpoint of interest, Δ refers to logarithm of hazard ratio (placebo vs. study drug) and N refers to number of events. While totality of data will be looked at closely, a Go decision to continue the program for later development in a Phase III confirmatory trial is generally made if the one-sided p-value from the POC trial is less than α favoring the study drug. Notice that the standard error for estimate of the treatment difference is $2 / \sqrt{N}$ which is equal to $\Delta/(Z_{1-\alpha}+Z_{1-\beta})$ from the sample size formula, the cutoff point for the minimum empirical treatment difference (empirical bar) relative to Δ in a Go decision (i.e., corresponding to one-sided p-value $< \alpha$) is $Z_{1-\alpha}/(Z_{1-\alpha}+Z_{1-\beta})$. Clearly, the empirical bar increases when Type I error rate decreases or when Type II error rate increases. It is >0.5 when $\alpha < \beta$ and >1 when $\beta > 50\,\%$.

In the oncology therapeutic area, a single confirmatory trial accompanied with a supportive POC trial usually meet the minimum requirements for regulatory registration purposes. Denote by C_2 the cost for a POC trial and by C_3 the cost for the future Phase III confirmation trial in the same population. In the first line lung cancer setting, a typical POC trial with $(\alpha, \beta) = (0.1, 0.2)$ for the detection of a 40 % hazard reduction in terms of progression-free-survival may need 100–150 patients with a minimum follow-up of 4–6 months. A confirmatory trial in the same setting with $(\alpha, \beta) = (0.025, 0.1)$ for the detection of a 25 % hazard reduction in terms of overall survival may need 600–800 patients with a minimum follow-up of 8–10 months. When cost is proportional to sample size, the relative cost of a POC trial to a confirmatory trial (i.e., C_2/C_3) is around 20 % in this setting. The Phase II to Phase III cost-ratio may be different in different settings. For simplicity, we consider C_3 to be fixed, i.e., design of the Phase III trial is independent of strength of signal from the POC trial. We leave the extension on non-fixed C_3 to Chap. 5, Sect. 5.2.3.

5.2.1   Design of a Single POC Trial

Let us start with a simple question. Given a fixed budget for conducting a typical POC trial with $(\alpha, \beta) = (0.1, 0.2)$ as described above, what is the optimal (α, β) to be most cost-effective? There are infinitely many ways to choose (α, β) as long as the choice satisfies the sample size constraint below.

$$Z_{1-\alpha} + Z_{1-\beta} = Z_{1-0.1} + Z_{1-0.2} \tag{5.2}$$

Each choice corresponds to a different Go–No Go criterion to confirmatory trial. A self-evident choice is $(0.2, 0.1)$ by the equivalence of (β, α) to (α, β) in Eq. (5.1). However, a Type I error rate of 20 % or indeed any number for this matter could easily be challenged. Many clinical researchers (Rubinstein et al. 2005; Simon et al. 2001; Estey and Thall 2003; Korn et al. 2001) have provided qualitative guidance for how to properly size POC trials and make Go–No Go decisions. Here we provide quantitative guidance. To answer the above question, let us assume that the true standardized effect size θ has a binary distribution in that the probability is p for $\theta = \Delta$ and $1-p$ for $\theta = 0$, and consider the following benefit–cost ratio function that involves design parameters $(p, \alpha, \beta, B, C_2, C_3)$:

$$R_1 = \frac{Bp(1-\beta)}{C_2 + C_3\left[p(1-\beta) + (1-p)\alpha\right]} \tag{5.3}$$

The numerator represents the benefit adjusted with probability-of-success (POS) and Type II error (the benefit of a truly inactive drug is assumed to be zero). It represents the expected number of active drugs correctly identified by the POC study, multiplied by the benefit per drug, and thus is a simple surrogate for overall benefit. The denominator represents the summation of the cost for the POC trial and the expected cost for the Phase III trial multiplied by the probability of a positive outcome, true or false, from the POC trial. Thus the denominator represents the total

Table 5.1 Optimal designs of a POC trial with fixed sample size under $(\alpha, \beta) = (0.1, 0.2)$

POS (p)	C_2/C_3	Optimal α (%)	Optimal β (%)	Empirical bar relative to Δ
0.1	0.2	6.7	26.7	0.71
0.1	0.3	8.8	22.0	0.64
0.1	0.4	10.7	18.9	0.59
0.2	0.2	7.2	25.3	0.69
0.2	0.3	9.6	20.7	0.62
0.2	0.4	11.5	17.8	0.56
0.3	0.2	8.0	23.7	0.66
0.3	0.3	10.4	19.3	0.59
0.3	0.4	12.6	16.4	0.54

expected cost of the overall late development program, where the Phase III trial happens if and only if the POC trial gives a true positive or a false positive outcome. Hence, the ratio-function defined in Eq. (5.3) directly measures the cost-effectiveness of the design. Maximization of R_1 is equivalent to maximizing of the return in benefit in the face of limited resources, rendering the design strategy the most cost-effective one from a portfolio management standpoint. When B is unknown (likely the case for most of the oncology drugs because it is driven by the drug activity that is hard to predict based on preclinical and early clinical data), it does not have any impact on optimization, making our proposed approach more robust to uncertainties in benefit assessment, in contrast to the decision-theoretic approach. In our illustration, we assume that C_2/C_3 is known so that the optimal choice of (α, β) can be easily obtained by maximizing R_1 subject to the sample size constraint (5.2) for fixed (p, C_2/C_3). In practice, actual values of (B, C_2, C_3) are relevant if the R_1 value is used for choosing which trials to conduct among many opportunities. Apparently, a minimum requirement for a trial to be included in a portfolio of trials is $R_1 > 1$ when B, C2, and C3 are determined reasonably accurately and expressed in comparable units.

Table 5.1 provides optimal design parameters for a typical POC with fixed sample size under $(\alpha, \beta) = (0.1, 0.2)$ for different POS levels and C_2/C_3 values. As expected, the empirical bar associated with optimal (α, β) decreases with increasing POS and C_2/C_3. In the first line lung cancer setting where C_2/C_3 is around 0.2, the optimal empirical bars are in the range of 0.66Δ to 0.71Δ, the optimal α levels are in the range of 6.7–8.0 % (one-sided) and the optimal β levels are in the range of 23.7–26.7 %. As a comparison, the starting point of $(\alpha, \beta) = (0.1, 0.2)$ would be approximately optimal at $C_2/C_3 = 0.3$ when POS is 30 %, and the associated optimal empirical bar for a Go decision would be lower at 0.60Δ.

5.2.2 Design of Multiple POC Trials

Let us consider a more complicated problem. Suppose that there is a fixed budget for conducting a certain number of POC trials with $(\alpha, \beta) = (0.1, 0.2)$. But there are more trials with different POS and benefit that are of similar interest. What is the optimal resource allocation strategy and optimal design parameters? These POC trials may be for the same drug or for different drugs. Let $(p_i, \alpha_i, \beta_i, B_i, C_{2i}, C_{3i})$ be the design parameters associated with the i-th trial $(i = 1,\ldots,k)$. Consider the following general version of the benefit–cost ratio function to Eq. (5.3)

$$R_2 = \frac{\sum_{i=1}^{k} B_i p_i (1-\beta_i)}{\sum_{i=1}^{k} \left\{ C_{2i} + C_{3i} \left[p_i (1-\beta_i) + (1-p_i)\alpha_i \right] \right\}} \tag{5.4}$$

From the expression of R_2, it is clear that only relative benefit is needed for optimization. When the actual values of $(p_i, B_i, C_{2i}, C_{3i})$ for all indications are available, the optimal (α_i, β_i) are obtained by maximizing in R_2 in Eq. (5.4). Let us illustrate under the simplified assumption that cost structure and treatment effect for detection are the same for the k POC trials. We further assume that the costs for the corresponding Phase III trials are also the same and fixed, i.e., $C_{3i} = C_3$ $(i = 1,\ldots,k)$. After the simplification, the optimal Type I/II error rates (α_i, β_i) and resource allocation ratio (C_{2i}/C_2) only depend on relative benefit B_i, probabilities of success p_i, and the ratio of total POC trial resources to cost of a single Phase III trial, C_2/C_3. They are solved by maximizing Eq. (5.4) subject to the following constraints $(i = 1,\ldots,k)$

$$Z_{1-\alpha_i} + Z_{1-\beta_i} = \sqrt{C_{2i}/C_2}\left(Z_{1-0.1} + Z_{1-0.2}\right) \tag{5.5}$$

$$\sum_{i=1}^{k} C_{2i} = C_2 \tag{5.6}$$

Once optimal Type I/II error rates are obtained, optimal empirical bars follow immediately.

In the first example, we assume that there is a budget for one typical POC trial under $(\alpha, \beta) = (0.1, 0.2)$ but there are two POC trials with $p_1 = 0.3$ and $p_2 = 0.2$ as well as $B_1 = B_2$ of interest. Figure 5.1 presents the optimal resource allocation ratio and empirical bar for the two POC trials as a function of C_2/C_3. Just as in the single-trial case, the empirical bar associated with optimal (α, β) decreases with increasing POS and C_2/C_3. The figure shows that if the budget for the POC trials is around 20 % that of a confirmatory trial as in the first line lung cancer setting both POC trials should be conducted with approximately 60 % of the resource allocated to the one with 30 % POS and the remaining 40 % of the resource to the one with 20 % POS. The corresponding (α, β) is (10 %, 32 %) for the trial with 30 % POS and is (5 %, 68 %) for the one with 20 % POS. This analysis suggests more and smaller trials with higher empirical bars to be more cost-effective in this setting. The cutoff point in terms of C_2/C_3 value for deciding whether to conduct one or two trials is at about 17 % (the cutoff point would be considerably lower if the two trials had the same POS level—results are not shown here). If the budget is lower than that, it is more cost-effective to just conduct the trial with higher POS. The results are sensible and consistent with intuition. However, intuition alone will not be able to pinpoint the optimal decision points.

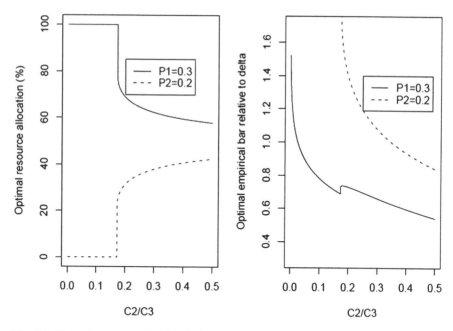

Fig. 5.1 Optimal resource allocation (*left panel*) and empirical bars for a Go decision (*right panel*) for two POC trials of different POS when there is budget for a typical POC trial under $(\alpha, \beta) = (0.1, 0.2)$. C_2 represents the cost for a POC trial and C_3 represents the cost for a Phase III trial

In the second example, we assume that there is a budget for two typical POC trials under $(\alpha, \beta) = (0.1, 0.2)$ but there are four trials with $p_1 = 0.4$, $p_2 = p_3 = 0.3$ and $p_4 = 0.2$ as well as $B_1 = B_2 = B_3 = 1$ and $B_4 = 2$ of interest. This represents a more complex situation than the first example. Figure 5.2 presents optimal resource allocation ratio and empirical bar for the four POC trials as a function of C_2/C_3. It shows that when the budget for two POC trials is over 40 % that of a single confirmatory trial as for the first line lung cancer setting, all four POC trials should be conducted. The trial with lowest POS (20 %) but highest benefit takes the largest share of resource at approximately 33 %. The trial with highest POS (40 %) is second at approximately 29 %. The remaining two trials with 30 % POS enjoy approximately 19 % each. In terms of empirical bar for a Go decision, it is highest for the two trials with 30 % POS followed by the trial with 20 % POS and the one with 40 % POS. Optimal number of trials and corresponding Go–No Go criteria depending on the C_2/C_3 value. When it is above approximately 18 %, all 4 trials should be conducted; when it is between approximately 12 and 18 %, the two trials with 40 % POS and 20 % should be conducted; otherwise, only the trial with 20 % POS (but highest benefit) should be conducted.

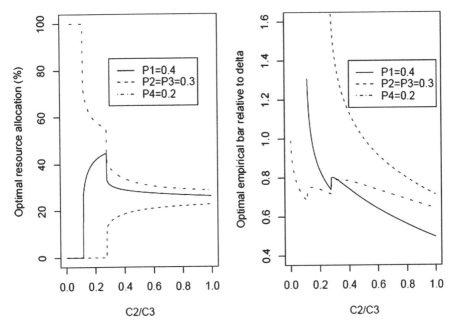

Fig. 5.2 Optimal resource allocation (*left panel*) and empirical bars for a Go decision (*right panel*) for four POC trials of different POS and benefit when there is budget for two typical POC trials under $(\alpha, \beta) = (0.1, 0.2)$. The benefit for the trial with lowest POS ($p_4 = 0.2$) is twice as high as for any of the three other trials. C_2 represents the cost for two POC trials and C_3 represents the cost for a single Phase III trial

5.2.3 Extensions

The proposed design strategy for POC trials can be easily extended to account for more complicated settings that may arise in oncology and other therapeutic areas. We show a few of them by considering the single-trial case as in Chap. 5, Sect. 5.2.1. Extensions to the multiple-trial case as in Chap. 5, Sect. 5.2.2 follow immediately.

General distribution for treatment effect: Instead of assuming that the true standardized effect size (θ) has a binary distribution, we may assume that it has a general distribution function, say $f(\theta)$, which might be estimated from previous trials on same drug or drugs with same mechanism of action. We may also assume the corresponding benefit to be $B(\theta)$. Observe that $B(\Delta) = B$ and $B(0) = 0$ for R_1 in Eq. (5.3). In this setup, a generalized version of R_1 is

$$R'_1 = \frac{\int B(\theta) f(\theta) \gamma(\theta) d\theta}{C_2 + C_3 \int f(\theta) \gamma(\theta) d\theta} \qquad (5.7)$$

where $\gamma(\theta)$ is the probability to Go when the treatment effect of the study drug is θ. Under the same assumption that the POC trial is sized at $(\alpha, \beta)=(0.1, 0.2)$ for an effect size Δ, $\gamma(\theta)$ satisfies

$$\left(Z_{1-\alpha} + Z_{\gamma(\theta)}\right)/\theta = \left(Z_{1-0.1} + Z_{1-0.2}\right)/\Delta \tag{5.8}$$

from the sample size formula in Eq. (5.1). Notice that $\gamma(\Delta)=1-\beta$ under the binary distribution. For ease of computation in practice, in absence of an objective continuous estimate for $f(\theta)$ we may assume a multinomial distribution which takes values at a set of discrete points, e.g., 0, 0.4Δ, 0.6Δ, 0.8Δ and 1.2Δ.

Adaptive design: Another extension is to adaptively size the Phase III trial based on the outcome from the POC trial. For example, the Go–No Go decision may be revised so that a Phase III trial at cost of C_3 will be conducted if the *p*-value from the POC trial is less than α but greater than α' ($\alpha'<\alpha$). But a smaller trial at cost of C_3' will be conducted if the *p*-value is less than α' (study drug is more active than initially expected). If the assumed benefit is B for *p*-value between α' and α, and B' for *p*-value less than α', the corresponding benefit–cost ratio function would be

$$R''_1 = \frac{\left[B'\left(1-\beta'\right)+B\left(\beta'-\beta\right)\right]p}{C_2 + C_3\left[p\left(\beta'-\beta\right)+\left(1-p\right)\left(\alpha-\alpha'\right)\right]+C'_3\left[p\left(1-\beta'\right)+\left(1-p\right)\alpha'\right]} \tag{5.9}$$

Notice that both (α, β) and (α', β') satisfy the sample size formula. One may find the optimal α and α' (i.e., Go–No Go criteria) for fixed C_3 and C_3'.

Multiple arms or endpoints: Some POC trials may have multiple arms for dose selection purpose or may have more than one endpoint (Sun et al. 2009). As long as the decision rule is quantifiable, our proposed approach can be applied with minimal modifications. Take a dose-selection POC study with two active arms and a placebo arm (1:1:1 randomization) for example. Let Z_1 and Z_2 be the two statistics for testing the treatment effect against placebo of the two dose levels with positive values corresponding to favorable outcomes for the study drug. Observe that Z_1 are Z_2 are normal variables with correlation 0.5. The decision rule is to carry the dose level with maximum Z-statistics (play the winner) to Phase III if it satisfies that $\Pr(\max\{Z_1, Z_2\}>0)<\alpha^*$. Let β^* be the Type II error rate corresponding to the maximum Z-statistics under a given alternative hypothesis. It has a more complex relationship with α^* under the sample size constraint. The optimization problem is more difficult than in Eq. (5.2) but certainly tractable.

Flexible budget: In the previous sections, a 2-arm trial under $(\alpha, \beta)=(0.1, 0.2)$ is used as reference for standard cost of a POC trial. Standardization of cost structure as such is a common practice in portfolio management. But the reference trial may use a different set of (α, β) in practice. Optimal designs will change accordingly. The changes will be more drastic when the budget for a POC trial is not fixed upfront and needs to be optimized. Chap. 4, Sect. 5.2.2 discussed the related example of allocating POC resources among competing programs. Details and associated program codes have been previously published (Chen and Beckman 2009a).

5.3 Optimal Futility Analysis Strategies

After a drug has passed POC evaluation, a natural follow-up is to conduct a Phase III confirmatory trial in the same population. Phase III oncology trials usually implement a group sequential design with a survival endpoint (Jennison and Turnbull 2000). To mitigate failure rate, a confirmatory trial has at least one futility interim analysis. The study prior to the interim analysis is sometimes called a Phase II part and the one afterwards a Phase III part, making the trial a Phase II/III combination trial. The Phase II part may involve dose selection, population selection and other conventional Phase II characteristics. In our discussion below, we consider a straight Phase III confirmatory trial without such Phase II features, which will be discussed in Chap. 4, Sect. 5.5. The example trial has one interim analysis and the endpoint for deciding whether to continue or not after the interim analysis is the same as the primary endpoint for the overall trial. The trial is designed for detecting a survival benefit of interest (e.g., 25 % hazard reduction in the first line lung cancer setting) at Type I error rate of 2.5 % (one-sided) and Type II error rate of 10 % (90 % power) prior to futility adjustment. The futility boundary is assumed to only impact the Type II error rate but not the Type I error rate (non-binding), a common assumption in the drug registration environment. As before, it is assumed that the Phase III trial costs C_3 if it runs to completion.

5.3.1 Futility Analysis of a Single Trial

Suppose that after cost C_{IA} is spent at the interim look, t fraction of survival information (proportion of events observed at interim analysis) is available for analysis. A Go decision will be made if the one-sided p-value from the analysis is less than α favoring the study drug and a No Go decision will be made otherwise (α is referred to be the futility boundary in p-value scale). Denote by β the Type II error rate spent at the interim analysis. How to appropriately choose (α, β) to make the Go–No Go decision the most cost-effective? Consider the following benefit–cost ratio function

$$R_3 = \frac{Bp(1-\beta^*)}{C_{IA} + (C_3 - C_{IA})\left[p(1-\beta) + (1-p)\alpha\right]} \tag{5.10}$$

where β^* is the overall Type II error rate, i.e., $1-\beta^*$ is the actual overall power after taking the futility analysis into account. This ratio function has similar if not identical interpretation as Eq. (5.3). Just as in the previous sections, the benefit term B is fixed and does not have an impact on the optimal choice of (α, β). Observe that the test statistics at information fraction t (denoted by X_t) and at final analysis (denoted by X) have correlation $\sqrt{t}$. The unconditional probability for X_t to cross

Table 5.2 Optimal futility boundaries at interim analysis after 50 % of budget is spent

POS (p)	Information fraction	Futility boundary in p-value (%)	Empirical futility bar relative to Δ	Beta-spent (%)	Overall power (%)
0.3	0.15	45.0	0.10	13.0	80.2
0.3	0.20	36.8	0.23	13.3	80.3
0.3	0.25	30.9	0.31	13.1	80.8
0.5	0.15	51.6	−0.03	9.8	82.8
0.5	0.20	42.5	0.13	10.4	82.6
0.5	0.25	35.5	0.23	10.6	82.8
0.7	0.15	61.6	−0.23	6.1	85.7
0.7	0.20	51.3	−0.02	6.9	85.3
0.7	0.25	43.2	0.11	7.4	85.2

the interim futility bar is $1-\beta$ and for X to demonstrate statistical significance at the final analysis is 90 %. The overall Type II error rate β^* for the trial satisfies the following relationship

$$\Pr\left(X_t > Z_\beta, X > Z_{0.1}\right) = 1 - \beta^* \tag{5.11}$$

From the sample (event) size formula, (α, β) satisfies

$$Z_{1-\alpha} + Z_{1-\beta} = \sqrt{t}\left(Z_{1-0.025} + Z_{1-0.1}\right) \tag{5.12}$$

Maximization of R_3 in Eq. (5.10) with respect to (α, β) subject to the constraints (5.11) and (5.12) yields the optimal design parameters for the futility analysis. As before, the empirical futility bar relative to Δ in a Go decision is $Z_{1-\alpha}/(Z_{1-\alpha}+Z_{1-\beta})$. The conditional power for a positive trial after successfully passing the futility analysis is

$$\Pr\left(X > Z_{0.1} \mid X_t > Z_\beta\right) = \left(1-\beta^*\right)/\left(1-\beta\right) \tag{5.13}$$

The first example illustrates how optimal futility boundaries change with information fraction and POS after 50 % of the budget is spent, i.e., $C_{IA} = 0.5C_3$ (Table 5.2). The empirical futility bar decreases with increasing POS level, rightfully reflecting the impact of prior information as expected. It increases with increasing information fraction, suggesting that a more definite decision can be made when more information becomes available. For trials of low POS, a mild to moderate positive trend in effect size should be observed before moving forward. But for trials with high POS level, even a slight negative trend could trigger the same decision. The optimal overall power ranges from 80–81 % at p=0.3 to 82–83 % at p=0.5 to 85–86 % at p=0.7 after accounting for the futility analysis. As a comparison, although the aforementioned sample size minimization approach may be able to find the optimal futility boundaries under a prespecified level of Type II error rate (or overall power), it cannot be used to decide which level to start with. This is something our proposed approach can naturally address. However, the sample size minimization approach is appropriate if it is the intention of the trial to maintain the overall Type II error rate at a prespecified level. Notice that, although the optimal overall power decreased by 4–10 % it can be easily seen from Eq. (5.13) that the conditional power for a positive trial after the futility analysis is generally higher than 90 %.

5.3.2 Futility Analyses for Multiple Trials

In a portfolio management of multiple confirmatory trials with different benefit and POS, how should one appropriately prespecify their futility boundaries? To answer this question, consider the following general version of the benefit–cost ratio function analogous to Eq. (5.10)

$$R_4 = \frac{\sum_{i=1}^{k} B_i p_i \left(1 - \beta_i^*\right)}{\sum_{i=1}^{k} \left\{ C_{IAi} + \left(C_{3i} - C_{IAi}\right)\left[p_i\left(1 - \beta_i\right) + \left(1 - p_i\right)\alpha_i\right]\right\}} \tag{5.14}$$

where subscript i is used to indicate the design parameters for the i-th trial. Maximization of R_4 with respect to (α_i, β_i) subject to same constraint as in Eq. (5.11) and (5.12) yields the optimal solution. The timing for each trial at the futility analysis can be totally different from each other.

Consider two Phase III trials with same total cost (i.e., $C_{31} = C_{32}$) but different benefit and POS. The first trial has lower POS but has a benefit twice as high as the second one. An interim futility analysis occurs after 50 % of the budget is spent, just as in the first example of Chap. 4, Sect. 5.3.1. Table 5.3 shows the optimal futility

Table 5.3 Optimal futility boundaries at interim analyses for two POC trials after 50 % of budget is spent for each when the benefit ratio is 2:1 between the two (p_1 vs. p_2)

		Trial with POS=p_1		Trial with POS=p_2	
POS (p_1/p_2)	Information fraction	Futility boundary in p-value (%)	Empirical futility bar relative to Δ	Futility boundary in p-value (%)	Futility boundary in empirical bar relative to Δ
0.3/0.5	0.15	50.8	−0.02	49.3	0.01
0.3/0.5	0.20	42.0	0.14	40.4	0.17
0.3/0.5	0.25	35.3	0.23	33.8	0.26
0.3/0.7	0.15	45.8	0.08	65.2	−0.31
0.3/0.7	0.20	37.9	0.21	55.3	−0.07
0.3/0.7	0.25	32.0	0.29	45.6	0.07
0.5/0.7	0.15	60.4	−0.21	55.4	−0.09
0.5/0.7	0.20	50.4	−0.01	45.7	0.09
0.5/0.7	0.25	42.7	0.11	37.3	0.20

boundaries for each trial at common information fraction under different POS assumptions. Just as in Table 5.2, the empirical futility bar generally increases with increasing information fraction but decreases with increasing POS level. The bars are comparable between the two trials when the POS is 30 % for the first one and 50 % for the second one. The bars become higher for the first one and lower for the second one when POS for the second trial is changed to 70 %, i.e., the benefit–POS balance favors the second one. The balance shifts back to the first one when its POS is changed to 50 %. This example provides important insight into the dynamic impact of POS and benefit on the cost-effectiveness of a Go–No Go decision in futility analysis.

5.3.3   Extensions

We have used the time-to-event survival endpoint (typical endpoint in oncology) for illustration, but the approach can be easily extended to any type of endpoint (e.g., continuous or binary endpoint in other therapeutic areas). We used 10 % for Type II error rate for illustration purpose. The approach can be easily revised to account for a different Type II error rate. The same extension as for POC trials can be made by assuming a general distribution function for true treatment effect as well as one for benefit. Observe that information on the survival endpoint is often collected in the POC trial preceding the Phase III trial. It provides an objective estimate of the distribution function for the true treatment. A similar adaptive design can be implemented by adopting a multitier decision rule (i.e., sample size and cost for the remaining trial is dependent upon the interim outcome). Further extensions specific to a Phase III trial may include the following.

Optimal timing of futility analysis: Optimal timing for futility analysis is a less explored topic in literature. Gould (2005) discusses this topic in the context of POC trials. Our proposed approach allows evaluation of timing. By comparing optimal R_3 or R_4 values at different time points of practical relevance, optimal timing for interim analysis can be determined. However, caution must be exercised in such analysis because timing is driven by other practical considerations as well. Moreover, if the curve of the efficiency function is broad and flat near the optimum, any choice within the range may be reasonable.

Multiple futility analyses: When there is a need (and it is feasible) to have more than one futility analyses, similar cost-effectiveness evaluation can be conducted for comparison of different futility boundaries. It becomes more complicated if an intermediate endpoint is used for an early futility analysis. However, it is tractable if the relationship between the intermediate endpoint and the clinical endpoint can be properly estimated.

5.4 Application to a Seamless Phase II/III Design

5.4.1 Study Design of the Motivating Example

The motivating example comes from the development of a drug candidate for platinum resistant ovarian cancer patients. By the time this test drug's MTD was defined, several competing drug candidates in the same class had completed single arm Phase II studies. To become commercially viable, a seamless Phase II/III design was considered to accelerate the program in that two doses will be studied in Phase II and only one will be carried to Phase III. The primary hypothesis of the pivotal trial is that:

- The test drug is non-inferior to the comparator (chemotherapy) in terms of overall survival (OS) at the 1.1 hazard ratio margin (and superior to the comparator in terms of safety profile).
- *OR* the test drug is superior to the comparator in terms of OS.

Hierarchy testing procedure will be used to control the type I error rate. That is, the non-inferiority will be tested first, and once passed, the superiority will be tested.

There are two types of seamless designs, inferentially seamless and operationally seamless. The inferentially seamless designs (Stallard and Todd 2003; Posch et al 2005) combine Phase II data and Phase III data with some multiplicity adjustment to control type I error rate in the final analysis. Although statistically valid, such designs are deemed to be less well understood adaptive designs by regulatory agencies. Operationally seamless designs only use Phase III data in the final analysis, but the enrollment is seamless between Phase II and Phase III. In addition to acceptance by regulatory agencies, several other factors led the development team to choose the operationally seamless Phase II/III design. One factor is the difficulty of using surrogate biomarker, in this case progression-free survival (PFS), to make GNG decision while the Phase III endpoint is OS. Another factor is about which decision body to make the dose selection based on Phase II data. If the inferentially seamless design is chosen, the dose selection has to be made by an external data monitoring committee (eDMC), because otherwise the Phase II data may be unblinded and cannot be utilized in the final analysis. Dose selection is usually a complicated decision. Even though the guidelines for dose selection can be prespecified in the study protocol, not all scenarios can be foreseen or simulated. Therefore, the development team preferred to make the dose selection by a joint effort of internal and external experts and chose an operationally seamless design over an inferentially seamless design.

The final design of the motivating example is shown schematically in Fig. 5.3 with GNG bars derived below. In the Phase II portion, patients will be randomized to three treatment groups with equal allocation: test drug at high dose, test drug at low dose, and control. The primary endpoint for Phase II is PFS. Phase II enrolls about 210 patients and completes after 135 PFS events have been observed to have sufficient power for each dose of the test drug to demonstrate superiority to the control in terms of PFS. The primary endpoint of Phase III is OS. Phase III enrolls

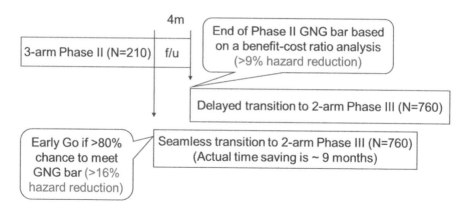

Fig. 5.3 Flowchart of the seamless Phase II/III study in platinum resistant ovarian cancer patients

about 720 patients and completes after 508 deaths have been observed to have sufficient power to demonstrate that the test drug is non-inferior to the control drug. This sample size also provides sufficient power (>95 %) to demonstrate that the test drug is superior to the control in terms of event rate for a safety endpoint.

In order to realize seamless transition, an interim analysis will be conducted in Phase II. The enrollment of Phase II will close when it is predicted that approximately 4 months after this time point there will be 135 PFS events. The interim analysis will take place approximately one month before the accrual completion. The purpose of this interim analysis is to determine whether Phase III enrollment can be initiated before final data of Phase II is available. If a Go decision is made, one arm of the test drug along with the control arm will be carried to Phase III. If a Go decision cannot be made at the interim analysis, Phase III will be on hold and a final decision will be made at end of Phase II. The Go criterion at this interim analysis is to have at least 80 % conditional power (as a team consensus) to make a Go decision at the final analysis of Phase II. Since it will take about one month to conduct the interim analysis and make a decision, the timing of this interim analysis is chosen so that Phase III accrual will potentially start seamlessly when Phase II accrual completes.

5.4.2 Incorporating Surrogate Biomarker Data in Go–No Go (GNG) Decision Making

The GNG decision for a drug candidate to move from Phase II to Phase III is a major decision in drug development. Ideally the decision should be made based on the data from the same endpoint which will be the primary endpoint of Phase III (i.e., OS in oncology or a composite cardiovascular event in cardiovascular disease). Since it usually takes long time to observe the clinical endpoint data, a common practice in drug development is to make GNG decision only based on the surrogate biomarker (i.e., PFS in oncology or blood pressure and glucose level in cardiovascular disease). However this approach often causes heated debate within the development team as what role the (limited) clinical endpoint data plays. In oncology, this often leads to a vague conditional requirement of "positive OS trend" before a Go decision can be made. In Chen and Sun (2011), it is proposed to combine the PFS data and OS data for decision making so that no information is wasted and a decision rule can be prespecified without ambiguity. Before we explain how to combine PFS and OS data, we first discuss how to use PFS data from Phase II to estimate OS treatment effect.

The relative effect size (γ) between a clinical endpoint and a surrogate endpoint in general holds the key in such estimation. Estimation of γ should be based on proper meta-analysis. In our motivating example, the ratio between OS and PFS (in log-hazard-ratio scale) is estimated to be 0.6 (Chen et al. 2013, Sun and Chen 2012). It implies that the treatment effect in OS is 60 % of the treatment effect in PFS, which represents a reasonable estimate based on published data of a variety of solid tumor in recent years. For example, if a drug has a treatment effect of hazard ratio (HR) = 0.8 in OS it is expected to have a treatment effect of HR = 0.69 in PFS. In other words, if the treatment effect in PFS is 31 % hazard reduction in Phase II, it implies that the treatment effect in OS is 20 % hazard reduction. Most GNG decisions between Phase II and Phase III in oncology drug development were made this way, even though often times the relative effect size were implicitly used and the decision makers may not even realize it. Is the translation from effect size in PFS to effect size in OS always a one-to-one translation? The answer is no. To adequately account for the uncertainty in effect size translation, we assume that the relative effect size (γ) has a normal distribution with mean of 0.6 and standard deviation of 0.2. This assumption covers a wide range of effect size ratio seen in the literature. With this variability, a 0.69 hazard ratio in PFS may translate into a range of hazard ratio in OS, and 95 % confidence interval of the estimated HR in OS fall between 0.69 and 0.93.

We then used a weighted method to combine the OS effect predicted from the observed PFS effect ($\gamma\Delta_{PFS}$) and the observed OS effect OS (Δ_{OS}), both in log-hazard-ratio scale, using the formula below (Chen and Sun (2011).

$$S = -\left(w\Delta_{OS} + (1-w)\gamma\Delta_{PFS}\right) \qquad (5.15)$$

With minus sign on the right-hand side, S is an approximate measure of hazard reduction, a parameter clinical researchers are more familiar with. Since the number of OS events in Phase II is relatively small compared to the number of PFS events, a weight of 0.15 (i.e., $w = 0.15$) is given to the observed OS effect in Phase II, and a weight of 0.85 is given to the predicted OS effect. This weight approximately minimizes the variance of S when the true treatment effect is in the parameter space of interest while the actual numbers of PFS and OS events are reasonably close to the target. The correlation between Δ_{PFS} and Δ_{OS}, and the variance of γ are all incorporated into the variance estimate of S. (See Chen and Sun 2011 and Sun and Chen 2012 for technical details of the characteristics of the test statistics.)

In the next section, we will discuss what value of S will constitute a GNG criterion between Phase II and Phase III using the same technique as developed in previous sections.

5.4.3   A Benefit–Cost Effective GNG Criterion

We denote the Go criterion from Phase II to Phase III to be $S > C$, where S is given in Eq. (5.15) and C is a critical value to be solved so that the return on investment can be maximized. $P(S > C)$ is the probability of Go from Phase II to Phase III.

We assume that the treatment effect has a discrete prior distribution, with π_1 probability of being superior the control with HR = 0.8, π_2 probability being equivalent to the control with HR = 1, and $(1 - \pi_1 - \pi_2)$ probability of being inferior to the control with HR = 1.1. We used $\pi_1 = \pi_2 = 1/3$ in our example, i.e., the test drug is assumed to have equal chance of being superior, equivalent, and inferior to the control drug. In this example, the Phase III is successful in two scenarios: (1) Superiority in efficacy is demonstrated; (2) Only non-inferiority is demonstrated. The regulatory approvability and benefits are different in these two scenarios. We incorporated this consideration into our benefit calculation. In our example, stakeholders and experts believe the relative approvability from health authority is 2:1 for scenario 1 vs. scenario 2, and the corresponding relative benefit is 5:1. Let V be the relative value of the two scenarios, then $V = 2 \times 5 = 10$.

With the above setup, let B be the predictive POS adjusted benefit of the program in the motivating example,

$$B = M_B \sum_{i=1}^{2} \pi_i p_i \left(V q_{S,i} + q_{NI,i} \right) \tag{5.16}$$

where

- M_B is an unknown constant. It is the overall benefit of the test drug when only non-inferiority in efficacy is demonstrated. Just like most of the oncology projects, it is extremely difficult to predict the benefit including commercial value. Fortunately, it does not have any impact on our analysis.
- π_i is the probability mass of the discrete prior distribution for the treatment effect (HR), $i = 1, 2, 3$. $\pi_1 + \pi_2 + \pi_3 = 1$. Because there is no value of the test drug when it is inferior to the control, we do not include $i = 3$ in the benefit calculation.
- p_i is the probability of Go from Phase II to Phase III under the ith value of HR in the discrete prior distribution. For example, p_1 is $P(S > C)$ under HR = 0.8.
- V is the relative value of demonstrating superiority in efficacy vs. demonstrating non-inferiority in efficacy and superiority in safety, and it is 10 in our case.
- $q_{S,i}$ is the probability of demonstrating superiority in Phase III under the ith value of HR in the discrete prior distribution.
- $q_{NI,i}$ is the probability of only demonstrating non-inferiority in Phase III under the ith value of HR in the discrete prior distribution.

- Let D be the cost of the development program for Phase II and Phase III portion.

$$D = M_C\left(R + \sum_{i=1}^{3}\pi_i p_i\right) \tag{5.17}$$

where

- M_C is a constant. It is the cost of the Phase III study, which just like M_B does not have any impact on our analysis.
- R is the relative cost of Phase II portion to Phase III portion. In the motivating example, the operation team's estimate of R is 0.4 including Phase III trial initiation and various other factors.

With the above setup, the optimal GNG bar C is obtained by maximizing the benefit–cost ratio B/D with respect to C whereas B and D are provided in Eqs. (5.16) and (5.17), respectively. The input variables that we need to give before solving for C are: the discrete prior distribution of treatment effect, the relative benefit of the superiority vs. non-inferiority Phase III results which is considerably easier to assess than the absolute benefits, and the relative cost of the Phase II portion vs. the Phase III portion. For the values of the input variables that we used in the motivating example, the optimal bar is $C=0.09$. Roughly speaking, this corresponds to a 9 % hazard reduction based on the joint estimate of the OS (S). The solid line in Fig. 5.4 illustrates how the benefit–cost ratio changes with C, which decreases when it moves farther away from the optimal value. This is typical in a

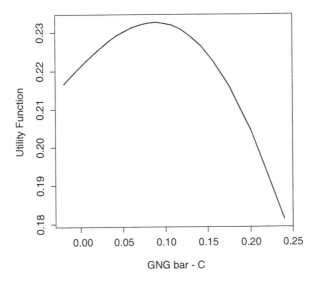

Fig. 5.4 Illustration of how the benefit–cost ratio (B/D) changes with the GNG Criterion (C) in the Phase II/III study in platinum resistant ovarian cancer patients

benefit–cost ratio analysis; the optimal design is unique and optimality is mathematically global.

When using the surrogate biomarker PFS data in decision making, we made an assumption about the relative effect size of PFS and OS. At the end of Phase II, to mitigate the risk of using a wrong assumption, we should check the relative effect size observed in Phase II. If the observed OS effect is smaller than the lower bound of the 95 % confidence interval (CI) for the predicted OS effect from PFS effect ($\gamma\Delta_{PFS}$), we would be concerned because it indicates that the observed OS effect is much smaller than the predicted effect from PFS data using the historical relationship of relative effect size. Therefore, our proposed GNG criteria at the end of Phase II are (1) the estimated OS effect (S) is greater than the optimal bar (~9 % hazard reduction based on benefit–cost ratio analysis); (2) the observed OS effect is greater than the lower bound of the 95 % CI for the predicted OS effect (to mitigate the risk of a wrong assumption on historical relationship of relative effect size). The dotted line in Fig. 5.5 shows the boundary for criterion (5.2). Overall, it is a Go decision if the observed PFS effect and OS effect from Phase II falls below both solid and dotted lines, and is a No Go decision otherwise.

Now we have the optimal GNG bar for the end of Phase II data, we can back-calculate the bar for the interim analysis (IA) in Phase II which gives 80 % conditional probability that the Go bar will be passed at the end of Phase II. The

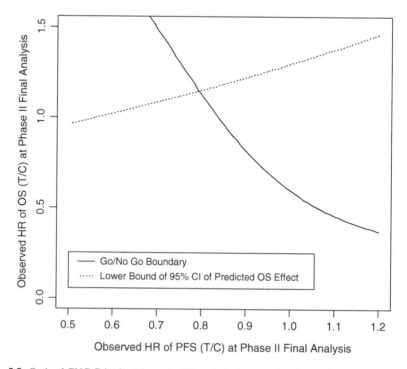

Fig. 5.5 Optimal GNG Criteria at the end of Phase II in the Phase II/III study in platinum resistant ovarian cancer patients. The lower bound of the 95 % CI of predicted OS effect is the upper bound of the 95 % CI in hazard ratio scale (test vs. control). The higher the HR the smaller the treatment effect

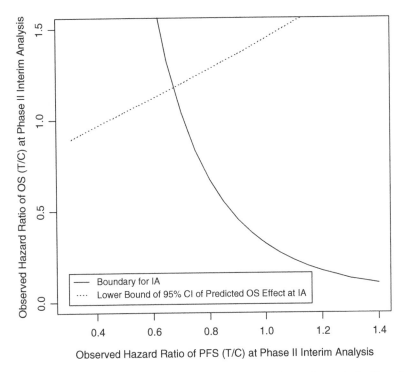

Fig. 5.6 Criteria at interim analysis of Phase II to trigger Phase III enrollment in the Phase II/III study in platinum resistant ovarian cancer patients. The lower bound of the 95 % CI of predicted OS effect is the upper bound of the 95 % CI in hazard ratio scale (test vs. control). The higher the HR the smaller the treatment effect

calculation shows that a seamless Phase III enrollment will be triggered if the following criteria are met for the interim analysis data.

(a) The estimated OS effect (S) is greater than 0.16 (~16 % hazard reduction).
(b) The observed OS effect at IA is greater than the lower bound of the 95 % CI for the predicted OS effect based on observed PFS effect at IA.

Figure 5.6 shows the boundaries for criterion (a) and (b). If the observed OS effect and PFS effect at IA fall below both solid and dotted lines, Phase III enrollment will be triggered while waiting for the Phase II data to become mature.

5.5 Conclusions

In this chapter, we have defined a benefit–cost ratio function for measuring efficiency of two Go–No Go decisions (Phase II POC to Phase III transition and futility analysis of a Phase III trial). Maximization of the benefit–cost ratio function leads to optimal cost-effective decisions. Both decision issues are complex in nature and each merits a separate treatment. They are bundled together in this chapter to demonstrate the broad applications of our proposed approach so that readers have a comprehensive appreciation. Some of the extensions mentioned in the chapter are being worked in greater depth and results will be presented in separate publications.

Our approach to the two decision issues is most appropriate when resources saved from a No Go decision after a POC trial or from early termination of a Phase III confirmation trial can be immediately redeployed to emerging projects of higher interest. Therefore, one major application of this approach is in, but certainly not limited to, portfolio management of a large and steady flow of drug candidates under fixed resource constraints. If the condition of an excess of development opportunities beyond available resources is not met, our designs may not be optimal. However, when there are not enough drug candidates lined up for development, our proposed approach helps set an upper limit on how high the cutoff point for a Go–No Go decision should be. Our approach is suitable when absolute benefit of drug candidates cannot be well assessed. Otherwise, the decision-theoretic approach may represent a viable alternative solution. As with any optimization problem, the curve for a utility function may be relatively flat at the optimum. When applying our method, practitioners need to make sure that the mathematically optimal solutions are also of practical relevance. Although we have used a prior POS estimate, we did not take a fully Bayesian approach to the decision issues. This is consistent with common practice in the drug development environment, and avoids complexity in presentation. Interested readers may consult Berry (2004) for possible Bayesian expansion.

The general method is simple to implement and easy to understand. It provides statisticians working in the late-stage development environment with a quantitative, objective approach to key clinical program design issues. The extensions discussed in previous sections may inspire expanded applications of this method.

In this chapter, we also used a motivating example in oncology to discuss and address a few challenging aspects in Phase II/III drug development: (1) How to use seamless design to accelerate development timeline? (2) How to explicitly incorporate surrogate biomarker data in decision making? (3) How to make objective GNG decision from Phase II to Phase III by maximizing the benefit–cost ratio? The example shows that the benefit of a seamless design can be fully realized in practice after proper risk mitigation.

Although our work is motivated by oncology drug development where cost-effectiveness of a Go–No Go decision is a major concern, the general method proposed in this chapter should be equally applicable to therapeutic areas with the same concern or to similar decision issues at any stage of drug development. These may include transition from earlier phases to Phase II, incorporation of a subpopulation (e.g., defined by a gene signature) hypothesis in a confirmatory trial, optimal alpha split between a full population and a subpopulation hypothesis in a confirmatory trial (Chen and Beckman 2009c), and many other possibilities.

References

Anderson KA (2006) Optimal spending functions for asymmetric group sequential designs. Biom J 48:1–9

Berry D (2004) Bayesian statistics and the efficiency and ethics of clinical trials. Stat Sci 19:175–187

Chen C, Beckman RA (2009a) Optimal cost-effective designs of proof of concept trials and associated Go-No Go decisions. J Biopharm Stat 19:424–436

Chen C, Beckman RA (2009b) Optimal cost-effective Go-No Go decisions in late-stage oncology drug development. Stat Biopharm Res 1:159–169

Chen C, Beckman RA (2009c) Hypothesis testing in a confirmatory phase III trial with a possible subset effect. Stat Biopharm Res 1:431–440

Chen C, Beckman RA (2014) Maximizing return on socioeconomic investment in phase II proof-of-concept trials. Clin Cancer Res 20:1730–1734

Chen C, Sun L (2011) On quantification of PFS effect for accelerated approval of oncology drugs. Stat Biopharm Res 3:434–444

Chen C, Sun L, Li C (2013) Evaluation of early efficacy endpoints for proof-of-concept trials. J Biopharm Stat 23:413–424

Estey EH, Thall PF (2003) New designs for phase 2 clinical trials. Blood 102:442–448

Gould L (2005) Timing for futility analyses for "proof of concept" trials. Stat Med 24:1815–1835

Jennison C, Turnbull BW (2000) Group sequential methods with applications to clinical trials. Chapman and Hall/CRC, London

Korn EL, Arbuck SG, Pluda JM et al (2001) Clinical trial designs for cytostatic agents: are new approaches needed? J Clin Oncol 19:265–272, 3154–3160 (correspondence)

Leung D, Wang Y (2001) A Bayesian decision approach for sample size determination in phase II trials. Biometrics 57:309–312

O'Hagen A, Stevens JW, Campbell MJ (2005) Assurance in clinical trial design. Pharm Stat 4:187–201

Patel NR, Ankolekar S (2007) A Bayesian approach for incorporating economic factors in sample size design for clinical trials of individual drugs and portfolios of drugs. Stat Med 26:4976–4988

Posch M, Koenig F, Branson M, Brannath W, Dunger-Baldauf C, Bauer P (2005) Testing and estimation in flexible group sequential designs with adaptive treatment selection. Stat Med 24:3697–3714

Rubinstein LV, Korn EL, Freidlin B et al (2005) Design Issues of randomized phase II trials and a proposal for phase II screening trials. J Clin Oncol 23:7199–7206

Simon R (1989) Optimal two-stage designs for phase II clinical trials. Control Clin Trials 10:1–10

Simon RM, Steinberg SM, Hamilton M et al (2001) Clinical trial designs for the early clinical development of therapeutic cancer vaccines. J Clin Oncol 19:1848–1854

Stallard N (1998) Sample size determination for phase II clinical trials based on Bayesian decision theory. Biometrics 54:279–294

Stallard N (2003) Decision-theoretic designs for phase II clinical trials allowing for competing studies. Biometrics 59:402–409

Stallard N, Todd S (2003) Sequential designs for phase III clinical trials incorporating treatment selection. Stat Med 22:689–703

Stallard N, Whiehead J, Cleall S (2005) Decision-making in a phase II clinical trial: a new approach combining Bayesian and frequentist concepts. Pharm Stat 4:119–128

Sun L, Chen C (2012) Advanced application of using progression-free survival to make optimal Go-No Go decision in oncology drug development. ASA Proceedings of the Joint Statistical Meetings 2012, Biopharmaceutical Section, Alexandria, VA: American Statistical Association

Sun Z, Chen C, Patel K (2009) Optimal two-stage randomized multinomial designs for phase II oncology trials. J Biopharm Stat 19(2):485–495

Chapter 6
Timing and Frequency of Interim Analyses in Confirmatory Trials

Keaven M. Anderson

Abstract In many pivotal clinical trials, timing and frequency of interim analyses are important for ethical treatment of patients and for practical and regulatory purposes. It is often desirable to evaluate a large trial of a new treatment that has some safety risk in order to stop or modify the trial based on the emerging risk–benefit profile compared to control treatment. Statistical considerations would suggest not stopping too soon in order to avoid large Type I or Type II error or basing a decision on inadequate data. Regulators often prefer to minimize interim analyses of efficacy due to presumed bias created by early stopping and an inability to adequately evaluate important secondary efficacy endpoints, safety, or the general risk–benefit profile for the new treatment. For practical purposes, analyses must be done soon enough to have a meaningful impact on the trial. For the same reason, limiting enrollment rates and ensuring prompt collection and analysis of data are important. We discuss tradeoffs between these factors in deciding when to perform interim analyses. In addition to formal evaluations for early positive efficacy findings, there are different considerations for trials early in the development process, for safety monitoring during a trial, and for futility analyses. We consider logistical and regulatory issues throughout.

Keywords Interim analysis • Timing • Frequency

K.M. Anderson (✉)
Merck Research Laboratories, UG1C-46, 351 North Sumneytown Pike,
North Wales, PA 19454-2505, USA
e-mail: Keaven_Anderson@merck.com

W. He et al. (eds.), *Practical Considerations for Adaptive Trial Design and Implementation*, Statistics for Biology and Health,
DOI 10.1007/978-1-4939-1100-4_6, © Springer Science+Business Media New York 2014

6.1   Introduction

There are a variety of unknown factors at the time of study design that can make it highly important to evaluate the risk–benefit of a new treatment during the course of a clinical trial. Patient safety is the most important of these factors, but safety monitoring is often done in a statistically informal way due to the lack of knowledge of what type of safety issues may arise or the frequency with which they may appear. More formal procedures are often set up for efficacy evaluation and many issues arise:

- Lack of knowledge of the treatment effect for efficacy of the new treatment under study.
- Lack of precise knowledge of the outcome distribution in the control group.
- Regulatory concerns of stopping a trial early for a positive efficacy finding or for doing multiple interim efficacy analyses.
- The ability to collect, enter, and analyze data in a timely fashion.
- Enrollment rates that allow interim analysis that is meaningful well before a trial is completed.
- Primary endpoints that are too far out in time to be evaluated at interim analyses.
- Use of surrogate endpoints for interim analyses.
- Ensuring that Type I error and Type II error associated with an interim analysis are adequately controlled. Other statistical properties such as the observed treatment effect required to stop a trial or a conditional power evaluation may also be considered.
- For more adaptive trials, selecting treatment arms to continue or adapting sample size can be challenging objectives.

We will discuss the above items largely through a series of examples. There is no pretense at completeness as there are many situations that have presented and will potentially present themselves. However, we hope the examples may provide a useful point of reference for many readers. Many of the examples are based on the practical experience of the author as opposed to, or in addition to, theoretical considerations. The organization of the chapter begins with a section on when strategies with frequent interim analyses might be used, followed by sections on interim analyses for futility and efficacy, and ending with a brief discussion.

6.2   Frequent Interim Analyses

In early development and in some cases in later development, frequent interim analyses may prove useful. Safety monitoring tends to be an ongoing process as a drug is first being studied. We will focus on more formal approaches where analyses are frequent. The FDA draft guidance on adaptive designs encourages more frequent adaptation and more innovative methods in early studies in development (Center for Drug Evaluation and Research and Center for Biologics Evaluation and Research 2010). Most typical are dose-finding trials with continuous or very frequent modeling. While these are addressed in other chapters, we mention a couple of specific approaches here.

For safety in oncology trials, the "3+3" design has a long history, but is often noted to have limitations in terms of accurately identifying a dose with a target toxicity level. Other approaches with frequent monitoring such as the continual reassessment method (CRM; O'Quigley et al. 1990) or variations such as the (modified) toxicity probability interval (Ji et al. 2010) can provide a more accurate method of dose-finding. These methods can formally adapt doses over longer sequences of patients, adapting to collect a suitable amount of data. The CRM method can sometimes be criticized as a 'black box' where the dose adaptations are not completely obvious. The mTPI is essentially a CRM method that has table that fully identifies the dose-adaptation rules, meaning that no computer program is required once the trial is enrolling. The speed of enrollment can be based on how close to an adaptation boundary the trial is at any point in time. That is, for lower-risk groups it may be possible to accelerate enrollment somewhat when not close to a toxicity bound.

For larger trials, including very large trials with rare, important safety events such as rotavirus vaccine trials evaluating intussusception (The REST Study Group 2006) or cardiovascular trials with intracranial hemmorhage risk, fully sequential methods can be useful. While group sequential methods are discussed elsewhere, fully sequential methods such as the sequential probability ratio test (SPRT, Wald 1945) or related methods (Siegmund 1985) are what we refer to here. For these examples, a formal evaluation of safety risk can be performed at the occurrence of each event. This has the advantage of stopping a trial as soon as a safety risk is reliably identified. For important risks identified prior to trial start, this formal approach can avoid an inappropriate early stop due to informal stopping decisions without evaluable operating characteristics.

Another early development area where adaptation is common is in Phase II, single arm efficacy evaluations of response rates. The Simon two-stage (Simon 1989) design provides a simple futility rule for an early stop in such trials. If this hurdle is passed, a fixed additional number of patients are evaluated. Without much change in operating characteristics, fully sequential monitoring can be performed with continuous monitoring to allow more flexibility in terms of when early decisions can be made between some minimum and maximum targeted number of observations using a truncated version of the SPRT (Wald 1945); this is implemented using the `binomialSPRT` routine in the gsDesign R package (Anderson 2014). Delaying the first analysis until some minimum sample size has been tested, consistent with the start of a Simon two-stage design, can reassure investigators that a trial will not be stopped too early. The continuous monitoring can reassure a sponsor that a formal futility stop or accelerated go to a next study can be adopted as soon as reasonably reliable conclusions can be made. Another alternative with more flexible timing based on Bayesian decision-making was developed by Lee and Liu (2008).

6.3   Futility Analyses

Futility analyses are interim analyses to consider stopping a trial early by examining signals for patient harm or lack of efficacy benefit. This can be considered the most effective way to save costs in a large portfolio of clinical trials typical in a large pharmaceutical company. The strategy may be less appealing to smaller companies with smaller product portfolios; it is also often unappealing to a 'product team' within a larger company which may have a large personal investment in a project. We will consider the topic of futility somewhat broadly in this discussion, including safety and risk–benefit considerations as well as efficacy. We will also briefly discuss the role of futility analyses in practical aspects of treatment selection.

Clearly, one of the most important aspects of early interim analyses is to monitor patient safety. In the previous section, we discussed the importance of ongoing safety monitoring. Another important type of safety interim analysis is to collect and analyze a uniform and systematic early review of safety to examine less obvious potential issues than those captured through ongoing safety monitoring. When there are potential safety issues, it is important to consider the risk–benefit tradeoff both for patients in the trial and for future patients who may receive benefit or harm from a new treatment. Some of these issues can only be addressed after a large trial is completed and will be discussed further in the following section. Others can be assessed for a tradeoff with potential positive efficacy findings during the course of a trial. The potential for more severe safety findings may drive an earlier interim analysis, while having more data for a careful tradeoff with efficacy benefit may suggest a delay in timing for any interim futility analysis. Often analyses of this nature are performed on a regular calendar basis, say every 3 or 6 months. Which of these analyses include efficacy analyses and to what extent is important for the control of Type I error will be discussed in the next section.

As noted by Bauer et al. (2010), a trial with an objective of treatment selection among multiple arms has a basic conflict between a desire to collect as much data as possible on a final treatment arm selected versus wanting as much data as possible to select between treatment arms. One issue this author has seen is an adaptive design where efficacy analysis of discontinued arms changes before a trial is completed since some patients on discontinued arms may not have had complete data at the time of an interim analysis. In the particular case of interest, in retrospect, a non-adaptive trial may have been preferable since the cost was not a major prohibition in Phase II, but having to reconsider multiple arms in Phase III was a major cost. That said, selecting between treatment groups at interim analyses is challenging in the absence of large differences in safety or efficacy, leading to a personal bias for this author to leave arms in a trial in absence of large differences. Another approach occasionally referred to by the FDA is to simply choose the highest dose that is safe at an interim analysis, along the lines of the Phase III (The PURSUIT Investigators 1998) trial of platelet inhibition in acute coronary syndromes. This allowed an analysis of a substantial number of patients to address a challenging dose selection question while not requiring completion of the entire the trial with two experimental arms.

The FDA draft guidance on adaptive design (Center for Drug Evaluation and Research and Center for Biologics Evaluation and Research 2010) provides only basic, general recommendations for futility analyses. While not directly commented on as a futility analysis, there are comments on monitoring enrollment and what criteria may be preventing timely enrollment of a trial. If this is done on a blinded basis, changes to enrollment criteria to speed timely completion may be considered. It is probably best to do this relatively early in the trial to ensure the majority of the trial is performed as uniformly as possible. Among the first considerations in performing an early futility analysis for efficacy is the tradeoffs between (1) setting a meaningful bound for clinical efficacy, (2) controlling the probability of stopping a trial for a drug that is truly useful (Type II error), and (3) performing any futility analysis at a time where stopping the trial or an arm in the trial can have a meaningful impact on the trial. We will discuss each of these topics separately, as well as the conflicts between these objectives.

We begin with the timing question as a futility analysis performed late in a trial may have a minimal impact on study costs relative to the impact it has on the simple interpretation of trial results achieved by running a trial to completion. The rates of enrollment versus collection of essential assessment data makes it impossible to perform interim futility analysis in many cases. If interim futility analyses are incorporated in such cases regardless of these considerations, it may mean that trial enrollment has to be halted prior to the futility being performed in order for the analysis to have an impact on the number of patients exposed to treatment. This can lead to many sites abandoning a trial in favor of other, actively enrolling trials— leading to the potential for substantial patient population differences before and after the interim analyses. If enrollment is not paused in these trials with fast enrollment relative to assessment, then the trial may be nearly completely enrolled prior to being able to actually perform the interim analysis. One consideration is to limit the number of sites enrolling patients until a futility analysis is performed; this can have a substantial impact on completing the trial. One could also consider performing a smaller trial initially to get a preliminary indication of efficacy, although a common reaction to this is that running two separate trials would substantially delay any possibility of bringing forward a new, potentially beneficial treatment to patients. The reader can see that tradeoffs are difficult under this type of scenario.

Next, we consider setting a clinically meaningful futility bound and control of Type II error. By "a clinically meaningful futility bound" we mean a bound that corresponds to requiring some positive indication of efficacy. With very little efficacy data, the estimate of treatment effect is highly variable and setting a clinically meaningful treatment bound results in substantial Type II error. Given the issues just noted with late interim futility analysis, finding the right tradeoff can be challenging. Generally, considering timing at 25–50% of data seems potentially useful. The earlier timing provides the potential of larger savings while requiring a "low clinical benefit bar" in order to avoid a steep power loss. The later timing requires particularly careful assessment of whether or not the interim analysis can be performed at a time when it has a meaningful impact on the trial. Another strategy that may be worth considering is lowering the desired power from a typical 90% (or more) to 85% or 80%, with the thought the most of the power loss will 'pay for' the ability to perform a meaningful early futility analysis. This also limits the increase in sample size that accompanies a strategy of a futility analysis with a stringent futility bar and high power.

All of the above reinforce the careful consideration of the tradeoffs between clinically meaningful futility bounds, meaningful timing for decisions and minimizing Type II error. One thing that makes this easier is if only substantial harm is considered sufficient justification for early futility stopping. If a futility analysis requiring some indication of clinical benefit cannot be performed, a futility analysis to react to harm in terms of the primary efficacy endpoint can still be highly important.

In order to try to get around some of the above tradeoffs, surrogate endpoints for the primary endpoint of interest are sometimes used for futility decisions. For many trials with longitudinal measures of an efficacy endpoint, it might be expected that efficacy at an early follow-up time point would be necessary for efficacy to exist at a later timepoint. For oncology trials, an early futility analysis based on progression free survival may be performed in a trial with an ultimate objective of showing a mortality benefit. While the impact of these strategies on power for the true endpoint of interest is difficult to assess, these are potentially important methods of realizing considerable savings in the conduct of a potentially large and expensive clinical trial.

Finally, we wish to mention that prior information on treatment effectiveness and risk–benefit has a substantial impact on consideration of a futility analysis. A drug that has a reasonably well-established safety and efficacy profile and is being studied in multiple related scenarios may not be an attractive candidate for futility analyses. As an example, an effective diabetes drug in Phase II may be studied in many Phase III indications and it may be desirable to get a complete assessment in each of the indications. In situations where a futility bar provides a first assessment of efficacy for any clinical indication for a compound, a futility bar may be considered more important, especially when the first indication studied is considered likely to provide the most promising population for the compound.

6.4 Efficacy Analyses

We begin this section with some regulatory considerations, followed by a discussion of study bounds and a discussion of calendar and information-based group sequential designs. We end with a brief discussion of blinded sample size re-estimation.

Early stopping for a positive efficacy finding can be a controversial topic. There may be pressures on a pharmaceutical company to bring a drug to market as soon as possible, making early establishment of efficacy attractive. These pressures can come not only from shareholders, but also from patient advocacy groups. However, the general regulatory and other societal perspectives require a careful assessment of the risk and benefit of a new drug before it is approved for human use (see, for example, ICH E9 or CFR312). As noted by Paul Canner in a review of interim monitoring of the coronary drug project (The Coronary Drug Project Research Group 1981), "...

decision making in clinical trials is complicated and often protracted...no single statistical decision rule or procedure can take the place of the well-reasoned consideration of all aspects of the data by a group of concerned, competent, and experienced persons with a wide range of scientific backgrounds and points of view." The FDA (CFR 312 part 21) notes that "Phase 3 studies...are intended to gather the additional information about effectiveness and safety that is needed to evaluate the overall benefit–risk relationship of the drug and to provide an adequate basis for physician labeling." These needs suggest that interim stopping criteria must go beyond any simple efficacy rule provided by, say, a carefully designed group sequential trial. My recent experience with FDA oncology regulators suggested no interim efficacy analyses until after 50 % of efficacy data have been collected. This runs counter to some previous experience where large treatment effects were observed early (e.g., EPILOG Investigators 1996; Demetri et al. 2006). The EPILOG trial (EPILOG Investigators 1996) may have been an exception since the drug studied was previously approved, the efficacy benefit was twice that observed in a previous trial, and previous safety concerns were substantially reduced; also, while the interim analysis was early in terms of the planned final information, there was already a large number of patients treated. In any case, the case for changing the prevalent treatment paradigm was compelling. In addition to FDA suggestions to limit early efficacy analyses, the European Medicines Agency (EMA) has also strongly suggested limiting the number of interim efficacy analyses.

Along with timing recommendations, the FDA sometimes suggests (e.g., Center for Drug Evaluation and Research and Center for Biologics Evaluation and Research 2010) O'Brien–Fleming-like criteria (O'Brien and Fleming 1979; Lan and DeMets 1983) for early stopping. While these are generally considered conservative criteria for stopping, we wish to note here that at 60 % of the final sample size for a group sequential trial designed with 90 % power and 2.5 % Type I error, 1 sided, the approximate treatment effect required to stop the trial early is approximately 1.04 times the treatment effect for which the trial is powered. Thus, even more stringent interim bounds may be desirable if there are substantial risk–benefit considerations beyond the primary endpoint. For instance, in an oncology trial with a primary progression free survival endpoint, as complete assessment as possible of overall survival can be an essential part of the evaluation of benefit; in this situation early stopping for efficacy should be done cautiously. For treatments of chronic conditions where evaluation of safety is particularly important for assessing risk–benefit tradeoffs, early stopping should consider the sample size needed for risk–benefit evaluation.

As discussed in the section on frequent interim analyses, calendar-based timing of analyses may be of use in efficacy evaluations for a drug. It is not uncommon for enrollment rates or event rates that vary from those used to plan a trial. If events occur slower than expected, there may be a much longer gap between planned efficacy analyses. If events occur faster than expected, the anticipated time between planned interim analyses can largely disappear. Information-based group sequential trials (Jennison and Turnbull 2000; Mehta and Tsiatis 2001; Scharfstein et al. 1997; Tsiatis 2006) adapt interim and final analysis boundaries based on the amount of statistical information available at an interim analysis. This is most commonly achieved through the use of error spending functions to establish and modify group sequential bounds (Lan and DeMets 1983). In these cases, a gap of more than 1 year or less than, say, 6 months, may be considered too long and too short of a time, respectively, between an evaluation of risk–benefit that includes an efficacy evaluation. For many trials, planning interim analyses at least partially on a calendar basis using a spending function approach can be essential to having an appropriate number of and timing of interim analyses.

6.5 Discussion

We have provided some considerations for timing and number of interim analyses that run from continuous analysis of important safety outcomes or early efficacy findings to a very limited number of efficacy evaluations in pivotal trials. All possibilities exist depending on the needs of a trial, and there are many statistical methods to deal with the many interim analysis issues that need to be addressed in a trial (Dragalin 2006). The general summary of timing and number of interim analyses is:

- Safety monitoring should be ongoing during a trial, often with systematic reviews of safety at interim analyses carried out at regular calendar intervals. Formal safety stopping rules may be considered for endpoints that are anticipated to potentially demonstrate a drug safety issue.
- Trials in early development may benefit from frequent analyses that allow altering or stopping a trial; this is actually encouraged by the FDA (Center for Drug Evaluation and Research and Center for Biologics Evaluation and Research 2010).
- Interim analyses for futility should carefully consider tradeoffs between the impact on power, the ability to stop a trial at a meaningful time and the approximate clinical benefit required to pass a futility bound. Earlier futility analyses can be meaningless in terms of establishing some sign of efficacy or can have a substantial power impact if made too stringent. Late interim analyses can minimize the ability to meaningfully impact the conduct of a trial.
- Efficacy interim analyses are often required to be very stringent, reasonably well into a trial, and infrequent. Careful risk–benefit evaluation should be considered in addition to any formal efficacy stopping bound.

References

Anderson KM (2012) gsdesign: Group sequential design. R package version 2.9.2

Bauer P, Koenig F, Brannath W, Posch M (2010) Selection and bias – two hostile brothers. Stat Med 29:1–13

Center for Drug Evaluation and Research and Center for Biologics Evaluation and Research (2010) Guidance for industry. Adaptive design clinical trials for drugs and biologics. Draft guidance.

United States Department of Health and Human Services, U.S. Food and Drug Administration, URL   http://www.fda.gov/downloads/Drugs/GuidanceComplianceRegulatoryInformation/Guidances/ucm201790.pdf

Demetri GD, van Oosterom AT, Garrett CR, Blackstein ME, Shah MH, Verweij J, McArthur G, Judson IR, Heinrich MC, Morgan JA, Desai J, Fletcher CD, George S, Bello CL, Huang X, Baum CM, Casali PG (2006) Efficacy and safety of sunitinib in patients with advanced gastro-intestinal stromal tumour after failure of imatinib: a randomised controlled trial. Lancet 368:1329–1338. doi: 10.1016/ S0140-6736(06)69446-4

Dragalin V (2006) Adaptive designs: terminology and classification. Drug Inform J 40:425–435. doi: 0092-8615/2006

EPILOG Investigators (1996) Platelet glycoprotein iib/iiia receptor blockade and low-dose heparin during percutaneous coronary revascularization. New Engl J Med 336:1689–1696

Jennison C, Turnbull BW (2000) Group sequential methods with applications to clinical trials. Chapman and Hall/CRC, Boca Raton

Ji Y, Liu P, Li Y, Bekele BN (2010) A modified toxicity probability interval method for dose-finding trials. Clin Trials 7:653–663. doi: 10.1177/ 1740774510382799

Lan KKG, DeMets DL (1983) Discrete sequential boundaries for clinical trials. Biometrika 70:659–663

Lee JJ, Liu DD (2008) A predictive probability design for phase ii cancer clinical trials. Clin Trials 5:93–106

Mehta C, Tsiatis AA (2001) Flexible sample size considerations using information-based interim monitoring. Drug Inform J 35:1095–1112

O'Brien PC, Fleming TR (1979) A multiple testing procedure for clinical trials. Biometrika 35:549–556

O'Quigley J, Pepe M, Fisher L (1990) Continual reassessment method for phase i clinical trials in cancer. Biometrics 46:33–48

Scharfstein DO, Tsiatis AA, Robins JM (1997) Semiparametric efficiency and its implication on the design and analysis of group-sequential studies. J Am Stat Assoc 92:1342–1350

Siegmund D (1985) Sequential analysis. Tests and confidence intervals. Spring, New York

Simon R (1989) Optimal two-stage designs for phase ii clinical trials. Contr Clin Trials 10:1–10

The Coronary Drug Project Research Group (1981) Practical aspects of decision making in clinical trials: The coronary drug project as a case study. Contr Clin Trials 1:363–376

The PURSUIT Investigators (1998) Inhibition of platelet glycoprotein iib/iiia with eptifibatide in patients with acute coronary syndromes. New Engl J Med 339:436–443

The REST Study Group (2006) Safety and efficacy of a pentavalent humaâĂŞbovine (wc3) reassortant rotavirus vaccine. New Engl J Med 354:23–33

Tsiatis AA (2006) Information-based monitoring of clinical trials. Stat Med 25:3236–3244. doi: 10.1002

Wald A (1945) Sequential tests of statistical hypotheses. Ann Math Stat 16:117–186. doi: 10.1214/ aoms/1177731118

Chapter 7
Approaches for Optimal Dose Selection for Adaptive Design Trials

David Lawrence and Frank Bretz

Abstract Adaptive designs use accumulating data to modify in a prospectively planned manner certain design aspects of a clinical study without undermining its validity and integrity. The aim of this chapter is to review adaptive design approaches for dose finding and optimal dose selection and to demonstrate that adaptivity is a fundamentally important concept, which can be applied to dose selection in different stages of clinical development. We review the major statistical methods available for planning and analyzing adaptive designs in Phase I, II, and III. To illustrate the ideas, we refer to examples and case studies from the literature, where available.

Keywords Dose selection • Maximum tolerated dose • Minimum effective dose • MCP-Mod • Dose limiting toxicity

7.1 Introduction

As outlined in Chap. 1 of this book, a major driver for adaptive designs is to increase the information value of clinical trial data to enable better decisions, leading to more efficient drug development processes and improved late-stage success rates. This is particularly true for optimal dose selection: A well-known problem of failed Phase III programs is often believed to be poor dose selection resulting from inappropriate knowledge of the dose–response relationship (efficacy and safety) at the end of

D. Lawrence (✉)
Novartis Pharmaceuticals Corporation,
One Health Plaza, East Hanover, NJ 07936-1080, USA
e-mail: david-1.lawrence@novartis.com

F. Bretz
Novartis Pharma AG, WSJ-27.1005, 4002 Basel, Switzerland
e-mail: frank.bretz@novartis.com

W. He et al. (eds.), *Practical Considerations for Adaptive Trial Design and Implementation*, Statistics for Biology and Health,
DOI 10.1007/978-1-4939-1100-4_7, © Springer Science+Business Media New York 2014

125

the learning phase of drug development, i.e., Phase II. Selection of a dose (or doses) to carry into confirmatory Phase III trials is among the most difficult decisions in drug development. Although the exact numbers are unknown, it is believed that the high attrition rate plaguing the pharmaceutical industry in Phase III studies are due, at least in part, to inadequate dose selection for confirming safety and efficacy in the intended patient population—doses that are too low to achieve adequate benefit, as well as doses that are too high and lead to dose-related safety events. There is also evidence that, even after registration, dose adjustments in the label continue to be required with some frequency (Cross et al. 2002; Heerdink et al. 2002). Given this context it is no surprise that dose finding has been described as "difficult, essential and often badly done" (Senn 1997). This chapter illustrates, with examples, some of the adaptive dose finding options that exist across the phases of drug development and may aid us in our understanding of the dose–response relationship and improve the probability of selecting the correct dose, or doses, to take to market.

7.2   Current Issues with Dose Ranging and Issues to Consider for Adaptive Dose Ranging

The basic difficulty in getting the right dose is the trade-off between wanted and unwanted effects. In the past, dose finding studies were often designed using a small number of doses and a narrow dose range, often focused on the upper end of the dose–response relationship. Only in recent years has there been a noticeable shift towards investigating the full dose–response relationship and estimating the so-called minimum effective dose (MED). The MED denotes the smallest dose achieving a prespecified clinical treatment effect. Knowing the MED is important, because it defines a lower bound for therapeutically useful doses.

One of the main issues with dose response is that many different profiles are possible. Figure 7.1 displays a non-exhaustive set of possible profiles that are often seen in clinical dose finding studies, together with the associated MED. In this example the MED occurs at an expected treatment effect of approximately 250 units implying that the threshold for clinical relevance is an improvement of 200 units over the placebo response (where the placebo, dose 0, response is approximately 50 points). As seen from Fig. 7.1, the MED depends quite strongly on the true, underlying dose response profile and can vary between 50 (for the emax1 model) and 350 (for the linear model).

An indication of the importance of properly conducted (and informative) dose response studies is the early publication of the ICH E4 guideline (ICH 1994), which is the primary source of regulatory guidance in this area. The guideline gets very specific already in the introduction when it motivates the importance of dose response information:

> Historically, drugs have often been initially marketed at what were later recognized as excessive doses ... This situation has been improved by attempts to find the smallest dose with a discernible useful effect or a maximum dose beyond which no further beneficial effects is seen...

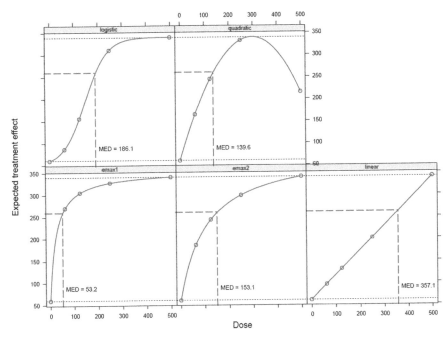

Fig. 7.1 Example dose response profiles often seen in clinical dose finding studies. *Open dots* indicate the expected responses at selected dose levels. The minimum effective dose (MED) is defined as the smallest dose achieving a prespecified clinical treatment

It becomes transparent from this quote, and the remainder of the ICH E4 guideline, that regulatory agencies recognize the need to obtain appropriate dose response information as a critical part of clinical drug development. But even if it is generally agreed that understanding the relationships among administered dose, drug-concentration in blood, and clinical response is important, setting the objectives for an actual trial may be subject to much debate and different questions might be of interest: (1) detecting a dose response signal, (2) identifying a predefined clinically relevant response within the observed dose range provided that a dose response signal has been established, (3) selecting a target dose to be further studied in late phase trials, and (4) estimating the dose response profile within the observed dose range (Bornkamp et al. 2007).

Typically, dose selection in a clinical program begins with the drug being first studied in man as single ascending doses, followed by multiple ascending doses in healthy volunteers. Initially we wish to establish both a "no effect" dose and a dose where subjects begin to experience "symptom-limiting" adverse events (the so-called maximum tolerable dose, MTD). This can then be followed by evidence that the drug has an effect on the disease being studied, often conducted by a dedicated proof-of-concept (PoC) study. Once PoC has been declared, dose ranging will be performed in a study containing multiple doses to identify the dose response shape and estimate the MED or other target doses of interest. The result of the dose response study will be used to inform the dose, or doses, to be taken forward into Phase III and ultimately to market. However, in many cases only a small amount of clinically-derived data are available to justify the dose selection and that data may be being used in a suboptimal fashion.

In contrast to standard dose finding, in adaptive dose finding prespecified adaptations allow modifications to the original study design as dose response information accrues. This information can be used to answer one or more of the four questions outlined above. Generally speaking, adaptive designs use accumulating data to modify aspects of the study in a prospectively planned manner without undermining the validity and integrity of the trial (Gallo et al. 2006). Validity involves the statistical properties of the trial related to inference and estimation, i.e., providing correct statistical inference by, for example, ensuring control of the Type 1 error rate, and the calculation of adjusted p-values, estimates, and confidence intervals, assuring consistency between different stages of the study and minimizing statistical bias. Trial integrity is primarily about transparency and trial conduct acceptable to the intended external audience, i.e., providing convincing results to a broader scientific community, by, for example, preplanning as much as possible, basing any study design changes on intended adaptations and maintaining confidentiality of data while the study is ongoing.

The majority of adaptive dose finding studies take place in Phase I and II and, thus, regulatory concerns often associated with adaptive trials in the confirmatory setting (Phase III) are less of an issue here. Adaptive dose finding designs should be considered as an effective learning paradigm for drug development where the risks of missing an accurate assessment of the true underlying dose response profile of an investigational treatment are borne by the sponsor. These plans would not require special approval from regulatory agencies. While trial designs for early phase drug development are under the purview of the sponsoring company as long as strict compliance to regulations around potential human risk and safety is maintained, a successful dose ranging trial brings major evidence to regulatory discussions such as End-of-Phase IIa or IIb meetings. It is also possible for investigation of dose to continue into Phase III and then there is additional regulatory concern. These issues will be discussed in Sect. 7.5. Nevertheless, to ensure the validity of the trial results, there has to be an implicit assumption that demographic and other relevant characteristics of the patients enrolled in the study remain relatively constant over time. As with any adaptive design, it is assumed that the efficacy response being measured is available in a sufficiently rapid time frame (relative to the enrollment period and the duration of the study) to allow for meaningful adaptations to occur. It is very common for an adaptive dose finding trial to use an endpoint different from the endpoint used in the confirmatory trial for regulatory approval because, for example, the registration endpoint takes too long to measure (e.g., a survival endpoint). In such situations, a validated biomarker with shorter duration may be introduced for the purpose of either proof-of-concept or adaptive randomization of patients. Lastly, it is assumed that the transmission of relevant information to the data analysis group is sufficiently rapid to allow adaptations to occur according to the prescribed methodology. Additional points to consider when designing an adaptive dose ranging study would be to ideally run the study in a small number of centers to limit issues with drug supply management. Of course the ability to produce enough dose levels (i.e., no manufacturing problems) must be present. Issues such as these must be taken into consideration before embarking on any adaptive dose finding study.

7.3 Phase I

When evaluating a new experimental treatment, the purpose of first-in-human studies is to identify the MTD. Phase I trials are typically adaptive whether they involve single or multiple ascending doses. In general, cohorts of healthy volunteers (e.g., six subjects on active and two on placebo) will enter the study and decisions will be made after each cohort on whether to initiate the next dose or possibly stop the trial altogether. These decisions will be based on safety, tolerability, pharmacokinetics, and pharmacodynamics.

The need for and acceptance of adaptive dose escalation designs is particularly well established in the area of Oncology. Here, MTD finding studies in Phase I frequently classify a patient's toxicity (safety) data into one of two levels: dose limiting toxicity or not. The purpose of MTD finding studies is then to estimate the dose which achieves a probability of toxicity close to a targeted level, frequently in the order of 25–35 %, although the actual level will be situational dependent. Adaptive dose escalation designs to estimate the MTD then allocate small cohorts of patients (typically of size 3) to a selected dose based on the available cumulative toxicity data, that is, the dose that is anticipated to achieve a degree of toxicity closest to the targeted level. The dose selection mechanism is therefore response adaptive: the cumulative knowledge is used to inform the actual dose allocated to the (future) next cohort of patients. This allocation can be informed by a number of methods, including Bayesian adaptive dose escalation designs, such as the continual reassessment method (CRM) proposed by O'Quigley et al. (1990). The original CRM chooses the first dose level based on some assumed dose response model. After each cohort of patients, the model is updated. The updated model is used to calculate the probability of dose limiting toxicity (DLT) at each dose of interest. The statistical dose recommendation for the next patient cohort is communicated to the clinical team, who decides on the next dose based on the statistical input as well as other relevant information (e.g., toxicities that do not qualify for a DLT). The basic CRM has led to much research (Garrett-Mayer 2006) and numerous extensions (Neuenschwander et al. 2008; Cheung 2011).

7.4 Phase IIa/IIb

The advantages of an adaptive dose ranging design in Phase II may be illustrated by an example of a combined Phase IIa/b study in dental pain (Vandemeulebroecke et al. 2010). The compound was developed as an analgesic for the treatment of chronic pain. In order to provide a scientific rationale for the clinical development in such a chronic indication, the potential benefit of the compound was first investigated in a proof-of-concept study for an acute pain indication. More specifically, a dental pain study was developed which looked for proof of analgesic efficacy after molar teeth were removed. In view of this clinical development plan and the possibility to apply the compound as a multiple dose therapy for chronic pain indications, it was imperative to collect conclusive dose response information for both efficacy and safety in the intended dental pain PoC study. More specifically, there was a need to determine:

- A safe dose range for testing in patients.
- Whether the efficacy signal observed was large enough to support further development.
- The dose–response relationship in order to select one or more doses for larger, later stage trials.

To aid these decisions and to accelerate the outlined development plan, the dental pain study considered here prospectively combined Phase IIa and Phase IIb by bridging PoC and dose finding into a single, adaptive study. The PoC part looked for proof of analgesic efficacy after molar teeth were removed. If PoC could be established, the study would seamlessly continue into a dose finding part, to provide dose ranging information for the further development of the compound in the chronic pain indication.

Accordingly, this dental pain study consisted of three parts A, B and C, see Fig. 7.2. Part A consisted of the first administration of the compound in patients. Its goal was to determine two safe doses for Part B (Low & High dose). Part B investigated PoC. It compared Low and High dose of the compound against placebo for PoC declaration, based on patients from Parts A and B. Only if PoC was declared, would the study continue with dose finding in Part C. The complete data from Parts A and B is used to optimize the design of Part C. The aim of Part C was to establish dose response information for both efficacy and safety. For example, it would be used to determine the MED, i.e., the smallest dose that achieves a clinically relevant effect. The final analysis would use the MCP-Mod approach (Bretz et al. 2005;

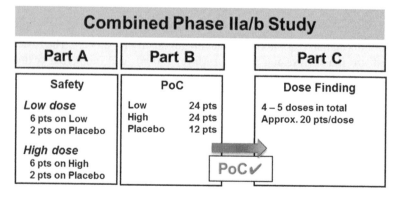

Fig. 7.2 Combined Phase IIa/b study bridging proof-of-concept and dose finding (pts = patients)

CHMP 2013), based on all data from Part A, B, and C. The MCP-Mod approach combines principles of *M*ultiple *C*omparisons *P*rocedures with *Mod*eling techniques to overcome some of the shortcomings of applying either approach alone. More specifically, it provides an efficient statistical methodology for model-based design and analysis of Phase II dose finding studies acknowledging model uncertainty through the following steps: (1) testing for the presence of a dose response signal, (2) selecting the best dose response model for the observed data out of a pre-specified set of candidate models, and (3) estimating target doses of interest (e.g., the minimum effect dose, MED) via modeling.

In a traditional drug development program, Parts B and C would be run as two separate studies. However, in this study design it was decided to use an adaptive design prospectively combining, PoC and dose finding, to more efficiently use the accumulating data across the three seamless parts of the study. It is an adaptive design because between Part B and C an interim analysis is performed to (1) assess PoC and possibly terminate the study early for futility, and (2) use the complete data from Parts A and B to optimize the design of Part C. The application of such an adaptive design was possible because of:

- The availability of a fast readout for a clinically relevant endpoint (reduction in pain intensity 72 h after removing the molar teeth).
- The possibility to conduct this study in very few centers, thus avoiding potential drug supply management issues.
- The ability to produce small enough dose levels (no manufacturing issues).
- The availability of a clinical team bridging Early and Full Development to prospectively plan an integrated PoC and dose finding study.

This trial design was well accepted by regulatory agencies and this case study shows how dose response information can be sequentially built up by combining PoC and dose finding in an adaptive manner and how this information may be used to select doses to be tested in later development stages.

7.5 Phase III

Although it would be preferable to learn about dose in early phase studies when decision making comes under the heading of "sponsor's risk," in certain situations it may be necessary to further investigate dose in Phase III. This is possible using a pivotal two-stage adaptive design with dose selection at interim. Such a design aims at addressing two objectives by a single, uninterrupted study conducted in two stages, which otherwise would have been addressed by two separate studies. Under the adaptive design, one (or more) dose level(s) are selected using data from the first stage reviewed at an interim analysis. These dose(s) are then carried forward to the second stage. The final analysis of the selected dose(s) includes data from both stages, and is performed in such a way that the validity of the conclusions is maintained (Bretz et al. 2009).

As this type of study is used for pivotal confirmation of efficacy and safety, it will be submitted to regulatory agencies. Regulatory agencies are more cautious about adaptive designs for confirmatory trials than for exploratory trials (CHMP 2007; FDA 2010). This arises from concerns over trial validity and integrity, for example due to potential information leak (i.e., unblinding of patients or investigators to study results before final database lock) due to the ensuing adaptations, introducing operational bias and therefore compromising trial integrity (Gallo 2006). This caution is understandable, since confirmatory trials assume a considerable body of pre-existing information and limit sponsor options in dealing with uncertainties. The adverse impact of moving forward (i.e., approval) with an ineffective or unsafe product is much greater at this stage than at earlier stages of drug development. As a result, regulators want scientific assurance that the proposed adaptive design has the desirable property of a confirmatory trial and is not proposed purely to save trial cost and time at the possible expense of scientific rigor. Both the European Medicines Agency (EMA) and the US Food and Drug Administration (FDA) have produced guidances on adaptive designs (CHMP 2007; FDA 2010) and are aligned with clear common areas for attention: Type I error rate control, rigorous planning, data confidentiality at interim analyses, as well as a limited number and frequency of adaptations (preferably limited to only one type of adaptation in a confirmatory trial). In the confirmatory setting, hypotheses about the potential beneficial effect for a new therapy have to be prespecified in the study protocol and need to be confirmed at the study end using proper statistical analysis methods (Bretz et al. 2009).

One example of a Phase III two-stage adaptive design is the INHANCE study (Donohue et al. 2010). Other examples of two-stage adaptive clinical trials with dose selection at the end of stage 1 are described in (Heritier et al. 2011; Chaturvedi et al. 2014). INHANCE was a multinational, multicenter, double-blind, double dummy, adaptive, parallel group study design with blinded formoterol and open label tiotropium as active controls in patients with chronic obstructive pulmonary disease (COPD). The study was split into two stages. In the first stage two of four indacaterol doses were selected at an interim analysis (based on data from the first 14 days of treatment, i.e., an early readout of the efficacy endpoints) to continue into a second stage where efficacy, safety, and tolerability of the two selected doses could be confirmed in comparison to active and placebo comparators over a total of 26 weeks. It was one of the pivotal trials used to support registration of indacaterol. The study design is shown in Fig. 7.3, where the two selected indacaterol doses in stage 2 (which could be any two of the four indacaterol doses from stage 1) are denoted as A and B.

A Data Monitoring Committee (DMC) of recognized experts in the respiratory and statistical field appointed by the sponsor but independent of study conduct reviewed efficacy and safety data at the interim analysis. Dose selection was primarily based on predefined criteria comparing the efficacy of indacaterol with placebo and the active controls. One of the most important issues in adaptive designs for confirmatory clinical trials is an adequate separation of the decision making committee (in this case, the DMC) from the project team, i.e., there should be no sponsor involvement in the decisions made at the end of stage 1 of a confirmatory two-stage adaptive design. Therefore, there is a need to prespecify the process by

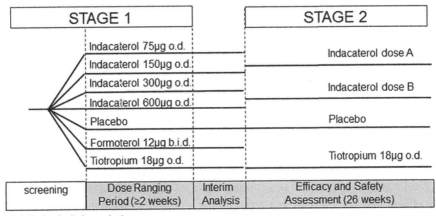

b.i.d=bis in die (twice a day)

Fig. 7.3 INHANCE—a Phase III two-stage adaptive design with dose selection (adapted from Lawrence et al. 2014)

which any decision will be made by this external, independent DMC, with an algorithm for determining the adaptation specified and agreed in advance. For the INHANCE study, a set of dose selection guidelines for a variety of possible interim analysis scenarios was compiled and included in the DMC charter. The DMC was asked to select two adjacent doses (i.e., either 75 µg and 150 µg, 150 µg and 300 µg, or 300 µg and 600 µg) based on trough Forced Expiratory Volume in 1 s (FEV_1) and FEV_1 area under curve ($AUC_{(1h-4h)}$) after two weeks of treatment. Safety data was also presented to the DMC to include in its deliberations.

In the confirmatory setting there are two key issues that are fundamental to the acceptability of an adaptive design: Type I error rate control and sponsor access to interim data. In the INHANCE study the final analysis consisted of comparing the two selected dose groups with placebo and tiotropium on a prespecified sequence of the primary, key and important secondary endpoints. Evidence from both stages was combined in a rigid statistical hypothesis-testing framework. In this study, a Bonferroni adjustment with a significance level $\alpha/4$ was used for comparing each of the two dose groups against placebo, since the study started with four indacaterol doses. Here, α denotes the usual study-wise Type I error rate acceptable for confirmatory trials (i.e., $\alpha=0.05$ for two-sided or $\alpha=0.025$ for one-sided hypotheses testing). The primary, key, and important study objectives were tested sequentially at level $\alpha/4$ in the prespecified hierarchy for each of the two selected doses (Maurer et al. 1995).

Current regulatory guidance in more traditional monitoring settings, such as group sequential designs, specifies that sponsors should not have access to interim data while trials are ongoing. One concern in the context of adaptive designs is that unanticipated complexities might not fit a prespecified algorithm, such as unexpected safety signals, lack of monotone dose response or potential stop for futility. Additionally, the interim decision could have major impacts on the sponsor's business, and it is therefore in the sponsor's interest to have some limited role pre-planned in the DMC charter. For the INHANCE study, the proposed interim decision rules were included in the DMC charter with the understanding that the DMC had the discretion to deviate from them as necessary. If the DMC were confronted with data that would result in a deviation from the dose selection guidelines, the DMC were able to confidentially discuss unblinded results with two senior members of the sponsor (who were identified by role in the company in the charter and were not otherwise involved in the study) to reach consensus on the doses chosen. If the consensus deviated from the guidelines, the DMC would document an explanation of the decision making for possible future reference by regulatory agencies, but that was to remain confidential while the trial was ongoing.

The results of the interim analysis of INHANCE have been published in full (Barnes et al 2010), as have those of the final analysis (Donohue et al. 2010). More details on the methodology employed in this trial can be found in Lawrence et al. (2014). INHANCE was included as a pivotal study in submissions to regulatory agencies globally and indacaterol is now approved in all major markets globally for once-daily maintenance bronchodilator treatment of airflow obstruction in adult patients with COPD. This example illustrates that in certain specific situations dose selection in Phase III is possible using adequate adaptive methods.

7.6 Discussion

Adaptive designs have a potential role in optimal dose selection. Integrating proof-of-concept and dose selection or the dose selection and confirmatory phases of drug development has a number of advantages, most obviously in the lack of delay between two subsequent phases and a faster overall drug development process. Adaptive designs make efficient use of resources by reducing patients' exposure to potentially less effective or unnecessarily high doses. For the selected doses, the data from both study stages contribute to the analysis of the overall study.

In a review of the PhRMA working group there was broad agreement that model-based adaptive designs in "Learn" phase have the potential to greatly improve the efficiency of learning about the dose response, thus leading to more reliable dose selection for Phase III (Krams et al. 2007). The PhRMA working group on adaptive dose ranging studies clearly indicated the superiority of adaptive methods. There is a consensus that detecting dose response is considerably easier than estimating it, or identifying the target dose to bring into the confirmatory phase. Sample sizes used for dose ranging studies based on power calculations to detect the presence of dose response, are likely to be inadequate for dose selection and actual dose response estimation. Adaptive dose ranging designs and methods clearly lead to gains in power to detect dose response and in precision to select target dose(s) and to estimate the dose response (Bornkamp et al. 2007). Clinical trials are not designed in a financial vacuum, so there may be resource constraints for Phase II programs that mean more than one dose may need to be brought forward to the next phase of development. Two-stage adaptive trials in Phase III may provide an opportunity to further refine the choice of dose, although these trials should be considered to belong in the realm of "Confirm." As such their applicability requires case-by-case consideration and discussion with regulatory agencies.

The advantages of adaptive dose ranging studies do not come without cost and one should balance the potential gains associated with adaptive dose finding designs against their greater methodological and operational complexity. Adaptive dose finding designs require substantial planning, using existing knowledge, and careful assessments of the properties of interim decisions and the related risks. They are likely to require additional resources during the planning phase. Additionally, the initial dose finding period needs to be long enough for a thorough evaluation of the treatment effects.

The adequacy of the interim dose selection procedure/PoC criterion is critical to the success of any such adaptive trial. Ideally, the endpoint(s) used at the interim analysis should be the same as or shown to be strongly correlated with the final study primary endpoint, and should be recognized and accepted (Chow and Chang 2008). As dose is a critical aspect and the knowledge generated from an adaptive dose ranging trial is crucial in taking the drug to approval even when the trial usually occurs in the early phase of the drug development it is important to include potential regulatory concerns as a part of the trial design considerations. The timing of initiating these regulatory discussions is also very important. Depending on the design features, it could occur as early as a pre-IND meeting if a Phase IIa/b seamless adaptive dose ranging trial is planned. Early discussion would have the further advantage of triggering much earlier internal discussion and potentially provoking more thorough modeling and simulation initiatives looking at many possible development options. This is likely to improve the quality of a development program whether an adaptive design is ultimately used or not.

7.7 Conclusions

It is seven years since the PhRMA white paper on innovative approaches for designing and analyzing adaptive dose ranging trials. This paper made clear that better dose response learning approaches exist and can produce substantial knowledge gains. However, while there is evidence that learning about dose has improved dose response still remains a difficult subject. Unfortunately there is no silver bullet approach to the dose finding conundrum. No design/method uniformly is best: relative performance depends on the specific scenario and assumptions made along with the learning priorities of the trial, e.g., dose selection vs. dose response characterization. Sample size calculations need to take account of these differing priorities and should also take into account the precision of estimated dose required. Adaptive designs have a major role to play in dose selection but it is not always best/necessary to use adaptive designs. Simulations should be used for protocol design to investigate the most appropriate approach in specific situations (adaptive, model-based, Bayesian, optimal design, etc). The most appropriate place to use adaptive designs in dose selection would appear to be in the early phases of drug development and combining proof-of-concept and dose selection into one seamless trial seems a learning space where major learning gains can be made. In certain situations it may be valid to select more than one dose for Phase III and couple this with an adaptive design.

Stephen Senn's observation that dose finding is "difficult, essential" remains true but with the use of model based approaches and adaptive designs we have the potential tools to make sure it is not "badly done."

References

Barnes PJ, Pocock SJ, Magnussen H, Iqbal A, Kramer B, Higgins M, Lawrence D (2010) Integrating indacaterol dose selection in a clinical study in COPD using an adaptive seamless design. Pulm Pharmacol Ther 23:165–171

Bornkamp B, Bretz F, Dmitrienko A, Enas G, Gaydos B, Hsu CH, Koenig F, Krams M, Liu Q, Neuenschwander B, Parke T, Pinheiro J, Roy A, Sax R, Shen F (2007) Innovative approaches for designing and analyzing adaptive dose ranging trials (with discussion). J Biopharm Stat 17:965–995

Bretz F, Pinheiro J, Branson M (2005) Combining multiple comparisons and modeling techniques in dose response studies. Biometrics 61:738–748

Bretz F, Koenig F, Brannath W, Glimm E, Posch M (2009) Adaptive designs for confirmatory clinical trials. Stat Med 28:1181–1217

Chaturvedi PR, Antonijevic Z, Mehta C (2014). Practical considerations for a two-stage confirmatory adaptive clinical trial design and its implementation: ADVENT trial. In W He, J Pinheiro, OM Kuznetsova, editors, Practical Considerations for Adaptive Trial Design and Implementation. Springer, New York, 77–93

Cheung YK (2011) Dose finding by the continual reassessment method. Chapman & Hall, New York

CHMP (2007) Reflection paper on methodological issues in confirmatory clinical trials with an adaptive design (CHMP/EWP/2459/02)

CHMP (2013) CHMP Draft Qualification Opinion of MCP Mod as an efficient statistical methodology for model-based design and analysis of Phase II dose finding studies under model uncertainty. EMA/CHMP/SAWP/592378/2013. http://www.ema.europa.eu/docs/en_GB/document_library/Regulatory_and_procedural_guideline/2014/02/WC500161027.pdf Accessed 24 Feb 2014

Chow S-C, Chang M (2008) Adaptive design methods in clinical trials—a review. Orphanet J Rare Dis 3:11

Cross J, Lee H, Westelinck A, Nelson J, Grudzinkas C, Peck C (2002) Postmarketing drug dosage changes of 499 FDA-approved new molecular entities, 1980–1999. Pharmacoepidemiol Drug Saf 11:439–446

Donohue JF, Fogarty C, Lötvall J (2010) Once-daily bronchodilators for chronic obstructive pulmonary disease: Indacaterol versus tiotropium. Am J Respir Crit Care Med 182:155–162

FDA (2010) Guidance for Industry: Adaptive design clinical trials for drugs and biologics (draft February 2010) www.fda.gov. Accessed 8 Feb 2011

Gallo P (2006) Confidentiality and trial integrity issues for adaptive designs. Drug Inf J 40:445–450

Gallo P, Chuang-Stein C, Dragalin V, Gaydos B, Krams M, Pinheiro J (2006) Adaptive designs in clinical drug development—An executive summary of the PhRMA Working Group. J Biopharm Stat 16:275–283

Garrett-Mayer E (2006) The continual re-assessment method for dose finding studies: a tutorial. Clinical Trials 3:57–71

Heerdink ER, Urquhart J, Leufkens HG (2002) Changes in prescribed dose after market introduction. Pharmacoepidemiol Drug Saf 11:447–453

Heritier S, Lô SN, Morgan CC (2011) An adaptive confirmatory trial with treatment selection: practical experiences and unbalanced randomization. Stat Med 30:1541–1554

ICH-E4 (1994) ICH Harmonized Tripartite Guideline. Topic E4: Dose response information to support drug registration. http://www.ich.org/products/guidelines/efficacy/efficacy-single/article/dose-response-information-to-support-drug-registration.html. Accessed 24 Feb 2014

Krams M, Burman C-F, Dragalin V, Gaydos B, Grieve A, Pinheiro J, Maurer W (2007) Adaptive designs in clinical drug development: opportunities, challenges, and scope. Reflections following PhRMA's November 2006 workshop. J Biopharm Stats 17:957–964

Lawrence D, Bretz F, Pocock S (2014) INHANCE: an adaptive confirmatory study with dose selection at interim. In: Trifilieff A (ed) Indacaterol—the first once-daily long-acting Beta2 agonist for COPD. Springer, Basel, pp 77–92

Maurer W, Hothorn L, Lehmacher W (1995) Multiple comparisons in drug clinical trials and preclinical assays: a-priori ordered hypotheses. In: Vollmar J (ed) Biometrie in der chemisch-pharmazeutischen Industrie. Stuttgart, Fischer Verlag, pp 3–18

Neuenschwander B, Branson M, Gsponer T (2008) Critical aspects to the Bayesian approach to phase I cancer trials. Stat Med 27:2420–2439

O'Quigley J, Pepe M, Fisher L (1990) Continual re-assessment method: a practical design for Phase I clinical trials in cancer. Biometrics 46:33–48

Senn S (1997) Statistical issues in drug development. Wiley, Chichester

Vandemeulebroecke M, Bornkamp B, Bretz F, Pinheiro J (2010) Adaptive dose ranging studies. In: Chow SC, Pong A (eds) Handbook of adaptive designs in pharmaceutical and clinical development. Chapman & Hall/CRC, Boca Raton, pp 11-1–11-22

Chapter 8
A Review of Available Software and Capabilities for Adaptive Designs

Yevgen Tymofyeyev

Abstract This chapter provides a brief review of methodologies and software solutions for several types of adaptive designs: the traditional and adaptive group sequential designs including sample size reestimation, multistage adaptive designs with arm and subpopulation selection at interim analyses, and adaptive designs for dose-finding studies.

Keywords Adaptive design software • Simulations • Group sequential • Many-to-one comparison • Arm selection • Population enrichment • Dose-ranging

Novel statistical methods for design and analysis of clinical trials seek to address the growing complexity of development programs for new drugs and devices and to improve study efficiency in general. Adaptive designs (AD) often present computational challenges which result in the need for robust software implementation. For example, group sequential methods require efficient numerical integration to define a study design. There are many cases where planning a trial using statistical simulations is the only feasible way to evaluate operating characteristics of the design under different scenarios. This chapter is intended to provide a review of the available AD software and their capabilities. Our focus is primarily on the methods for Phase 2 and Phase 3 clinical studies. The description of the AD methodologies is intrinsic for the presentation of the implementations' capabilities and uses. So a fair amount of the material presented in this chapter is a concise overview of how a particular method works and what it does. The intent was to highlight the working principles and paradigms. Software that would be referred to as an implementation of a particular method or procedure typically contains very extensive manuals, sometimes thousands pages long. Some software packages are very comprehensive,

Y. Tymofyeyev (✉)
Model Based Drug Development Department, Janssen Research and Development,
Titusville, NJ 08560, USA
e-mail: ytymofye@its.jnj.com

W. He et al. (eds.), *Practical Considerations for Adaptive Trial Design and Implementation*, Statistics for Biology and Health, DOI 10.1007/978-1-4939-1100-4_8, © Springer Science+Business Media New York 2014

so listing their capabilities and features would be beyond the scope of this chapter. We are going to use a method-centric way of material arrangement without providing a qualitative comparison of the various software packages. Whenever some comparison is presented, it serves as an example of the evaluation process that a designer might want to consider.

Section 8.1 describes the traditional and adaptive group sequential designs along with implementations for a single hypothesis test framework. Adaptive study designs with multiple hypotheses either due to several treatment arms or subpopulations are considered in Sect. 8.2. Section 8.3 contains a review of methods and software for adaptive dose-finding studies. The chapter concludes with a discussion of the current state of available AD implementations and future trend

8.1 Traditional and Adaptive Group Sequential Designs

Group sequential designs are well-established methods that are commonly used in clinical trials where repeated significance testing is done during interim analyses (IA) of an ongoing study. Numerical computations for the methods are primarily based on application of recursive integration techniques by Armitage et al. (1969), originally developed for the sequential testing procedure. The applicability of group sequential methods is very broad because the methodology covers practically all possible statistical testing situations resulting from different trial designs and analysis types. We refer the reader to the excellent textbook by Jennison and Turnbull (2000) for a comprehensive review of this topic. The following canonical form of the group sequential testing framework is used to embed a wide variety of designs, at least asymptotically. Throughout this section we consider methods that are known to control the Type I error rate based on theoretical justifications.

Consider the hypothesis testing problem for the parameter of interest θ and assume that the joint distribution of the test statistics Z_1, Z_2, ..., Z_K at the K planned analyses (interim and final) follows the multivariate normal distribution with the increasing sequence of statistical information denoted by $\{I_1, I_2, ..., I_K\}$ such that

1. $E(Z_j) = \theta \sqrt{I_j}$
2. $Cov(Z_i, Z_j) = = \sqrt{I_i}/\sqrt{I_j}, \ 1 \leq i \leq j \leq K.$

The statistical information about θ is proportional to the sample size (or to the number of events for time-to-event data) and is the reciprocal of the variance of the θ estimate.

The landmark tests of Pocock and O'Brien-Fleming introduced in the 1970s were originally developed for a fixed number of equally spaced information levels. Although there are techniques that extend the traditional "fixed" boundary group sequential designs to cases with unequal and different than originally planned increments of information, (see Emerson and Fleming (1989) and Pampallona and Tsiatis (1994)), the practical popularity of the group sequential methods is probably due to the error spending function approach proposed by Lan and DeMets (1983) and Kim and DeMets (1987). This approach allows flexibility for the number and timing of interim analyses. It can accommodate irregular and unplanned analyses provided that future analyses do not depend on previous estimates of θ, and the maximum statistical information about θ is fixed upfront. This is different for adaptive group sequential designs, where future analyses are flexible and can be data-driven. In particular, the future analyses can be determined using the unblinded treatment effect. Originally introduced by Bauer (1989), the adaptive designs approach has received considerable attention in the literature (e.g., refer to Bauer et al. (2001) and Posch et al. (2003)).

Here, we discuss software solutions available for the group sequential designs including the adaptive aspect just described. We restrict our attention to the two stand-alone commercial implementations—EAST™ 6.2 by Cytel Inc. and ADDPLAN™ v6.0 by Aptive Solution Company. We also consider the implementation programmed as a module within the R programming language, called the gsDesign package (available from CRAN; http://www.cran.r-projects.org). The gsDesign package comes with the simple graphical user interface program called gsDesing-Explore. Many other solutions are available (e.g., PASS 11 and SAS v9.2 SEQDESIGN). Recent reviews that the author is aware of are manuscripts by Wassmer and Vandemeulebroecke (2006) and Zhu et al. (2011).

The early versions of EAST handled the traditional group sequential method. Starting from version 5, the adaptive group sequential design module was offered. ADDPLAN software has a somewhat different paradigm as it is based on the weighted combination test principle of Lehmacher and Wassmer (1999). It is similar to the method proposed by Cui et al. (1999) to control the type I error rate when adaptive sample size reestimation is performed at the interim analysis. The combination test is defined in terms of the stage-wise p-values from the K stages by $\rho(p_1,\ldots,p_K)=\sum_{j=1}^{K} w_j \Phi^{-1}(1-p_j)$, where $\Phi^{-1}(.)$ is the inverse of the standard normal cumulative density function, and $\sum_{j=1}^{K} w_j^2 = 1$. The recursive integration framework is also valid for this formulation, and the critical values for the traditional fixed information group sequential designs can be computed (including the alpha spending function method) by adjusting the stage weights to

$$w_j = \sqrt{n_j \left(n_1 + \ldots n_K\right)^{-1}},$$ where n_j is the planned sample size (information) at stage

j, $j = 1,\ldots K$. The predefined and fixed weights ensure the control of the Type I error rate even in the presence of data-driven adaptations, provided that stage-wise p-values are stochastically independent under the null hypothesis. For example, this condition holds if the stage-wise p-values are computed from separate subject cohorts that constitute study stages. For trials with a survival endpoint, the study stages are formed by the calendar time. Wassmer (2006) showed that the inverse normal combination method is also applicable for censored survival endpoints.

Both ADDPLAN and EAST support the adaptive design methodology based on (a) the weighted combination method and (b) the conditional type I error approach by Muller and Schafer (2001) and Brannath et al. (2002), also referred to as "the recursive combination approach" in the literature. The latter method is very general. It allows for data-driven change of an entire design, e.g., study size, timing of IA, spending functions, and population enrichment. It can be applied recursively multiple times during the study.

The core functionality of the R package gsDesing by K. Anderson is the quantification of group sequential design boundaries and properties. The package also includes useful utility routines for binary and time-to-event study planning. It has a very rich preprogrammed collection of the spending functions and provides an excellent platform to optimize study design with respect to α- and β-spending functions (see Anderson (2007)). Anderson and Clark (2010) showed examples where the study design requirements are better met by considering the spending functions' families with more than one parameter (which is not available in EAST or ADDPLAN).

Zhu et al. (2011) provided a detailed side-by-side comparison of the capabilities of East v.5.2, ADDPLAN v5.0, gsDesign R package, and SAS v9.2 SEQDESIGN and SEQTEST implementations for traditional group sequential methods. Although there are some differences in capabilities and features, it would be fair to say that all platforms provide functionalities that are adequate to cover most practical situations.

Programming language environments like SAS or R are highly customizable for performing design simulations and actual analyses during study monitoring and final reporting. It is interesting that EAST opened a door for additional customizations through calls to user written routines in the R language. Also, design features like the lag in subjects' response, accrual, and dropout were added for normal and binary endpoints to facilitate the quantification of potential resource savings due to early stopping of AD studies. This is useful for comparison of the traditional and adaptive group sequential designs, as the benefits of early stopping with the traditional group sequential methods are reduced by the so-called the "pipeline" effect (when subjects are already enrolled by not evaluable for analysis).

ADDPLAN 6.0 and EAST 6.2 software have benefits due to the graphical user interface (GUI) and the extensive collections of step-by-step wizard navigations for many testing problems that cover normal, binomial, survival data types. Also, tools for the creation, review and comparison of multiple design scenarios are provided. EAST 6.2 provides a richer collection of features and capabilities in the opinion of the author. In addition to design and simulation modules, ADDPLAN and EAST are equipped with the analysis GUI for study monitoring and calculation of confidence intervals and p-values. Nevertheless, execution of interim analysis outside of a fully automated system like SAS is undesirable as manual data transfer prompts potential errors. A remark regarding challenges of an analysis execution is that, if an adaptive design method requires stage-wise data analysis, one needs to plan on how subjects with partial data at the time of the IA are handled, e.g., in trials where there are multiple observations per subject.

The decisions to stop early in group sequential trials are defined by the stopping boundaries that can be expressed in different scales, e.g., Z-, p-, and B-values. One scale, the conditional power (CP) value, deserves special attention because it requires assumptions about the future data (see Lachin (2005)). The conditional power is the probability of getting statistically significant positive results in the ongoing study given the interim analysis data. CP often serves as the main criterion for the sample size reestimation. Depending on the assumptions about the future data, CP would have a very different numerical value for the same observed at the interim data. EAST, ADDPLAN, and gsDesign allow for relatively easy translation of one boundary scale to another including the observed IA effect size scale, which is useful for communication purposes. Besides different boundary scales, it is important to consider how the interim decision rules would play out under different scenarios for the true parameter θ. An example is the evaluation of the probability to increase the sample size in an AD study, if the true value of θ is half of what has been originally used to power the fixed sample size design study.

Next, we move to the setup when an additional level of complexity is considered—multiple hypotheses due to the presence of several treatment arms or several subpopulations in the study.

8.2   Confirmatory Adaptive Multistage Designs with Multiple Hypotheses

This section focuses on confirmatory multistage designs, specifically, the adaptive seamless designs (ASDs) that integrate Phase II and Phase III trials into one trial, the so-called seamless Phase II/III design. One example of the seamless Phase II/III design is when doses are selected at IA after the completion of the Phase II portion, and, after that, subjects are randomized only to the selected doses and the control arm in the confirmatory Phase III portion of the trial. The final comparison of the selected doses to the control includes data before and after dose selection. The adaptive multistage procedure for the just described "many-to-one" comparison setting is extensively studied in the literature (e.g., refer to Bretz et al. (2009) for an overview). Another important application of ASDs is referred to as the patient enrichment or population enrichment design (see Temple (1994, 2005)). There, at an interim adaptation point, some selection of patient subpopulations (typically based on a predictive model of response) is done, and the enrollment is limited to the selected subpopulations in the remainder of the trial. In both examples, proper control of the type I error is required to adjust for multiple hypotheses testing and adaptive treatment arms (subgroups) selection at IA. Often, ASDs also incorporate early stopping for efficacy or futility as well as sample size reestimation. Statistical methodologies need to account for all potential sources of the Type I error rate inflation in such designs.

Due to the complex nature of ADs with multiple hypotheses involved, it is difficult to derive operating characteristics of such methods analytically. Instead, simulations are typically used to investigate and optimize design properties. The typical objectives of a trial simulation include: (a) computation of the essential operating characteristics such as power to demonstrate that the design adequately meets requirements; (b) comparison of alternative designs, in particular, the conventional design where Phase II and Phase III studies are done separately; (c) identification of the optimal design parameters such as sample sizes, timing of interim analyses, analysis methods, and rules that drive selection and early stopping at adaptation points.

The commercial software implementation for the multistage adaptive seamless designs is provided by ADDPLAN™ 6.0 in two modules—MC and PE. The latter module covers patient enrichment designs and the former is for multiple comparisons in multistage studies. The R package we are aware of is called "asd" (available from CRAN; http://www.cran.r-projects.org) described in Parsons et al. (2012).

We briefly review the statistical methodology of ASDs next.

8.2.1 Classical Multiplicity Adjustment Method

A simple approach is to adjust for the original number of hypotheses involved using the conventional multiplicity adjustments, although just a subset of these hypotheses would be tested at the final analysis as some hypotheses were unselected at interim. The closure test principle by Marcus et al. (1976) is a fundamental method used to control the family-wise Type I error rate in many-to-one comparisons. An individual null hypothesis is rejected at the global level α only if all intersection hypotheses from the closed system that involve the individual hypothesis are rejected by a local α-level test. There is flexibility as for the choice of a method to be used for testing the intersection hypotheses (e.g., the commonly used tests are Dunnett, Sidak, Simes, and Bonferroni procedures). Koenig et al. (2008) described how conventional methods could be modified to account for the treatment selection procedure. Note that this simple method does not allow for adaptations other than arm selection (i.e., no early stopping or sample size recomputation).

8.2.2 Adaptive Dunnett Test Procedure

Proschan and Hunsberger (1995) proposed the adaptive two stage test for a single null hypothesis based on the *conditional error function*. This concept was generalized in Muller and Schafer (2001). The method is based on preserving the conditional Type I error rate. The null hypothesis H can be rejected at the final analysis controlling the Type I error at α if the p-value from the second stage, p_2, is less than $A(p_1)$, where p_1 is the p-value from the first stage, and A is any non-increasing function such that $\int A(p)dp = \alpha$.

Koenig et al. (2008) developed the adaptive two stage test in the context of many-to-one treatment arm comparison where the conditional type I error is computed for the Dunnett test (this is known as the *Adaptive Dunnett Test Procedure*). For this procedure the variance is assumed to be known, so it should be used in studies with a large sample size in order for the approximation to be valid. No formal early stopping rules are developed within this procedure, so it can be used only for treatment selection and sample size reestimation for a single interim analysis.

8.2.3 Design Based on Combination Test Approach

The approach based on a combination test function applied together with the closed test principle described above provides plenty of flexibility for ASDs while controlling Type I in a strong sense. Several authors suggested this approach for the adaptive treatment arm selection design (refer to Bauer and Kieser (1999); Kieser et al. (1999); Posch et al. (2005)). Using this framework, the multistage adaptive study selection process of multiple arms (subpopulations) at an interim time can also incorporate the adaptive early stopping and sample size reestimation. Furthermore, the selection rule is very flexible; in particular, the number of arms selected after interim analyses does not have to be prespecified. The statistical methodology for the adaptive enrichment design where prespecified subpopulations or the full population is selected at the interim analysis is similar to the arm selection case (see Brannath et al. (2009) and Wang et al. (2009)).

Friede and Stallard (2008) compared performance of the three methods described above and the method proposed by Stallard and Friede (2008) for treatment selection. For the latter method, the critical value is derived from the test statistic which is the sum of the largest test statistics based on the data from each stage of the trial. Therefore, the number of treatment arms present in the trial at each stage needs to be prespecified. Their results suggested similar power properties for the three adaptive design methods.

ADDPLAN 6.0 software provides a comprehensive simulation platform for the multi-armed seamless designs and adaptive population enrichment designs in the MC and PE modules, respectively. There are many common features and functionalities between the MC and PE modules, but some aspects, such as the specification of subpopulations and logical structure among hypotheses, (e.g., the concept of the full population in the enrichment designs), segregate the modules. The R package asd implements only the adaptive selection of arms at the single interim analyses using the combination function approach applied together with Dunnett's procedure. An interesting feature of the package is that the selection could be based either on the actual primary endpoint of interest or the early outcome correlated with the primary endpoint (see Friede et al. (2011)). Among others, both software solutions implement the following selection rules: the best performing arm; several best arms; all arms with the response no worse than a given threshold difference from the best arm; and all arms with the response greater than a given absolute response.

In general, the choice of an optimal design is likely to depend on the specifics of a particular study and in many circumstances the methods have similar power. The following table aggregates some rules of thumb features of the considered methods.

Method	Advantages	Disadvantages
Adaptive dunnett	Good power properties. Allows for sample size reestimation (SSR) and arbitrary arm selection rules	No early stopping; applicable for large sample sizes (assumes response variance is known); complex; requires special software
Combination test applied together with closed testing principle	Good power; flexible methods (early stoppings, SSR, selection rules)	Complex; requires special software; Inference is based on weighted test statistics, not usual sufficient test statistics
Classical multiplicity adjustment, e.g., Dunnet procedure	Simple conservative approach; no special software is required	Less powerful in cases when the sample size for stage 1 is small
Separate phase 2/3	Simple approach	Substantial drop in power if sample size for stage 1 is large

Method	Advantages	Disadvantages
Group sequential based on the sum of stage-wise maximum of tests, by Stallard and Friede (2008)	Good power; Inference is based on the usual sufficient test statistics (cutoff values are prespecified)	No SSR; need to prespecify number of arms present at stages; no commercial software is currently available

8.3 Adaptive Designs for Dose-Ranging Studies

In this section we consider designs and implementation software for adaptive dose-ranging studies. We will differentiate between the ADR design with a few interim analyses and the designs from the large class of methods that utilizes the so-called *frequent adaptation scheme*. For this class, it is typically assumed that time to observed response is short relative to the whole trial duration; therefore, changes in subject allocation ratio could appear after observing responses from each small cohort of subjects. In cases where time to observed response is relatively long, longitudinal modeling to predict final response based on early readouts can be considered. There is a wide variety of designs that fall into this framework available in the literature. Bornkamp et al. (2007) and Dragalin et al. (2010) report on the two evaluation studies done by the PhRMA Working Group on Adaptive Dose-Ranging Studies to compare different approaches.

The general algorithm utilized in ADR designs is the following:

- Fit a model using all available data at an adaptation point.
- Based on the fitted model, optimize allocation for the next cohort of subjects to maximize some utility function, for example, information at the target dose or the minimal dose that provides the specified response relative to placebo.
- Repeat above steps at each adaptation point using accumulating subject responses.

The ADR designs can incorporate other types of adaptation, e.g., early dose (study) stopping or arm selection. Therefore, the considerations provided in Sects. 8.1 and 8.2 are applicable here as well. We briefly describe several adaptive design methods next.

8.3.1 Bayesian Parametric Designs

The Bayesian parametric designs assume that responses follow some functional model which captures potential dose–response profiles. For example, consider the four parameter logistic model specified by the equation for the expected response value,

$$E(Y \mid D) = \beta + \delta \Big/ \big(1 + \exp\big((\theta - D)/\tau\big)\big)_{,}$$

where D is a dose level and Y is the response. For the continuous response, the observational error is assumed to be normally distributed with mean 0 and variance σ^2. For the binary case, $Y = 1$ indicates a "response" and $Y = 0$ indicates "no response." Here δ is the absolute range of values of the response Y, β is the minimum or maximum value of the response depending on whether δ is positive or negative, respectively, θ is the value of dose D that achieves half of δ (i.e., the dose that gives an expected response that is midway between the minimum and maximum responses), and τ is proportional to the slope of the dose response curve at $D = \theta$. The restriction that $\tau > 0$ is necessary for unique identification of the parameters. The four parameters β, δ, θ, and τ (and σ^2 for the continuous case) are treated as random variables with user-specified prior distributions. Once responses are measured on a cohort, the posterior distribution of the parameters is calculated and used in an allocation (decision) rule. For example, the rule that seeks to minimize a weighted average of the posterior response variance at prespecified percentiles of the dose–response curve. There is no closed form solution for the posterior distributions, so computationally intensive Bayesian techniques are employed.

Alternate parameterizations of the above model or models with fewer parameters can be used.

8.3.2 Normal Dynamic Linear Models

Berry et al. (2002) proposed using Normal Dynamic Linear Models (NDLM) in the dose–response setting. A dynamic linear model is typically defined in terms of a system of equations specifying how observations of a process are stochastically dependent on the current process state and by how the process parameters evolve in time (refer to West and Harrison (1997)). In the dose–response setting, the role of time is played by the dose variable. NDLM does not require a monotonic dose–response relationship assumption; only the assumption about dose ordering is necessary. This allows flexibility in the shape and form of the response. NDLM can be viewed as a smoothing technique that is applied to estimate the response at each dose level by sharing information across doses. The degree of smoothing is controlled by a parameter, and its misspecification might result in an inadequate fit. At extreme values of the smoothing parameter, the NDLM estimate approaches the simple mean estimate. Note that as with any smoothing technique, an NDLM fit results in some bias in the response estimate at a dose level.

As an example, consider the following simple model formulated in terms of a set of equations where the doses are indexed by j and subjects are indexed by k:

$$Y_{jk} \mid dose Z_j = \theta_j + v_{jk}, \quad v_{jk} \sim N\left(0, \sigma^2\right)$$
$$\theta_j = \theta_{j-1} + \delta_{j-1} + w_j, \quad w_j \sim N\left(0, W\sigma^2\right)$$
$$\delta_j = \delta_{j-1} + \varepsilon_j, \quad \varepsilon_j \sim N\left(0, W\sigma^2\right)$$

In this model, the parameter W defines smoothness, and can be estimated from the data if some assumption is made regarding its relationship with the observation error σ^2. Different NDLM implementations might vary with respect to how to control the smoothness.

At each adaption point, an NDLM is fitted using all available data, and the posterior probability of the response is computed. Based on the fit, randomization of subjects to treatments (including placebo) is done sequentially in cohorts by optimizing some utility function defined according to study objectives. The Bayesian formulation is useful in the interim analysis decision making process. For example, the posterior probability that response exceeds some threshold can drive an early dose or study stopping decision.

8.3.3 "Up-and-Down" Designs

The so-called "up-and-down" methods belong to the class of model-free adaptive designs for dose-finding. This methodology has broad application. It often used in early phase toxicity clinical trials. A comprehensive review of the topic is given by Ivanova (2006). Suppose that the goal of the study is to estimate a dose that provides the targeted prespecified probability of response. Cohorts of subjects are treated sequentially during the study. The subsequent cohort receives the next lower or next higher dose (if available) than the previous cohort depending on responses observed thus far. Up-and-down designs are easy to understand, as intuitively it is clear that the assigned doses migrate to and cluster around the target dose of interest. The design minimizes observations at doses that are too low or too high in comparison to a completely randomized design. These designs can be used in the combined proof-of-concept and dose-finding trials. There are modifications of the up-and-down designs that use information from all previous cohorts of subjects, not only the most recent cohort (see the t-statistic design by Ivanova et al. (2008)).

8.3.4 Fixed Dose Ranging Design

It is important to compare performance characteristics of an adaptive design relative to the fixed-sample design. The latter are typically easier to implement than adaptive designs. Usually, equal allocation is used, but it worth considering unequal allocation when optimizing power of test procedures. The following two fixed design analysis approaches are often adopted.

8.3.4.1   ANOVA Method

- Compare each dose to placebo using some adjustment for multiplicity (e.g., the Dunnett (1955) procedure). If there is at least one significant difference from placebo, conclude that dose response is established.
- The smallest significant dose that meets the minimal clinical effect requirement is selected as the target dose.
- The dose–response relationship can be modeled as just a simple estimation of means at each dose, by isotonic regression, or by other model fitting techniques.

For details on the estimates based on isotonic regression refer to Robertson et al. (1988). The isotonic estimators are the maximum likelihood estimates under the assumption of monotonicity of response. No particular parametric model is necessary, only the response ordering assumption is required. In many situations it is natural to restrict attention to the monotonic (or unimodal) dose–response relationship to improve mean square errors of the estimators compared to the simple mean estimates.

8.3.4.2   MCPmod Approach

Bretz et al. (2005) proposed the procedure that utilizes both multiple comparisons and modeling techniques, hence the name MCPMod, for use in the dose-finding study design and analysis. First, the set of plausible dose–response profiles, (e.g., "Emax," exponential or quadratic models) needs to be identified as the candidate models. After that, the optimal contrast tests and the corresponding critical value, which takes into account correlation among tests, are computed to handle multiplicity in establishing the dose–response. This is similar to the trend test analysis introduced by Tukey et al. (1985). Next, to estimate the target dose or the minimum efficacious dose, the model that best fits the data (based on the AIC or BIC criteria) is selected. Alternatively, the model corresponding to the most extreme contrast test statistic can be used as well. The precision of the dose estimation can be assed using bootstrapping techniques. This methodology is implemented in the R package "DoseFinding" (refer to Bornkamp et al. (2009)). Also, the ADDPLAN™ DF modular provides a standalone software implementation.

8.3.5   Two Stage (Multistage) Adaptive Design

The methods discussed in Sect. 8.2 (implemented in ADDPLAN 6 MC) are clearly applicable in the dose-ranging studies as well. For that, each dose is viewed as a separate treatment arm. In principle, dose–response modeling can be used for a dose selection rule and COMPASS™ software has such functionality.

Another example is the MCPmod method extended to the adaptive design framework by Bornkamp et al. (2011). The adaptive version of this approach incorporates determination of the optimal design that aims to change subject allocation depending on responses observed at interim analyses. Interestingly, it was noted by the authors that most benefits from the adaptations in terms of improved operating characteristics would come within just a few interim analyses. The results from the Bornkamp et al. (2007) and the Dragalin et al. (2010) simulation studies also seemed to be in concordance with this remark. The same conclusion can be drawn from the example of the simulation study presented in the subsection below.

The designs with few interim analyses for dose selection are common in practice. Also, a reasonably large sample size for the initial stage is usually recommended for the adaptive designs with the frequent adaptation scheme described above in order to reduce "wandering" on the dose levels adjusting for early noisy data.

When the trial execution complexity is weighted against the benefits from interim adaptations, the designs with a single or few IAs can be a good middle-ground approach between the fixed-sample design and the designs with frequent changes to the allocation ratio during the trial.

8.3.6   Implementation Software, a Simple Example of the Simulation Study for the Designs Comparison

As an example of the simulation study that one might need to conduct in order to decide on the most appropriate method for a particular trial, consider the following evaluation strategy. We restrict attention to some methods described above and with implementations available in commercial software by COMPASS™ by Cytel Inc. and FACTS™ by Tessella and Berry Consultants. The point of this exercise is not to identify the best procedure or implementation but rather to demonstrate the evaluation practice. We are not optimizing the tuning parameter for each method here, nor are we using the full capability of simulation features (e.g., longitudinal response modeling, early stopping etc.). In a particular clinical trial, these choices should be made by balancing on relative priorities and importance of specific dose-finding objectives on the basis of operating characteristics.

The designs' performances were explored under two sets of conditions: (1) moderate or large number of dose levels in a trial; (2) different numbers of equally spaced interim analysis (adaptations) conducted during a trial. The true underlying

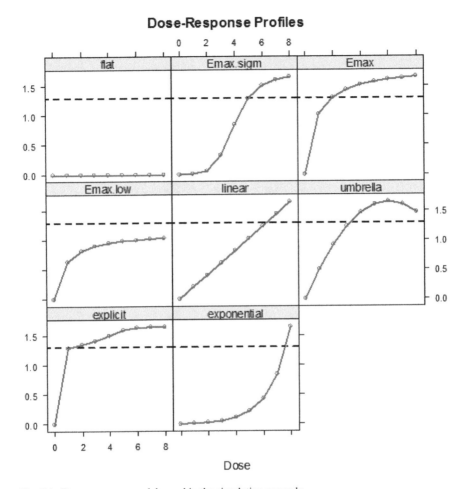

Fig. 8.1 Dose–response models used in the simulation example

dose–response curves used to simulate data are presented in Fig. 8.1. We consider the following methods and implementation versions:

1. Fixed-sample design (implemented in R)

    (a) Equal allocation to all doses and placebo (dose 0)
    (b) Placebo skewed allocation (about twice as many subjects on placebo than on each dose)

2. FACTS software

    (a) Normal Dynamic Linear Model (NDLM)
    (b) No model (simple mean estimates at each dose level)

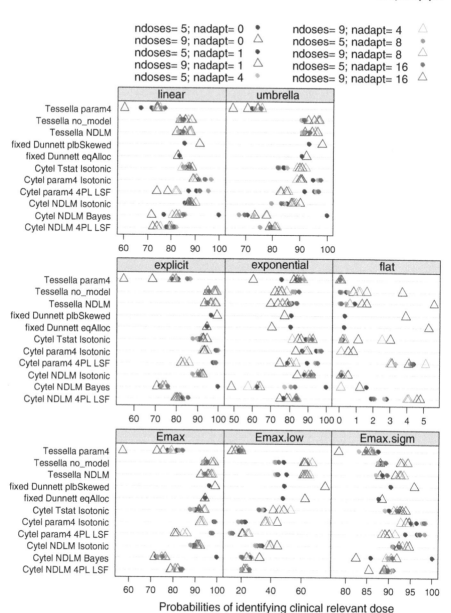

Fig. 8.2 An example of the side-by-side method comparison by looking at the probability of identifying clinical relevance

(c) Bayesian parametric model ("Emax" curve with four parameters)

3. COMPASS software

(a) Bayesian parametric model (four parameter logistic curve)
(b) NDLM considering Bayesian modeling, isotonic regression or the least square error fit (LSF) based on four parameter logistic model
(c) T-statistic design ("up-and-down")

Figure 8.2 reports the probability of identifying clinical relevance defined as the probability of finding a dose with the effect size greater than or equal to the target response after establishing POC (proof-of-concept) where different methods are compared side-by-side for different configurations of the number of active doses and number of interim analyses in the trial. The figure was generated in R by loading saved simulation results, so the comparison could be done across two platforms. Both software platforms have convenient GUI to set up simulations and process results from different scenarios and design versions covering a very extensive list of capabilities and methods. The reader is referred to http://www.cytel.com/software/compass for the details on COMPASS design software. More information about FACTS can be found at http://www.smarterclinicaltrials.com/what-we-offer/facts/ .

8.4 Discussion

The current state of available commercial implementations of adaptive designs covers substantial practical needs. Furthermore, there is the dynamic ongoing development of tools and methodologies to close the gaps that still remain. One example of a gap is the implementation of the adaptive arm selection based on an endpoint different from the endpoint planned for the final analysis (e.g., an early readout for the primary endpoint). On the other hand, there are also practical situations where a need exists for custom-made programming to satisfy requirements and special features of a particular study or program. Such cases are hard to envision up-front in order to warrant a commercial off-the-shelf tool. An example could be a study with multiple doses of the active drug, multiple comparators and several primary endpoints, where the corresponding multiple tests can be organized into some logical structure resolved by the application of a gatekeeping-type of procedure (e.g., see Dmitrienko and Tamhane (2009)), to address the multiple testing problem. Adding adaptive aspects to this type of study will likely require new implementation solutions. Still, the already available off-the-shelf tools can be useful to get a sense of potential problems. Judging from the software development history, one might predict that future commercial programs are heading in the direction of providing consolidated solutions on a single platform (perhaps formed by a union of multiple modules that share common functionality). While this chapter deals with adaptive designs, the tools discussed are very useful in planning fixed design studies. Furthermore, fixed design studies can benefit from statistical simulations as well.

Acknowledgments The author would like to thank Steve Ascher for his help with writing this chapter.

References

Anderson KM (2007) Optimal spending functions for asymmetric group sequential designs. Biom J 49(3):337–345

Anderson KM, Clark JB (2010) Fitting spending functions. Stat Med 29(3):321–327

Armitage P, Mcpherson CK, Rowe BC (1969) Repeated significance tests on accumulating data. J Roy Stat Soc A 132:235–244

Bauer P (1989) Multistage testing with adaptive designs. Biom Inform Med Biol 20:130–148

Bauer P, Kieser M (1999) Combining different phases in the development of medical treatments within a single trial. Stat Med 18:1833–1848

Bauer P, Brannath W, Posch M (2001) Flexible two stage designs: an overview. Methods Inf Med 40:117–121

Berry SM, Carroll RJ, Ruppert D (2002) Bayesian smoothing and regression splines for measurement error problems. J Am Stat Assoc 97:160–169

Bornkamp B, Bretz F, Dmitrienko A, Enas G, Gaydos B, Hsu CH, Koenig F, Krams M, Liu Q, Neuenschwander B, Parke T, Pinheiro J, Roy A, Sax R, Shen F (2007) Innovative approaches for designing and analyzing adaptive dose-ranging trials (with discussion). J Biopharm Stat 17:965–995

Bornkamp B, Pinheiro JC, Bretz F (2009) MCPMod: an R package for the design and analysis of dose-finding studies. J Stat Software 29(7):1–23

Bornkamp B, Bretz F, Dette H, Pinheiro JC (2011) Response-adaptive dose-finding under model uncertainty. Ann Appl Stat 5:1611–1631

Brannath W, Posch M, Bauer P (2002) Recursive combination tests. J Am Stat Assoc 97:236–244

Brannath W, Zuber E, Branson M, Bretz F, Gallo P, Posch M, Racine-Poon A (2009) Confirmatory adaptive designs with Bayesian decision tools for a targeted therapy in oncology. Stat Med 28:1445–1463

Bretz F, Pinheiro J, Branson M (2005) Combining multiple comparisons and modeling techniques in dose–response studies. Biometrics 61:738–748

Bretz F, Koenig F, Brannath W, Glimm E, Posch M (2009) Adaptive designs for confirmatory clinical trials. Stat Med 28:1181–1217

Cui L, Hung HMJ, Wang S-J (1999) Modification of sample size in group sequential clinical trials. Biometrics 55:853–857

Dmitrienko A, Tamhane AC (2009) Gatekeeping procedures in clinical trials. In: Dmitrienko A, Tamhane AC, Bretz F (eds) Multiple testing problems in pharmaceutical statistics. Chapman and Hall/CRC Press, New York, NY

Dragalin V, Bornkamp B, Bretz F, Miller F, Padmanabhan SK, Perevozskaya I, Pinheiro J, Smith JR (2010) A simulation study to compare new adaptive dose-ranging designs. Stat Biopharm Res 2:487–512

Dunnett CW (1955) A multiple comparison procedure for comparing several treatments with a control. J Am Stat Assoc 50:1096–1121

Emerson SS, Fleming TR (1989) Symmetric group sequential test designs. Biometrics 45:905–923

Friede T, Stallard N (2008) A comparison of methods for adaptive treatment selection. Biom J 50:767–781

Friede T, Parsons N, Stallard N, Todd S, Valdes-Marquez E, Chataway J, Nicholas R (2011) Designing a seamless phase II/III clinical trial using early outcomes for treatment selection: an application in multiple sclerosis. Stat Med 30:1528–1540

Ivanova A (2006) Escalation, up-and-down and A+B designs for dose-finding trials. Stat Med 25:3668–3678

Ivanova A, Bolognese JA, Perevozskaya I (2008) Adaptive dose finding based on *t*-statistic for dose–response trials. Stat Med 27:1581–1592

Jennison C, Turnbull BW (2000) Group sequential methods with applications to clinical trials. Chapman & Hall/CRC, Boca Raton

Kieser M, Bauer P, Lehmacher W (1999) Inference on multiple endpoints in clinical trials with adaptive interim analyses. Biom J 41:261–277

Kim K, DeMets DL (1987) Design and analysis of group sequential tests based on the Type I error spending rate function. Biometrika 74:149–154

Koenig F, Brannath W, Bretz F, Posch M (2008) Adaptive Dunnett tests for treatment selection. Stat Med 27:1612–1625

Lachin JM (2005) A review of methods for futility stopping based on conditional power. Stat Med 24:2747–2764

Lan KKG, DeMets DL (1983) Discrete sequential boundaries for clinical trials. Biometrika 70:659–663

Lehmacher W, Wassmer G (1999) Adaptive sample size calculations in group sequential trials. Biometrics 55:1286–1290

Marcus R, Peritz E, Gabriel KR (1976) On closed testing procedures with special reference to ordered analysis of variance. Biometrika 63:655–660

Muller H-H, Schafer H (2001) Adaptive group sequential designs for clinical trials: combining the advantages of adaptive and of classical group sequential approaches. Biometrics 57:886–891

Pampallona S, Tsiatis AA (1994) Group sequential designs for one-sided and two-sided hypothesis testing with provision for early stopping in favor of the null hypothesis. J Stat Plann Infer 42:19–35

Parsons N, Friede T, Todd S, Valdes-Marquez E, Chataway J, Nicholas R, Stallard N (2012) An R package for implementing simulations for seamless phase II/III clinical trials using early outcomes for treatment selection. Comput Stat Data Anal 56:1150–1160

Posch M, Bauer P, Brannath W (2003) Issues in designing flexible trials. Stat Med 22:953–969

Posch M, Koenig F, Branson M, Brannath W, Dunger-Baldauf C, Bauer P (2005) Testing and estimation in flexible group sequential designs with adaptive treatment selection. Stat Med 24:3697–3714

Proschan MA, Hunsberger SA (1995) Designed extension of studies based on conditional power. Biometrics 51:1315–1324

Robertson T, Wright FT, Dykstra RL (1988) Order restricted statistical inference. Wiley, New York, NY

Stallard N, Friede T (2008) A group-sequential design for clinical trials with treatment selection. Stat Med 27:6209–6227

Temple R (1994) Special study designs: early escape, enrichment, studies in non-responders. Comm Stat Theor Meth 23:499–531

Temple R (2005) Enrichment designs: efficiency in development of cancer treatments. J Clin Oncol 23:4838–4839

Tukey JW, Ciminera JL, Heyse JF (1985) Testing the statistical certainty of a response to increasing doses of a drug. Biometrics 41:295–301

Wang S-J, Hung HMJ, O'Neill RT (2009) Adaptive patient enrichment designs in therapeutic trials. Biom J 51(2):358–374

Wassmer G (2006) Planning and analyzing adaptive group sequential survival trials. Biom J 48:714–729

Wassmer G, Vandemeulebroecke M (2006) A brief review on software developments for group sequential and adaptive designs. Biom J 48(4):732–737

West M, Harrison J (1997) Bayesian forecasting and dynamic models, 2nd edn. Springer, New York, NY

Zhu L, Ni L, Yao B (2011) Group sequential methods and software applications. Am Stat 65(3):127–135

Chapter 9
Randomization Challenges in Adaptive Design Studies

Olga M. Kuznetsova

Abstract Adaptive design studies often face randomization challenges. Adaptive dose-ranging studies require randomization techniques that, in a small cohort, approximate reasonably well an inconveniently skewed allocation ratio to several treatment arms. When a small interim analysis sample needs to be balanced in several important predictors, dynamic allocation might be required to achieve this goal. Accelerated drug development often necessitates a large number of centers to speed up the study enrollment. When the drug is limited or costly, as is often the case with adaptive design studies conducted early in drug development, advanced randomization techniques are needed to efficiently manage the drug supplies in multicenter trials. In open-label adaptive design trials randomization procedures less predictable than permuted block randomization help reduce potential for selection bias. Randomization techniques developed for equal allocation to several treatment arms help dealing with the randomization challenges in equal allocation adaptive design studies. When these techniques are expanded to unequal allocation common to adaptive designs, care should be taken to preserve the allocation ratio at every allocation step. In this chapter we review randomization techniques useful in adaptive design studies, including those developed in recent years to specifically address the needs above.

Keywords Adaptive randomization • Brick tunnel randomization • Wide brick tunnel randomization • Unequal allocation minimization • Modified Zelen's approach • Allocation ratio preserving unequal allocation • Randomization • Allocation • Dose-ranging study • Covariate-adaptive allocation • Minimization • Allocation ratio • Unequal allocation • Multicenter study • Open-label study • Permuted block

O.M. Kuznetsova (✉)
Clinical Biostatistics, Merck Research Laboratories, RY34-A316, 126 Lincoln Avenue, Rahway, NJ 07065, USA
e-mail: olga_kuznetsova@merck.com

W. He et al. (eds.), *Practical Considerations for Adaptive Trial Design and Implementation*, Statistics for Biology and Health,
DOI 10.1007/978-1-4939-1100-4_9, © Springer Science+Business Media New York 2014

randomization • Selection bias • Dynamic allocation • Variations in allocation ratio • Expansion of allocation procedure to unequal allocation • Central randomization • Forced allocation • Randomization in multicenter trials • Divergence of the drug ID sequences • Double-permuted drug codes • Scrambled drug codes

9.1   Introduction

Widespread adaptive design trials revealed the need to address a number of unresolved randomization issues. In recent years, solutions for many of these issues have been found and implemented.

In the settings of adaptive dose-ranging studies randomization techniques that, in a small sample of subjects, approximate reasonably well an unbalanced allocation ratio to several treatment arms were lacking. Sophisticated methods are employed to derive the allocation ratio for the next cohort of subjects that works best for the specified goals of the dose-finding (Chap. 17). However, after the best allocation ratio is derived, patients are commonly randomized to multiple dose arms independently or using a permuted block schedule with a block size far exceeding the size of the cohort. As a result, the observed allocation ratio in the next cohort of subjects might differ a lot from the targeted one.

Kuznetsova and Tymofyeyev (2009, 2011a) offered a way to generate a small allocation sequence that keeps the allocation ratio close to the targeted one throughout the enrollment. They called their restricted randomization procedure the Brick Tunnel Randomization. This procedure can be used with a cohort of any size—an important requirement for adaptive dose-ranging studies where cohorts could vary in size depending on the screening pattern. The important property of the brick tunnel randomization is that the allocation ratio is the same for every allocated subject, regardless of his place in the allocation sequence. The allocation sequence can be generated automatically and made a part of the algorithm that derives the allocation ratio and the sequence of treatment assignments.

In adaptive design studies with an interim analysis performed on a small sample, an imbalance in a strong predictor of the response among the treatment groups makes the study results hard to interpret. When balance in several important predictors is required, the best if not the only randomization solution involves some form of dynamic allocation (Rosenberger and Lachin 2002; Taves 1974; Pocock and Simon 1975; Heritier et al. 2005; Signorini et al. 1993; Morrissey et al. 2010).

Dynamic allocation techniques might also be needed in multicenter adaptive design studies to efficiently manage limited or expensive at an early stage of development drug supplies. Accelerated drug development often requires studies with large number of centers which might be impossible to adequately supply for central randomization to multiple treatment arms.

The use of dynamic allocation techniques when coupled with the frequent need for unequal allocation in adaptive design studies presented theoretical challenges.

The problem was first identified by Proschan et al. (2011) who pointed out that in certain examples of minimization expansion to unequal allocation the re-randomization difference in the treatment group means is shifted away from 0. Kuznetsova and Tymofyeyev (2012) explained this phenomenon by changes in the allocation ratio from allocation to allocation in the described expansion of minimization to unequal allocation as well as in other examples of unequal allocation (Han et al. 2009). They derived the asymptotic value of the shift in the re-randomization difference in the treatment group means through the sequence of allocation probabilities at the i-th allocation ($i = 1, 2, \ldots$). They also showed that the asymptotic shift is 0 for procedures that preserve the allocation ratio at every allocation step. Avoiding variations in allocation ratio from allocation to allocation is also important because such variations can lead to selection and observer's bias even in double-blind studies; they can also lead to an accidental bias.

Kuznetsova and Tymofyeyev offered an easy way to expand any dynamic allocation procedure to unequal allocation while preserving the allocation ratio at every allocation step (Kuznetsova and Tymofyeyev 2011b, c, 2012). They applied their approach to expand a range of dynamic allocation procedures needed in adaptive design studies: those that provide balance in baseline covariates (minimization (Taves 1974; Pocock and Simon 1975; Kuznetsova and Tymofyeyev 2012), dynamic hierarchical schemes (Heritier et al. 2005; Signorini et al. 1993; Kuznetsova and Tymofyeyev 2011a, 2014b)), those that lead to efficient drug use in multicenter studies (modified Zelen's approach and dynamic allocation with partial blocks sent to centers (Morrissey et al. 2010; Kuznetsova and Tymofyeyev 2011b, c) and hybrid procedures that combine within-center balancing with balancing on important baseline predictors (Akazawa et al. 1991; Nishi and Takaishi 2003; Kuznetsova and Tymofyeyev 2014b).

Some adaptive design studies conducted early in drug development are open-label and thus require allocation procedures that reduce potential for selection bias. While a number of such allocation techniques are available for studies with equal allocation, they were lacking for studies with unequal allocation. Kuznetsova and Tymofyeyev offered a solution to his problem called Wide Brick Tunnel randomization (Kuznetsova and Tymofyeyev 2013b, 2014a) that preserves the allocation ratio at every step while keeping the allocation ratio close to the targeted one, but not as close as with the Brick Tunnel randomization to reduce the predictability of the next assignment.

In addition, often special precautions have to be taken in adaptive design studies when implementing an allocation or generating drug packaging codes. In a seamless Phase II/Phase III study the decision to drop a treatment arm will become apparent if the allocation numbers that correspond to this treatment arm remain unassigned on the allocation schedule generated at study initiation. In other examples, gaps in the original allocation schedule can unblind the study personnel to the actual treatment assignments. The sequences of the drug codes could be also unblinding with regard to treatment assignments when the drug use ratio changes across the study—which can be helped by using scrambled sequences of drug codes (Kuznetsova 2001; Lang et al. 2005).

In this chapter, we describe randomization challenges in adaptive design studies and solutions developed to overcome those. In Sect. 9.2 we describe Brick Tunnel randomization that keeps an allocation ratio close to the targeted one in a small cohort of subjects. In Sect. 9.3 we discuss the expansion of the covariate-adaptive procedures to unequal allocation that preserves the allocation ratio at every step. Section 9.4 is dedicated to the allocation procedures (fixed as well as dynamic) that facilitate efficient drug use in multicenter studies. In Sect. 9.5 we describe the techniques that help reduce potential for selection bias in open-label studies, including those with unequal allocation. In Sect. 9.6 we discuss implementation techniques that prevent unblinding with respect to adaptive decisions or treatment assignments through the sequence of allocation numbers or drug codes. Discussion concludes the chapter.

Response-adaptive allocation used in adaptive design studies is described in Chap. 10 of this book and is not discussed in present chapter. The only link to response-adaptive allocation is the description of the technique that implements the randomization in the adaptive design dose-ranging studies (Sect. 9.2).

9.2 Approximating Inconvenient Allocation Ratio in a Small Cohort with Brick Tunnel Randomization

In adaptive design dose-finding studies (Gaydos et al. 2006), small cohorts of subjects are typically randomized to several doses of the experimental treatment and placebo. The allocation ratio for the next cohort is determined by the performance of the doses in the earlier cohorts and desired distribution of subjects across the doses at the end of the study. In some studies, the cohort size is fixed, while in other studies the cohort sizes can vary.

The methods employed to derive the best ratio for the next cohort often result in an inconvenient allocation ratio, for example, 20:0:19:22:31:8 allocation to placebo and five doses of the experimental drug. Permuted block randomization will not match the target allocation well in a small cohort of subjects when the required block size is large (as 100 in the example above). In fact, permuted block allocation in this example will not be much better than independent allocation (complete randomization) often used in dose-ranging studies.

In studies where the cohort size is fixed at M subjects, the allocation ratio can be optimized over the range of the allocation ratios that can in fact be achieved in a cohort of M subjects. This approach will not work for studies where the size of the next cohort is not known in advance.

In studies where placebo arm is assigned to the same fraction of subjects in all cohorts, the allocation ratio to placebo vs. experimental drug can be better targeted with partial blocking (Parke 2008). It works in such a way that if the permuted block size is 20 and Placebo should be assigned to 20 % of subjects, one placebo allocation is randomly selected within each of the four consecutive sub-blocks of five subjects. This method ensures that placebo allocations are spread evenly across the block of 20 subjects; however, it does not help to approximate the targeted allocation among the doses of the experimental treatment.

Fig. 9.1 The allowed space for the 19:22:31 Brick Tunnel randomization to Treatment 1, Treatment 2, and Treatment 3, pictured within the allowed space for 19:22:31 permuted block randomization

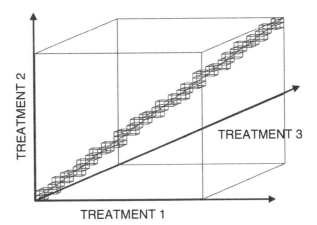

Kuznetsova and Tymofyeyev (2009, 2011a, b, c) introduced Brick Tunnel randomization that executes allocation to $K \geq 2$ treatment groups in $C_1{:}C_2{:}...{:}C_k$ ratio while keeping the allocation ratio close to the targeted one throughout the enrollment—in particular, in small cohorts of subjects.

To describe this procedure, it is helpful to visualize the allocation sequence in a study with K treatment groups as a path along the integer grid in the K-dimensional space where each of the axes represents one of the treatment groups. The allocation path starts at the origin and with each allocation moves one unit along the axis that corresponds to the assigned treatment (Berger et al. 2003). In a study with permuted block allocation to $K \geq 2$ treatment groups $G_1, ..., G_k$ in a $C_1{:}...{:}C_k$ ratio (where C_1, ..., C_k are integers that have no common to all of them divisor), at the end of each permuted block the allocation path returns to the allocation ray $AR = (C_1u, C_2u, ..., C_ku)$, $u \geq 0$, that represents the exact allocation ratio. Within the block, the allocation path can venture anywhere within the k-dimensional parallelepiped with the sides $C_1, C_2, ..., C_k$—which could be too far from the allocation ray for a small cohort.

The Brick Tunnel randomization restricts the allocation space by requiring the allocation path to be confined to the set of the k-dimensional unitary cubes pierced by the allocation ray $AR = (C_1u, C_2u, ..., C_ku)$, $u \geq 0$ (the "brick tunnel"). The important property of the Brick Tunnel randomization is that the transition probabilities at each node within the tunnel are defined in such a way that the allocation ratio is the same for every allocation step (Kuznetsova and Tymofyeyev 2009, 2011a).

Figure 9.1 illustrates the advantage of the Brick Tunnel randomization over the permuted block randomization in the example of the allocation in 19:22:31 ratio to Treatment 1, Treatment 2, and Treatment 3. Instead of occupying the whole parallelepiped of $19 \times 22 \times 31$ as is the case with permuted block randomization, allocation sequences are constrained to a chain of unitary cubes along the allocation ray $AR = (19u, 22u, 31u)$ when the Brick Tunnel randomization is used. Thus, even a short cohort of 10–15 subjects allocated along such sequence will have an observed allocation ratio reasonably close to 19:22:31.

For two groups, the allocation space for $C_1:C_2$ Brick Tunnel randomization $(C_2 \geq C_1)$ consists of the allocation sequences contained within the strip $\pm b_{BT}$ in height around the allocation ray $AR = (C_1u, C_2u)$, $u \geq 0$, where $b_{BT} = (C_2 - 1)/C_1 + 1$. Thus, in the two-group case the set of the Brick Tunnel allocation sequences is the same as the set of allowed sequences in Salama et al. (2008) expansion of the maximum procedure to unequal allocation that covers the strip $\pm b$ in height around the allocation ray, with $b = b_{BT}$. However, in Salama et al. expansion all allowed sequences are assigned equal probabilities, which leads to variations in the allocation ratio from allocation to allocation (Kuznetsova and Tymofyeyev 2009, 2011a). In contrast, the Brick Tunnel randomization preserves the allocation ratio at every step and its allocation sequences are not equiprobable.

The transition probabilities for the two-group Brick Tunnel randomization are uniquely determined, while for more than two treatment groups the Brick Tunnel allocation sequences could be made to stay closer to the targeted allocation ratio or allowed to deviate more from it while still contained within the brick tunnel.

The algorithm to generate the Brick Tunnel allocation sequences could be programmed—easily in the case of the 2-group studies and with more complex derivations for $K > 2$ treatments. The generation of the Brick Tunnel allocation sequence can be incorporated into a module that analyzes the dose–response data, derives the allocation ratio, and generates the allocation schedule for the next cohort.

While adaptive dose-ranging studies with common to them inconvenient allocation ratio and small cohorts provide the most direct use for the Brick Tunnel randomization, unequal allocation arises in other types of adaptive studies. Multi-arm studies with sample size reestimation and two-stage studies where the second stage allocation ratio differs for new arms and old arms may also end up with an inconvenient allocation ratio and thus a large block size. BT randomization can be used in these studies to better approximate the targeted allocation ratio at the end of enrollment and make the allocation more balanced in time and thus less prone to an accidental bias associated with a time trend.

9.3 Covariate-Adaptive Allocation That Balances Treatment Groups in Important Baseline Covariates at the Interim Analysis

In adaptive design studies, the interim analysis is often performed on a moderate size sample. An imbalance in a strong predictor at the interim stage might lead to biased or unconvincing results and because of that to an incorrect interim decision. In a moderate size sample, randomization that does not explicitly enforce balance in known predictors might lead to an undesirable imbalance in some of them. Thus, the incentives to balance randomization on important predictors in adaptive design studies are strong.

While balance in a small number of predictors (1–3) could be typically achieved with stratified randomization (Zelen 1974; Rosenberger and Lachin 2002), with a large number of predictors stratification often fails to provide desired balance due to a large number of incomplete blocks (Therneau 1993). Dynamic allocation procedures, such as minimization (Taves 1974; Pocock and Simon 1975) or dynamic hierarchical schemes (Heritier et al. 2005; Signorini et al. 1993) can be successfully used to balance the treatment groups in a large number of predictors even in a small study (Therneau 1993; Scott et al. 2002; McEntegart 2003; Rosenberger and Lachin 2002). Usually the versions of these procedures that include a random element are recommended over largely deterministic versions (ICH 1998; CPMP 2003; Kuznetsova 2010).

Often the need to balance randomization within centers—either because of expected differences across centers or to efficiently manage the drug supplies—excludes stratification as a balancing tool since the strata become too small. Covariate-adaptive procedures that provide balance within study centers with or without balancing on other baseline predictors will be discussed in more detail in Sect. 9.3.

However, in studies with unequal allocation common for adaptive design studies, a proper expansion of dynamic allocation procedures to unequal allocation should be used. If the naïve expansion is undertaken, as in minimization examples considered in (Proschan et al. 2011) or version of unequal allocation minimization proposed by (Han et al. 2009), the allocation ratio varies from allocation to allocation (Kuznetsova and Tymofyeyev 2009, 2011a, b, c, 2012). This provides potential for accidental bias (especially in studies with allocation stratified by center) as well as selection and evaluation bias (even in double-blind studies).

Proschan et al. (2011) considered expansion of the biased coin randomization and minimization to 1:2 allocation where variations in allocation probabilities were confounded with a temporal trend so that one treatment had a higher probability to be assigned at the positions where patients were healthier. As a result, the Type I error of the Z-test was inflated. This type I error inflation is a direct consequence of the variations in the allocation ratio and would not happen with unequal allocation procedures that preserve the allocation ratio at every allocation.

Additionally, Proschan et al. (2011) pointed out that in the considered examples of minimization expansion to two-group unequal allocation the re-randomization difference in the treatment group means is shifted away from 0. The shift in the re-randomization distribution lowers the power of the randomization test.

Kuznetsova and Tymofyeyev (2012) showed that the shift phenomenon is not peculiar to minimization or dynamic allocation, but instead is common to all unequal allocation procedures, fixed or dynamic, that have changes in the allocation ratio from allocation to allocation. They derived the asymptotic value of the shift in the re-randomization difference in the treatment group means through the sequence of allocation probabilities at the i-th allocation ($i = 1, 2, \ldots$). They also showed that the asymptotic shift is 0 for procedures that preserve the allocation ratio at every allocation step. More on the randomization test with allocation procedures that do not preserve the allocation ratio at every step can be found in (Kaiser 2012; Han et al. 2013; Kuznetsova and Tymofyeyev 2013a; Kuznetsova 2012).

Kuznetsova and Tymofyeyev offered an easy way to expand any allocation procedure (fixed or dynamic) defined for equal allocation to several treatment arms, to unequal allocation while preserving the allocation ratio at every allocation step (Kuznetsova and Tymofyeyev 2011b, c, 2012).

Suppose the expansion of the allocation procedure to allocation to $K \geq 2$ treatment groups G_l, $l = 1, \ldots, K$ in $C_1 : C_2 : \ldots : C_k$ ratio is desired, where $S = C_1 + C_2 + \ldots + C_k$. First, an equal allocation to S "fake" treatment arms $F_1, F_2, \ldots, F_s$ is executed following the algorithm defined for equal allocation to S arms. Then the first C_1 "fake" treatment arms $F_1 - F_{C_1}$ are mapped to Treatment G_1; the next C_2 "fake" treatment arms $F_{C_1+1} - F_{C_1+C_2}$ are mapped to Treatment G_2; and finally, the last C_k "fake" treatment arms $F_{C_1+\ldots+C_{k-1}+1} - F_S$ are mapped to Treatment G_k. Due to symmetry, such procedure will provide equal allocation to S "fake" treatment arms $F_1, F_2, \ldots, F_s$ at every allocation. Thus, it would automatically provide $C_1 : C_2 : \ldots : C_k$ allocation ratio to treatment groups G_l, $l = 1, \ldots, K$, at every allocation step.

This approach was applied by Kuznetsova and Tymofyeyev to expand to unequal allocation fixed and dynamic allocation procedures, such as biased coin randomization, minimization (Kuznetsova and Tymofyeyev 2012), modified Zelen's approach and dynamic allocation with partial block supplies sent to centers introduced for equal allocation by Morrissey et al. (2010) (Kuznetsova and Tymofyeyev (2011b, c)), and hierarchical allocation procedures that incorporate modified Zelen's approach at center level (Kuznetsova and Tymofyeyev 2014b). This approach works well when the block size is small—for example for 1:2, 1:3, or 2:3 allocation ratios common in clinical trials.

However, when the block size is large, such as 60 in the 14:21:25 allocation example considered in the section on the BT, the balance in treatment assignments overall or within a level of a covariate will not be better than the one provided with the permuted block randomization. In this case, other approaches can be used. For procedures based on modified Zelen's approach, modified Zelen's approach can be replaced with the dynamic allocation based on partial block supplies sent to the centers.

For biased coin randomization with $C_1 : C_2$ (or with probabilities p_1 and p_2, $p_1 < p_2$) allocation to treatment groups G_1 and G_2 the allocation ratio can be made constant in the following way. We will consider allocation to G_1 a preferred allocation after i allocations if

$$N_2 > N_1 \times C_2 / C_1$$

Let us fix the probability to assign G_1 when it is a non-preferred treatment for all allocations at $p_{nonpref} < p_1$. Let us denote by S_i the probability that after i allocations G_1 is the preferred treatment for the $(i+1)$-th allocation. Then the probability $p_{(i+1)\_pref}$ to assign G_1 at $(i+1)$-th allocation when it is a preferred treatment is derived from the equation

$$S_i \, p_{(i+1)\_pref} + (1 - S_i) \, p_{nonpref} = p_1.$$

With this choice of $p_{(i+1)\_pref}$, the probability to assign treatment G_1 at $(i+1)$-th allocation is preserved at p_1. The probabilities $p_{(i+1)\_pref}$ are calculated iteratively. With increasing i, the S_i and p_{i_pref} sequences converge to a periodic pattern with period $C_1 + C_2$. Lower $p_{nonpref}$ results in higher variations in p_{i_pref} across the allocations. Similar approach, with increased complexity, can be used for $C_1{:}C_2$ minimization with large block size.

Extensive simulations show that covariate-adaptive procedures provide good balance in several factors in small and moderate size studies (Taves 1974; Pocock and Simon 1975; Therneau 1993; Begg and Iglewicz 1980; Birkett 1985; Zielhuis et al. 1990; Weir and Lees 2003; Kuznetsova and Tymofyeyev 2012) and thus, meet the needs of adaptive designs.

Likelihood-based methods can be used in the analyses of the data from trials with covariate-adaptive randomization (Rosenberger and Lachin 2002; Rosenberger and Sverdlov 2008). It is recommended to include the factors that randomization balances on in the analysis model to preserve the Type 1 error (Kalish and Begg 1985, 1987); however, it might not be practical when the number of factors is large. In the past, the Type I error rates with covariate-adaptive procedures and the impact of omitting the covariates from the analysis model were studies through simulations. Forsythe (1987) and Weir and Lees (2003) demonstrated that Type I error is preserved when the covariates are included in the analysis of covariance model; for linear models, omission of covariates was shown to lead to conservative Type I errors (Birkett 1985; Weir and Lees 2003).

Recently, important theoretical developments were made by Shao et al. (2010) who established that a test procedure valid for simple randomization is valid for covariate-adaptive randomization provided that the model is specified correctly and includes the covariates used in the randomization procedure. Moreover, they proved that the two-sample t-test (test with omitted covariates) is conservative with covariate-adaptive biased coin randomization and derived bootstrap test that preserves the Type I error with this randomization procedure. Shao and Yu (2013) further advanced the statistical theory of inference with covariate-adaptive randomization by establishing asymptotic results for covariate-adaptive biased coin randomization under generalized linear models with possibly unknown link functions. They showed that for these models the t-test is conservative and constructed a valid test using bootstrap. They illustrated the theory with the examples of binary responses and event counts under the Poisson model as well as exponentially distributed continuous responses.

Furthermore, Ma and Hu (2013) showed that for a large class of covariate-adaptive designs the hypothesis testing is usually conservative and more powerful than with complete randomization.

Excellent review of the latest theoretical developments in the field of covariate-adaptive allocation is provided in Hu et al. (2014).

With advancing understanding of validity of covariate-adaptive allocation, these techniques can find a wider use in adaptive design trials when balance in several important predictors is needed for an accurate interim analysis decision.

9.4 Randomization Techniques That Promote Efficient Drug Use in Multicenter Trials and Better Approximate Targeted Allocation Ratio Within Centers

Adaptive designs are often used early in the drug development, when the drug supplies are scarce or expensive. At the same time, accelerated drug development often necessitates large number of centers to speed up the enrollment in the study. Each center requires its own initial stock of drug supplies to start randomization and additional drug shipments to replenish the drug supplies as subjects continue to be randomized. Thus, the allocation techniques that facilitate economical drug use in the multicenter trials can be very useful in adaptive design trials.

9.4.1 Stratified by Center Fixed Allocation

Stratified by center fixed allocation, where an allocation schedule (typically, a permuted block sequence) is predefined for each center provides full predictability of the required drug supplies. With predictable treatment assignments, each center needs the drug supplies only for the next few subjects on its own allocation schedule, while without such predictability each center needs the drug supplies for all possible combinations of the treatment assignments the next few subjects can get. For example, if in a study with equal allocation to six treatment arms a center requires drug supplies for the next three subjects, with predictable allocation the center needs three randomization drug kits at any point of enrollment compared to $3 \times 6 = 18$ drug kits for unpredictable allocation. This leads to large savings in drug supplies, especially in studies with multiple treatment arms, studies with unequal allocation, and studies where randomization visit drug supplies cannot be reused for later visits and thus are wasted at the end of enrollment.

Stratifying randomization by center might also be required when centers are expected to vary in response due to differences in subject population, medical practice, experience or other reasons.

However, stratified by center allocation becomes problematic if centers are small (which is common at the time of the interim analysis) and the block size is large (due to a large number of arms or unequal allocation common in adaptive design studies). In this case most of the blocks on the randomization schedule have just a couple of subjects at the time of the interim analysis and the treatment group totals might be out of balance for equal allocation studies or deviate from the targeted totals for unequal allocation studies. Incomplete blocks cause even a bigger problem when the randomization needs to be stratified by other baseline factors, thus breaking each center into several strata.

Balance in treatment assignments in studies with large number of centers can be improved if the center-specific permuted blocks are balanced across the centers (Kuznetsova and Ivanova 2006; Song and Kuznetsova 2003; Kuznetsova 2008;

Morrissey et al. 2010). Specifically, in a study with equal allocation to K treatment arms, $K \times K$ Latin squares with columns representing permuted blocks of K allocations are randomly generated. The columns of the first Latin square are sent to the first K centers (centers 1 through K) as the center-specific allocation schedules for the first K subjects enrolled at a center; the columns of the second Latin square are sent to centers $(K+1)$ to $2K$, and so on. When the first K centers have each at least j subjects enrolled, there will be a balance in treatment assignments across the filled rows of the Latin square, that is across the subjects allocated first, second, ..., and j-th in their respective centers. Thus, when all center-specific permuted blocks are barely filled, the balance in treatment assignments is improved through balancing across the centers more than through the balancing within the centers.

Balancing of permuted blocks across centers can be done for unequal allocation as well. When unequal allocation leads to a large block size, constrained permuted blocks (Youden 1964, 1972; Kuznetsova and Ivanova 2006; Song and Kuznetsova 2003; Kuznetsova 2008) that provide a better approximation of the targeted allocation ratio among the first few allocations can be used as the columns of the Latin squares. The task of constructing an unequal allocation Latin square with constrained permuted block columns can be very taxing on a statistician. An easier solution can be found in balancing the center-specific incomplete blocks across centers (Kuznetsova and Ivanova 2006; Song and Kuznetsova 2003; Kuznetsova 2008).

Consider an example of a 6-group study with a 2:3:3:4:4:4 allocation to groups A, B, C, D, E, and F (block size of 20) where the allocation needs to be stratified by center. The centers are expected to enroll up to 20 subjects each and an interim analysis is expected to include on average five subjects per center. Thus, each center needs a block of 20 allocations. To keep an allocation ratio among the first five subjects at a center close to the targeted allocation ratio, the block of 20 allocations is broken into four reasonably balanced incomplete blocks of 5 allocations of the following types: Type 1 = ABDEF, Type 2 = ACDEF, Type 3 = BCDEF, and Type 4 = BCDEF. Next, a random 4×4 Latin square that determines the sequence of four Types of incomplete blocks for each of the first 4 centers is randomly generated. Random permutation of the five treatment assignments within each incomplete block completes the generation of the 20-allocation permuted block schedules for each of the first four centers. Together, the allocations of the first 5 subjects in each of the first 4 centers comprise a complete block of 20. The procedure is repeated for the next four centers and so on. Thus, for studies with a large block size building an allocation schedule of incomplete permuted blocks balanced across centers keeps a within-center allocation ratio close to the targeted one and better approximates the overall allocation ratio at the time of the interim analysis compared to a regular stratified by center permuted block allocation.

Another option of dealing with a large block size in a multicenter study with small centers is the partial block center stratification described for studies with equal allocation to several treatment arms in (Morrissey et al. 2010). With this technique, the allocation schedule is cut into segments smaller than the block size that are distributed across centers at the study initiation. When a center is known to soon approach the end of its first allocation segment, the next segment is assigned to the center.

When all initial segments are filled, the allocation ratio among the subjects allocated using the initial segments is very close to the targeted one. As a result, even when subsequent segments are only partially filled, the overall balance in treatment assignments improves compared to regular stratified by center randomization. When applied to studies with unequal allocation, this technique will result in an overall balance similar to the one achieved with incomplete blocks balanced across centers, but will not necessarily provide a good within-center balance in treatment assignments.

Although these fixed allocation techniques help to improve balance in multicenter studies with stratified by center allocation, they do not provide an exact balance in smaller studies (or at the interim stage) and cannot accommodate several other stratification factors.

9.4.2   Central Randomization

Central randomization where subjects are allocated along the same allocation sequence regardless of their center, provides an excellent balance in treatment assignments and can be stratified by several factors. Central randomization is routinely used in adaptive design dose-ranging studies, where the cohorts are small and stratification by center is hardly an option, and is the most common randomization choice in other types of adaptive design studies. However, it generally demands larger stocks at the sites and might result in within-center imbalance in treatment assignments. When the drug is scarce, automatic support of resupplies through standard triggers (Chap. 15) is often supplemented by micro-management of limited supplies with close stock monitoring and manual shipment orders for faster enrolling sites.

The drug volume required to support central allocation can be reduced if, when a center is out of the drug that a subject is supposed to be allocated to, a subject is allocated to the next treatment on the schedule available at the center [forced allocation (McEntegart 2002)]. This option is offered by all IVRS providers and is often used in clinical trials. When forced allocation is allowed, the sites are stocked and resupplied with enough drug to result in a small percentage of forced allocations. In more complicated cases, the required stock levels and resupply trigger parameters are estimated through simulations (Chap. 15). Allowing small percentage of forced allocations considerably reduces the drug volume in an adaptive design study.

Forced allocation performed automatically by IVRS and concealed from anyone involved in the study prevents possible unblinding at the sites that might happen when the site learns that the subject cannot be allocated because the assigned drug is not available at the site. Additionally, forced allocation allows dealing with unforeseen delays in getting the drug to the sites, lost shipments, drug spoilage, and other problems. It is essential that the sites promptly acknowledge the drug shipments they receive, or else IVRS might unnecessarily force allocate subjects. For example, if the randomization visit shipment is not acknowledged at the site that has a large stock of placebo run-in supplies, IVRS might force allocate several subjects in a row to the placebo arm at that center.

There are no theoretical grounds to justify "maximum allowed" percentage of forced allocations. Although the practice of using forced allocation is widespread and it is believed that small percentage of forced allocations is acceptable to regulatory agencies (McEntegart 2002), there is no clear regulatory guidance on this very helpful for adaptive design studies technique.

Labeling of the drug supplies with central randomization in a study that uses unequal allocation has to be carefully considered when the sites are stocked with drug kits in a ratio different from the allocation ratio. In this case, the double-permuted drug kit labeling (not universally available) must be used as otherwise the partial unblinding of the treatment assignments through divergence in the drug ID labels could arise (Kuznetsova 2001; Lang et al. 2005; Byrom et al. 2011; He et al. 2012). This issue will be considered in more detail in Sect. 9.5.

9.4.3 Dynamic Allocation Procedures That Provide Within-Center Balance, Promote Balance in Other Covariates, and Reduce the Required Volume of Drug Supplies

Where non-dynamic allocation techniques fail to provide required balance in important baseline predictors (that might include center) or cannot support central randomization in a multicenter study with limited drug supplies, dynamic allocation procedures can be used to fulfil these needs.

Modified Zelen's approach described for studies with equal allocation in (Zelen 1974; McEntegart 2008; Morrissey et al. 2010) is the dynamic allocation that provides an excellent within-center balance and overall balance in treatment assignments. It can be stratified by other baseline factors (Zelen 1974) or incorporated in covariate-adaptive (Akazawa et al. 1991; Nishi and Takaishi 2003) or hierarchical allocation procedures (Kuznetsova and Tymofyeyev 2011b, c, 2014b) to provide balance in covariates other than center.

In studies with equal allocation to several treatment arms the simplest version of the modified Zelen's approach works in the following way. At study initiation a full block of treatment assignments is made available for allocation at each center; accordingly, a full block of randomization drug supplies is sent to each center. If a center is expected to enroll more than one block of subjects, the second block of allocations (and respective randomization drug supplies) will be later provided to the center. However, the second block of treatment assignments will not be made available for randomization at the center until the first block of randomization assignments is completely used. The central allocation schedule is prepared for the study and the subjects are allocated to the first unused treatment assignment on the central schedule available for randomization at their center. The gaps on the allocation schedule formed when a center cannot allocate a subject to the next treatment on the randomization sequence are filled in by the subjects allocated later at other centers. Thus, at the time of the interim analysis the randomization schedule will mostly consist of filled blocks providing an excellent balance in treatment assignments (Morrissey et al. 2010) even when centers have just one or two subjects each.

When stratification by baseline factors is required, a separate central allocation schedule is prepared for each stratum and subjects are allocated to the first unused treatment assignment on the schedule for their stratum available for randomization at their center.

The logistics or drug resupplies with this version of modified Zelen's approach is very simple, as the resupplies are sent in complete blocks regardless of what was used in the center.

With the described version of the modified Zelen's approach the sequence of treatment assignments at any given center is a permuted block sequence; however, this sequence is not prespecified in advance, but is instead determined by the order of subjects' entry into the study and the central randomization schedule. In studies with equal allocation to two arms or open-label studies, a permuted block sequence with the smallest block size S might be considered to have too many predictable allocations. In this case, one can use the version of the modified Zelen's approach where the imbalance in treatments assignments at a center (the range of the within-center treatment totals) is allowed to exceed 1, but is not allowed to exceed a pre-specified threshold M. This version requires larger volume of drug in circulation as M blocks of treatment assignments are available for allocation at any time. Thus, M blocks of randomization drug kits are sent to every center at study initiation. The $(M+1)$-th block of allocations is made available at a center when the first block of M allocations is completely used; by that time, the $(M+1)$-th block of randomization drug supplies should be received by the center.

When in a study with equal allocation the number of treatment arms is large and the centers are small, sending a whole block of supplies to each center could be wasteful. To reduce the drug waste, Morrissey et al. (2010) proposed to use a dynamic allocation procedure with partial block of supplies sent to the centers. This procedure is similar to modified Zelen's approach, except that partial blocks and not complete blocks of allocations are assigned to the centers. For example, in a study with seven arms where most centers are expected to enroll two to three subjects, partial blocks of three will be assigned to the centers. The subjects will then be allocated along the central allocation schedule—to the first treatment available for allocation at their center. As Goodale and McEntegart (2013) point out, this technique generally reduces the potential for selection bias as the contents of the incomplete blocks is unknown at the site.

These dynamic allocation procedures developed for studies with equal allocation could be even more useful in studies with unequal allocation where drug supplies issues are especially challenging. However, similar to minimization, these procedures need to be expanded to unequal allocation in a way that preserves the allocation ratio at every allocation (Kuznetsova and Tymofyeyev 2011b, c). If the modified Zelen's approach is naively generalized by making a permuted block of allocations (and drug kits) available at the study centers [as in (Frane 1998)], the achieved allocation ratio will vary depending on the order of allocation within a center. In the example of 2:1 allocation to Active and Control treatments, the probability of Control allocation will exceed 1/3 for the first and third allocations in center-specific blocks of three subjects, and will be below 1/3 in the second allocation in the block (Kuznetsova and Tymofyeyev 2011b, c). This problem is also observed with naïve expansion of the dynamic allocation with partial block supplies sent to the centers (Kuznetsova and Tymofyeyev 2011b, c).

Kuznetsova and Tymofyeyev (2011b, c) expanded these dynamic allocation procedures to unequal allocation following the allocation ratio preserving approach described in Sect. 9.2. For the partial block dynamic allocation an extra step is required: to define acceptable partial blocks of the drug supplies that preserve the symmetry with respect to the S fake treatments. A way to define such blocks is described in detail in (Kuznetsova and Tymofyeyev 2011b, c).

Using the partial block dynamic allocation in adaptive design dose-finding studies might reduce the amount of drug required to support the unknown allocation ratio in the next cohort. Indeed, this approach will not require all treatments to be available at every site. However, a valid drug resupply strategy for such studies and implementation aspects of this approach in dose-finding studies need to be further developed.

When randomization needs to be balanced on more baseline factors than stratified modified Zelen's approach can handle, modified Zelen approach at a center level can be successfully incorporated in a minimization-type covariate-adaptive procedure (Akazawa et al. 1991; Nishi and Takaishi 2003) or a hierarchical dynamic balancing scheme (Kuznetsova and Tymofyeyev 2011b, c, 2014b). For studies with unequal allocation, an expansion that preserves the allocation ratio at every allocation should be used.

Overall, a variety of advanced allocation techniques can be used in adaptive design multicenter studies to help reduce the required volume of drug while providing a good balance in treatment assignments in a small interim sample. When the within-center balance as well as balance in several important baseline covariates is required, dynamic allocation techniques based on modified Zelen's approach or partial blocks of supplies sent to the centers often perform much better than fixed allocation procedures, especially in studies with several treatment arms or large block size.

9.5 Allocation in Open-Label Adaptive Design Studies

Some randomized adaptive design studies conducted early in drug development are open-label—often because blinding is very difficult and thus is not considered practical in a non-pivotal study. Predictability of upcoming treatment assignments is a problem in open-label studies (mostly, in single-center studies or multicenter studies with randomization stratified by center where the investigator knows the complete sequence of treatment assignments) and might lead to a selection bias. Permuted block randomization commonly used in clinical trials is partially predictable because the allocation sequence is known to achieve the exactly targeted allocation ratio at the end of each block. Thus, the allocation procedures less predictable than permuted block randomization help reduce the potential for selection bias in open-label studies.

A number of allocation procedures that do not require reaching the exact allocation ratio at any point of randomization were developed for two-group studies with 1:1 allocation. Complete randomization (Rosenberger and Lachin 2002), where each subject is allocated independently in 1:1 ratio, is absolutely unpredictable, but can result in a notable imbalance in treatment group totals, especially in smaller studies. Biased Coin randomization where a subject is allocated with higher probability to the underrepresented group (Efron 1971) generally provides a good balance in treatment assignments throughout the enrollment. However, there exists a small probability that it will result in a relatively large imbalance in a small sample (Markaryan and Rosenberger 2010).

When the imbalance in treatment totals in a two-arm study with equal allocation needs to be tightly controlled, one of the allocation procedures that limit the imbalance in treatment assignments at a prespecified level can be used. Among these procedures are the replacement randomization (Pocock 1979), modified replacement randomization (Abel 1987), maximal procedure (Berger et al. 2003), Soares and Wu (1983) big stick design, Chen's biased coin design with imbalance tolerance (Chen 1999), Ehrenfest urn design (Chen 2000), and Baldi Antognini and Giovagnolli's (2004) adjustable biased coin design (with limited allowed imbalance). These procedures restrict the set of allowed allocation sequences to those for which the absolute imbalance in assignments to Treatments A and B after i allocations does not exceed prespecified threshold b: $|N_{Bi} - N_{Ai}| \leq b$, $i = 1, 2, \ldots$. Here N_{Ai} and N_{Bi} are the numbers of subjects allocated to treatments A and B, respectively, within the first i allocations. The procedures above differ in how they assign the probabilities to the allowed sequences.

In spite of being well described and studied in statistical literature, these procedures remain under-used in open-label studies, as they are typically not included in the standard randomization tool kit.

In most cases, these procedures can be easily expanded to an equal allocation to $K > 2$ treatment arms, with the imbalance in treatment totals across K arms after i allocations defined as the range of the treatment totals N_{ji}, $j = 1, \ldots, K$. Expanding these procedures to unequal allocation is a different matter.

For $C_1 : C_2$ $(C_1 \neq C_2)$ allocation to Treatments A and B the absolute imbalance in treatment assignments after i allocations is commonly defined as $|N_{Bi} - N_{Ai} \times C_2/C_1|$ (or proportional to this difference) (Salama et al. 2008; Han et al. 2009). Until recently, the problem of designing an unequal allocation procedure that includes all sequences that comply with a prespecified imbalance threshold $|N_{Bi} - N_{Ai} \times C_2/C_1| \leq b$ and preserve the allocation ratio at every allocation was not resolved. Existing allocation procedures either did not preserve the allocation ratio at every allocation (Salama et al. 2008) or did not include all allocation sequences that comply with the prespecified imbalance threshold (Zhao and Weng 2011).

Kuznetsova and Tymofyeyev offered a solution to this problem: the Wide Brick Tunnel randomization for $C_1 : C_2$ $(C_1 \neq C_2)$ allocation to Treatments A and B (Kuznetsova and Tymofyeyev 2014a). The procedure starts with the Brick Tunnel randomization which represents the sets of sequences that comply with the smallest possible imbalance threshold $b_{BT} = (C_2 - 1)/C_1 + 1$. Then selected pairs of consecutive treatment assignments of the Brick Tunnel sequences are switched places with probability $0 < \delta < 1$, thus expanding the set of allowed allocation sequences. The switches proceed until the set of allowed sequences includes all sequences that satisfy the imbalance requirement $|N_{Bi} - N_{Ai} \times C_2/C_1| \leq b$. The implementation details are described in (Kuznetsova and Tymofyeyev 2014a). Since Brick Tunnel randomization preserves the allocation ratio at every step and adding a random switch of consecutive allocations to this procedure leaves the allocation ratio intact, the Wide Brick Tunnel allocation keeps the allocation ratio constant at all allocations.

The main application of the Wide Brick Tunnel allocation is in two-arm open-label studies with unequal allocation. When the block size is large, the Wide Brick Tunnel randomization keeps the allocation ratio reasonably close to the targeted allocation (much closer than the permuted block schedule but not as close as the BT schedule), while reducing predictability compared to the Brick Tunnel randomization. Wide Brick Tunnel randomization might also be used to construct a randomization procedure for an unequal allocation in an open-label study with >2 arms [see examples in (Kuznetsova and Tymofyeyev 2014a)].

The switch technique could be used on its own to reduce the selection bias, in particular, in studies with equal allocation to >2 treatment arms. Often an adaptive design dose-finding study starts with an equal allocation to all arms to accumulate response information before the adaptive allocation begins. As the number of treatment arms is typically large—for example, placebo, active control, and six active doses—the permuted block schedule with the smallest block size S ($S=8$ in our example) is used to allocate subjects. Due to a large number of arms, most of the treatment assignments in an open-label study are not fully predictable—except the treatment assignments at the ends of the permuted blocks. The switch of the mS-th and the $(mS+1)$-th treatment assignments on a permuted block schedule (the last treatment in the m-th block and the first treatment in the $(m+1)$-th block) with probability $0 < \delta < 1$ makes the last assignment in the m-th block unpredictable. The switch could be executed for all permuted blocks on the schedule.

To reduce the potential for selection bias in open-label adaptive design trials with equal or unequal allocation, permuted block randomization can be replaced with one of the less predictable allocation procedures.

9.6 Avoiding Unblinding of the Adaptive Decisions or Treatment Assignments Through Allocation Numbers or Drug Codes

9.6.1 Avoiding Unblinding of the Adaptive Decisions Through Allocation Numbers

A common adaptive two-stage design includes Stage I with a large number of arms followed by Stage II where some of the treatment arms, for example, less efficacious doses of the experimental treatment, might be discontinued (Chaps. 4 and 14). If a common allocation schedule is prepared for both stages with the option to cross out the dropped arms for Stage II randomization, the possibility to unblind the adaptive decision through the allocation schedule arises (Byrom et al. 2011). Indeed, anyone with access to Stage II sequence of allocation numbers will see what fraction of allocation numbers remains unfilled on the Stage II schedule and deduce how many arms were dropped in reversed engineering (see Chap. 14). Moreover, if Stage I schedule had unequal allocation, it might be possible to identify the dropped arms.

The adaptive decision could be easily disguised by generating a separate schedule for Stage II. It could also be disguised with a single schedule for both Stages if the allocation numbers are kept blinded until the data base lock and the subjects are followed by their baseline numbers. Alternatively, subjects could be assigned sequential allocation numbers in order of randomization (as with a dynamic allocation) or scrambled (non-sequential) allocation numbers. Byrom et al. (2011), however, warn of other pitfalls of modifications to the original schedule.

9.6.2 Unblinding Through the Divergence of the Drug ID Sequences

Adaptive design studies with changes to the allocation ratio across randomization cohorts provide potential for partial unblinding of the treatment assignments through the drug kit labels. Indeed, if the drug ID codes are generated using a common permuted block schedule, the sequences of the drug IDs diverge with time (Kuznetsova 2001; Lang et al. 2005; Byrom et al. 2011, He et al. 2012). In some cases, all types of drug could be identified late in the study.

A simple solution is to randomly permute the sequence of drug codes within each drug type (Kuznetsova 2001; Lang et al. 2005), a technique often referred to as "double-randomized" or "double-permuted" or "scrambled" drug codes. Byrom et al. (2011) note that leaving the gaps in the drug code schedule allows one to use the reserved codes to introduce new treatments. Double-permuted drug IDs could also be used to package the drug supplies shareable across several studies with the same product. Sharing the drug supplies across the studies allows pursuing several indications with limited drug supplies early in the drug development, where Phase IIa/IIb adaptive design studies would fit.

However, drug management with double-permuted drug codes is not uniformly available and often costly, thus the need for it should be evaluated during the study design. Below we will consider several examples of the adaptive design studies where unblinding through divergence in drug IDs can occur and describe the extent of such unblinding.

9.6.2.1 Adaptive Design Dose-Finding Study with a Single Image or a Double-Dummy Masking Strategy

A typical example of an adaptive design study with changes to the allocation ratio is an adaptive design dose-finding study. In such studies the allocation ratio for the next cohort is determined by the performance of the dose arms in the previous cohorts and is not known in advance. The allocation algorithm is designed to allocate more subjects to the doses of most interest. The placebo arm is commonly allocated at the same ratio in all cohorts. The allocation schedule for the next cohort is prepared when the required allocation ratio becomes known.

When a study uses the same image tablets for all doses and placebo (a single image masking), typically a common permuted block drug ID schedule is prepared for all doses. Since the placebo arm is allocated at the same ratio in all cohorts, its drug IDs will increase at a steady pace. However, the drug IDs for the doses that enroll more subjects in the later cohorts will grow faster than the placebo ID, while the drug IDs for less used doses will grow slowly.

In some cases, the pattern of divergent drug IDs allows personnel to link the drug IDs to specific treatment arms. For example, consider a study where four doses of the experimental drug and placebo have the same image tablets. The drug ID schedule is prepared in equal ratio with the block size 5. Subjects are randomized in cohorts of 20; in each cohort placebo is assigned to exactly 20 % of subjects (four subjects). If the study design allows stopping enrollment in one or two lowest doses should they be found inefficient, one will know if one or both doses were stopped by the number of drug IDs left unused in each block as the randomization proceeds. The CIDs will also reveal if there is a group that performs better than others (and thus, has more subjects enrolled into it) and how many such groups there are. When the drug ID sequences diverge, the groups of subjects randomized to the same arm will be easily identified. In some cases, it will be possible to identify the arms—for example, placebo arm, or the high dose arm when the dose response is known to be monotone.

When in a dose-finding study tablets of different doses have different images, the double-dummy strategy is often employed to mask the treatment. To that end, a matching image tablet is prepared for each of the doses; each subject gets an active tablet for the dose he is allocated and a placebo tablet for each of the remaining doses. Typically, a separate drug ID schedule is prepared for each pair of tablets— an active tablet and a placebo tablet—corresponding to the same dose.

Consider the same example of the dose-ranging study with four active doses of the experimental drug and the placebo arm that now employs a double dummy strategy. Since each subject will receive one active tablet for the dose he is allocated to and three placebo tablets for the remaining doses, three times more placebo tablets than active tablets are packaged for each dose. Four separate drug ID schedules are prepared in 1:3 (Active to Placebo) ratio for each of the four doses.

With double-dummy blinding and separate schedules for each dose, stopping enrollment into a certain dose will be immediately obvious. Indeed, the placebo drug IDs on that dose schedule will continue to grow, while the gaps in the schedule corresponding to the Active tablets will remain unfilled. The arm with low enrollment will be manifested by having ¾ of the drug IDs in the blocks growing fast (Placebo drug IDs), while the remaining ¼ of the drug IDs (Active drug IDs) will lag behind and fill in at a slower pace. Similarly, the arm with high enrollment will have ¼ of its drug IDs (Active) filling in fast, and the rest of the drug IDs (Placebo) lagging behind. Thus, if there is a dose–response, the double-dummy blinding strategy with separate drug ID schedules for each dose will eventually unblind the performance of each dose through divergent drug IDs of active and placebo drug types. The individual allocations of the subjects in later cohorts will also be unblinded.

The problem remains if a single schedule is used for all doses.

9.6.2.2 Two-Stage Study with Stage II Allocation Ratio Unknown in Advance

Another potentially unblinding scenario common for adaptive design studies is when the allocation ratio is constant throughout a stage of the study, but is unknown in advance. For example, in two-stage trials with new doses included in Stage II, the allocation ratio for Stage II is often unequal as it differs for the old doses included in Stage I and the new doses added in Stage II. In addition, this ratio might depend on the actual numbers of subjects enrolled in Stage I arms before the randomization into Stage I was stopped. As the Stage II drug needs to be packaged before the exact allocation ratio for Stage II becomes known, the drug ID schedule is generated in the drug ratio somewhere in the middle of the possible range. Discrepancy between the actual allocation ratio and the drug packaging ratio provides a potential for partial, and in some cases, full unblinding.

9.6.2.3 Multicenter Study Where Drug Supplies Are Packaged in a Ratio Different from the Allocation Ratio

Divergence of drug IDs can also occur in an adaptive design multicenter study with unequal allocation ratio even when the allocation ratio remains constant throughout the study. Often in a multicenter study with a skewed allocation ratio and central allocation the drug supplies are packaged in a ratio different from the allocation ratio. This is done to provide the sites with enough of the "low ratio" treatment kits to minimize the chance of a site running out of these kits in the event a few "low ratio" treatment assignments in a row are made at the site. This typically results in the smaller groups being overstocked and the bigger groups being understocked in the set of supplies sent to the sites initially and maintained at the sites. This leads to a more "balanced" drug ratio of the site stocks, and thus, the packaged drugs, compared to the allocation ratio.

For example, in a 200-center study with 7:3:1 allocation to Experimental Drug, Active Control, and Placebo, where centers are expected to enroll about 6 subjects each, the initial pack might include four Experimental, three Active Control, and two Placebo drug kits. Most likely, this drug packaging ratio would be derived through informal considerations along the following lines. If a block of $7+3+1$ drug kits is sent to each site, there is a chance that at one of the sites the first two subjects are both allocated to Placebo. To avoid drug shortage in this case, two placebo kits instead of one are sent to each site. Also, there is no need to send seven Experimental drug kits to each site: four Experimental drug kits are sufficient as there will be enough time to send in replacement kits for the first couple of subjects before the fifth subject is allocated to Experimental Drug at the site. Formal considerations to justify this approach can be based on the acceptable probabilities of a stock-out for the resupply strategy used in the trial.

However, packaging the drug in 4:3:2 ratio will lead to the divergence of the drug ID sequences. Indeed, suppose a permuted block drug ID schedule was prepared in

4:3:2 ratio (block size 9). The randomization schedule, nevertheless, is a permuted block schedule with the allocation ratio of 7:3:1 (block size 11). At the study start, a block of nine drug kits is sent to each center and maintained through resupplies. A total of 200 blocks are sent out at study initiation. Thus, when randomization starts, the resupplies from blocks 201 and above on the drug ID schedule are sent out.

When the first 55 subjects are randomized into the study (5 blocks of 11), there are 35 subjects allocated to Experimental Drug, 15 subjects allocated to Active Control, and 5 subjects allocated to Placebo. That far into randomization, it is clear that the replacement drug kits sent to the sites are coming from different blocks on the replacement part of the drug ID schedule. If the 56th subject is allocated to Experimental Drug, the replacement drug ID will come from block 209 on the drug ID schedule; if he is allocated to Active Control the replacement drug ID will come from block 206; if he is allocated to Placebo the replacement drug ID will come from block 203.

Thus, if the drug IDs are not scrambled, the drug IDs for replacement kits will allow one to distinguish kits for arms A, B, and C very early in randomization. Someone with access to the complete sequence of the drug IDs received by all centers will be able to identify the treatment groups corresponding to the replacement kits in the considered example. In other examples, when some of the treatment arms have the same allocation ratios (as in 2:2:5:5 allocation), such observer will be able to differentiate large groups from the small ones, but not to distinguish between the two groups with the same ratio.

Study personnel that have access only to the drug IDs at their own site might or might not be unblinded or biased through the drug IDs they see.

In addition to considered examples, differences in the dropout rates among the treatment groups as well as up- or down- titration for efficacy or safety reasons can also provide the potential for unblinding through drug codes.

9.7 Discussion

There is a wide opportunity for the use of advanced randomization techniques in adaptive design studies. In dose-ranging studies, an inconvenient allocation ratio in a small cohort is better targeted with the Brick Tunnel randomization than with permuted block or complete randomization. In open-label adaptive design studies the allocation techniques less predictable than permuted block randomization help reduce the selection bias.

Dynamic allocation techniques are often required in adaptive design trials. Covariate-adaptive allocation can ensure balance in a large number of important predictors in a small interim analysis sample and thus reduce the risk of biased results leading to a wrong interim decision. In multicenter adaptive design trials, dynamic allocation methods provide within-center balance in treatment assignments and, if needed, balance in other important predictors. They also help efficiently manage limited and expensive drug supplies and reduce the required volume of drug supplies and the number of resupplies shipments.

In adaptive design studies IVRS that governs the complicated trial logistics is already in place (Chap. 12). Many IVRS providers have solid experience using dynamic allocation techniques, with all quality control steps [validation, testing as described in (Downs et al. 2010)] in place. Nevertheless, dynamic allocation remains underused in adaptive design studies in the pharmaceutical industry, even when it is clearly advantageous. As a result, the examples of studies with imbalance in one of the known important predictors large enough to question the study results are not uncommon (Rosenberger and Sverdlov 2008; Pond et al. 2010).

The major reason for reluctance to use dynamic allocation techniques is the uncertainty of regulatory acceptance of such techniques. While ICH Guidelines list covariate-adaptive allocation among other accepted allocation methods, its use was discouraged by the Points to Consider on Adjustment for Baseline Covariates (EAEMP CPMP 2003). This opinion was much debated in the literature (see Rosenberger and Sverdlov 2008; Buyse and McEntegart 2004) and the language that discouraged the use of dynamic allocation was removed from the latest Draft Guideline on Adjustment for Baseline Covariates (EMA CHMP 2013).

More positive regulatory views and better understanding of dynamic allocation due to recent advances in theory of inference following covariate-adaptive randomization (Shao et al. 2010; Shao and Yu 2013; Ma and Hu 2013; Hu et al. 2014) are likely to lead to a wider use of these procedures in adaptive design trials.

References

Abel U (1987) Modified replacement randomization. Stat Med 6:127–135

Akazawa K, Odaka T, Sakamoto M, Ohtsuki S, Shimada M, Kamakura T, Nose Y (1991) A random allocation system with the minimization method for multi-institutional clinical trials. J Med Syst 15(4):311–319

Antognini AB, Giovagnoli A (2004) A new 'biased coin design' for the sequential allocation of two treatments. J Roy Stat Soc C 53:651–664

Begg CB, Iglewicz B (1980) A treatment allocation procedure for sequential clinical trials. Biometrics 36:81–90

Berger VW, Ivanova A, Knoll M (2003) Minimizing predictability while retaining balance through the use of less restrictive randomization procedures. Stat Med 22:3017–3028. doi:10.1002/sim.1538

Birkett NJ (1985) Adaptive allocation in randomized controlled trials. Control Clin Trials 6:146–155

Buyse M, McEntegart D (2004) Achieving balance in clinical trials: an unbalanced view from EU regulators. Appl Clin Trials 13:36–40

Byrom B, McEntegart D, Nicholls G (2011) Adaptive infrastructure. In: Pong A, Chow S-C (eds) Handbook of adaptive designs in pharmaceutical and clinical development. Taylor and Francis Group, London, pp 20-1–20-25

Chen YP (1999) Biased coin design with imbalance tolerance. Comm Stat Stoch Model 15:953–975

Chen YP (2000) Which design is better? Ehrenfest urn versus biased coin. Adv Appl Probab 32:738–749

Committee for Proprietary Medicinal Products (CPMP) (2003) Points to consider on adjustment for baseline covariates. European Medicines Agency, London

Downs M, Tucker K, Christ-Schmidt H, Wittes J (2010) Some practical problems in implementing randomization. Clin Trials 7:235–245

Efron B (1971) Forcing a sequential experiment to be balanced. Biometrika 58:403–417

EMA Committee for Medicinal Products for Human Use. Guideline on adjustment for baseline covariates. Draft. 26 Apr 2013

Forsythe AB (1987) Validity and power of tests when groups have been balanced for prognostic factors. Comput Stat Data Anal 5:193–200

Frane JW (1998) A method of biased coin randomization, its implementation, and its validation. Drug Inf J 32:423–432, 0092-8615/98

Gaydos B, Krams M, Perevozskaya I, Bretz F, Liu Q, Gallo P (2006) PhRMA working group on adaptive designs: adaptive dose–response studies. Drug Inf J 40:451–461

Goodale H, McEntegart D (2013) The role of technology in avoiding bias in the design and execution of clinical trials. Open Access J Clin Trials 5:13–21

Han B, Enas NH, McEntegart D (2009) Randomization by minimization for unbalanced treatment allocation. Stat Med 28:3329–3346. doi:10.1002/sim.3710

Han B, Yu M, McEntegart D (2013) Weighted re-randomization tests for minimization with unbalanced allocation. Pharm Stat 12:243–253. doi:10.1002/pst.1577

He W, Kuznetsova OM, Harmer MA, Leahy CJ, Anderson KM, Dossin DN, Li L, Bolognese JA, Tymofyeyev Y, Schindler JS (2012) Practical considerations and strategies for executing adaptive clinical trials. Drug Inf J 46:160–174. doi:10.1177/0092861512436580

Heritier S, Gebski V, Pillai A (2005) Dynamic balancing randomization in controlled clinical trials. Stat Med 24:3729–3741. doi:10.1002/sim.2421

Hu F., Hu Y, Ma Z, Rosenberger WF (2014) Adaptive randomization for balancing over covariates. Wiley Interdisciplinary Reviews: Computational Statistics, 6, 288–303

ICH (1998) ICH Topic E9: statistical principles for clinical trials, available at http://www.ich.org/LOB/media/MEDIA485.pdf

Kaiser LD (2012) Dynamic randomization and a randomization model for clinical trials data. Stat Med 31:3858–3873. doi:10.1002/sim.5448

Kalish LA, Begg CB (1985) Treatment allocation methods in clinical trials: a review. Stat Med 4:129–144

Kalish LA, Begg CB (1987) The impact of treatment allocation procedures on nominal significance levels and bias. Control Clin Trials 8:121–135

Kuznetsova OM (2001) Why permutation is even more important in IVRS drug codes schedule generation than in patient randomization schedule generation. Control Clin Trials 22:69–71, Letter to the Editor

Kuznetsova OM (2008) Randomization schedule. In: D'Agostino R, Sullivan L, Massaro J (eds) Wiley encyclopedia of clinical trials. Wiley, Hoboken, NJ. doi:10.1002/9780471462422. eoct314, Published Online: 19 Sep 2008

Kuznetsova OM (2010) On the second role of the random element in minimization. Short communication regarding the short communication by D. Taves on "The Use of Minimization in Clinical Trials". Contemp Clin Trials 31:587–588. doi:10.1016/j.cct.2010.07.010

Kuznetsova OM (2012) Considerations in the paper by Proschan, Brittain, and Kammerman are not an argument against minimization. In response to Vance W Berger 'Minimization: not all it's cracked up to be', Clin Trials 2011; 8: 443. Clin Trials 9:370

Kuznetsova OM, Ivanova A (2006) Allocation in randomized clinical trials. In: Dmitrienko A, Chuang-Stein C, D'Agostino R (eds) Pharmaceutical statistics using SAS. SAS Press, Cary, NC, pp 213–236

Kuznetsova OM, Tymofyeyev Y (2009) Brick tunnel randomization—a way to accommodate a problematic allocation ratio in adaptive design dose finding studies. ASA proceedings of the joint statistical meetings. American Statistical Association, Alexandria, VA, pp 1356–1367

Kuznetsova OM, Tymofyeyev Y (2011a) Brick tunnel randomization for unequal allocation to two or more treatment groups. Stat Med 30:812–824. doi:10.1002/sim.4167

Kuznetsova OM, Tymofyeyev Y (2011b) Expansion of the modified Zelen's approach randomization and dynamic randomization with partial block supplies at the centers to unequal allocation. ASA proceedings of the joint statistical meetings. American Statistical Association, Miami Beach, FL

Kuznetsova OM, Tymofyeyev Y (2011c) Expansion of the modified Zelen's approach randomization and dynamic randomization with partial block supplies at the centers to unequal allocation. Contemp Clin Trials 32:962–972. doi:10.1016/j.cct.2011.08.006

Kuznetsova OM, Tymofyeyev Y (2012) Preserving the allocation ratio at every allocation with biased coin randomization and minimization in studies with unequal allocation. Stat Med 31:701–723. doi:10.1002/sim.4447

Kuznetsova OM, Tymofyeyev Y (2013a) Shift in re-randomization distribution with conditional randomization test. Pharmaceut Stat 12:82–91. doi:10.1002/pst.1556

Kuznetsova OM, Tymofyeyev Y (2013b) Expanding brick tunnel randomization to allow for larger imbalance in treatment totals in studies with unequal allocation. Proceedings of the joint statistical association 2013 meetings, Montreal, QC, Canada, 4–8 Aug 2013

Kuznetsova OM, Tymofyeyev Y (2014a) Wide Brick tunnel randomization—an unequal allocation procedure that limits the imbalance in treatment totals. Stat Med 33:1514–1530. doi:10.1002/sim.6051

Kuznetsova OM, Tymofyeyev Y (2014b) Hierarchical dynamic allocation procedures based on modified Zelen's approach in multi-regional studies with unequal allocation. J Biopharm Stat 24:1–17

Lang M, Wood R, McEntegart D (2005) Protecting the blind. GCPj p. 10 Nov 2005 14/11/05 3:39 pm

Ma W, Hu F (2013) Hypothesis testing of covariate-adaptive randomized clinical trials under generalized linear models. Paper presented at Joint Statistical Association 2013 Meetings, Montreal, Canada, 4–8 Aug 2013

Markaryan T, Rosenberger WF (2010) Exact properties of Efron's biased coin randomization procedure. Ann Stat 38:1546–1567. doi:10.1214/09-AOS758

McEntegart D (2002) Forced randomization when using interactive voice response systems. Appl Clin Trials 12(10):2–10

McEntegart D (2003) The pursuit of balance using stratified and dynamic randomization techniques: an overview. Drug Inf J 37:293–308

McEntegart D (2008) Blocked randomization. In: D'Agostino R, Sullivan L, Massaro J (eds) Wiley encyclopedia of clinical trials. Wiley, Hoboken. DOI:10.1002/9780471462422.eoct301. Accessed 13 June 2008

Morrissey M, McEntegart D, Lang M (2010) Randomisation in double-blind multicentre trials with many treatments. Contemp Clin Trials 31:381–391. doi:10.1016./j/cct/2010.05.002

Nishi T, Takaishi A (2003) An extended minimization method to assure similar means of continuous prognostic variable between treatment groups. Jpn J Biomet 24:43–55

Parke T (2008) Adaptive clinical trials in the real world. Paper presented at Massachusetts Biotechnology Council, 23 Apr 2008, Cambridge, MA

Pocock SJ (1979) Allocation of patients to treatment in clinical trials. Biometrics 35:183–197

Pocock SJ, Simon R (1975) Sequential treatment assignment with balancing for prognostic factors in the controlled clinical trial. Biometrics 31:103–115

Pond GR, Tang PA, Welch SA, Chen EX (2010) Trends in the application of dynamic allocation methods in multi-arm cancer clinical trials. Clin Trials 7(3):227–234

Proschan M, Brittain E, Kammerman L (2011) Minimize the use of minimization with unequal allocation. Biometrics 67(3):1135–1141. doi:10.1111/j.1541-0420.2010.01545.x

Rosenberger WF, Lachin JM (2002) Randomization in clinical trials. Wiley, New York, NY

Rosenberger WF, Sverdlov O (2008) Handling covariates in the design of clinical trials. Stat Sci 23:404–419

Salama I, Ivanova A, Qaqish B (2008) Efficient generation of constrained block allocation sequences. Stat Med 27:1421–1428. doi:10.1002/sim3014

Scott NW, McPherson GC, Ramsay CR, Campbell MK (2002) The method of minimization for allocation to clinical trials: a review. Control Clin Trials 23:662–674

Shao J, Yu X (2013) Validity of tests under covariate-adaptive biased coin randomization and generalized linear models. Biometrics 69:960–969. doi:10.1111/biom.12062

Shao J, Yu X, Zhong B (2010) A theory of testing hypotheses under covariate adaptive randomization. Biometrika 97:347–360

Signorini DF, Leung O, Simes RJ, Beller E, Gebski VJ (1993) Dynamic balanced randomisation for clinical trials. Stat Med 12:2343–2350

Soares JF, Wu CF (1983) Some restricted randomization rules in sequential designs. Comm Stat Theor Meth 12:2017–2034

Song C, Kuznetsova OM (2003) Implementing Constrained or Balanced Across the Centers Randomization with SAS v8 Procedure PLAN, PharmaSUG 2003 proceedings, Miami, FL, pp. 473–479. Accessed 4–7 May 2003

Taves D (1974) Minimization: a new method of assigning subjects to treatment and control groups. Clin Pharmacol Ther 15:443–453

Therneau TM (1993) How many stratification factors are "too many" to use in a randomization plan? Control Clin Trials 14(2):98–108

Weir CJ, Lees KR (2003) Comparison of stratification and adaptive methods for treatment allocation in an acute stroke clinical trial. Stat Med 22:705–726

Youden WJ (1964) Inadmissible random assignments. Technometrics 6:103–104

Youden WJ (1972) Randomization and experimentation. Technometrics 14:13–22

Zelen M (1974) The randomization and stratification of patients to clinical trials. J Chronic Dis 27:365–375

Zhao W, Weng Y (2011) Block urn design—a new randomization algorithm for sequential trials with two or more treatments and balanced or unbalanced allocation. Contemp Clin Trials 32(6):953–961

Zielhuis GA, Straatman H, van'T Hof-Grootenboer AE, van Lier HJJ, Rach GH, van den Broek P (1990) The choice of a balanced allocation method for a clinical trial in otitis media with effusion. Stat Med 9:237–246

Chapter 10
Response-Adaptive Randomization for Clinical Trials

Lanju Zhang and William F. Rosenberger

Abstract Response-adaptive randomization in clinical trials uses accumulated patient response data to adjust the allocation probability for the next patient, so that a particular objective, for example, more patients assigned to the better performing treatment arm, can be achieved. This ethically appealing randomization procedure has gained significant attention in academia, regulatory agencies, and industry in light of widespread of adaptive clinical trial designs with the FDA's Critical Path Initiative (FDA: Innovation or stagnation: challenge and opportunity on the critical path to new medical products, 2004). However, this procedure has also generated unmatched controversy since its first application in the ECMO trial (Bartlett et al., Pediatrics 76:479–487, 1985). In this chapter, we will describe response-adaptive randomization procedures from both frequentist and Bayesian perspectives and provide a comprehensive assessment on situations where such procedures should be applied.

Keywords Bayesian response-adaptive randomization • Benefit–risk assessment • Optimal allocation procedures • Response-adaptive randomization • Urn models

L. Zhang (✉)
Data and Statistical Sciences, Abbvie Inc., One North Waukegan Road,
R436/AP9A-LL, North Chicago, IL 60064, USA
e-mail: lanju.zhang@abbvie.com

W.F. Rosenberger
Department of Statistics, George Mason University, 4400 University Drive,
MS 4A7, Fairfax, VA 22030, USA
e-mail: wrosenbe@gmu.edu

10.1 Introduction

Most clinical trials are comparative studies where two or more treatments (or placebo) are administered to human subjects and their effectiveness is evaluated and compared. For instance, one may want to compare an investigational drug A to standard of care drug B in terms of blood pressure reduction in hypertensive patients. An ideal experiment or trial for this comparison is one in which all patients are exactly the same in all aspects except that they may have received different treatments, thus creating a state of "all other things being equal." Then the treatment effect, or the difference in blood pressure reduction between two groups of patients, can be evaluated without bias and attributed only to the treatment difference. However, such an ideal experiment will never happen in practice and randomization is used to design a trial or experiment so that it is as close to the ideal as possible.

Randomization as an experimental design principle did not originate in medical research. Its application was pioneered in 1920s by Ronald Fisher while he was working at Rothamsted Experimental Station, and popularized by his book (Fisher 1935). As mentioned above, the ideal state of "all other things being equal" cannot be achieved in practice; however, randomization can help to average out effect of factors between two treatment groups that may confound the treatment effect, and thus make a close to ideal comparison. On the other hand, statistical analysis of the experimental results usually demands that experimental outcomes are independently distributed. This assumption cannot be verified statistically; instead, it can only be substantiated through random sampling procedure (through randomization). Because of its role in reducing bias and providing valid basis for statistical analysis, randomization has become the cornerstone of experimental design.

10.1.1 Randomization in Clinical Trials

In clinical trials, the same principles apply and are well recognized in regulatory guidelines. For example, it is stated in ICH guidance E9 (ICH 1998) that, "The most important design techniques for avoiding bias in clinical trials are blinding and randomization, and these should be normal features of most controlled clinical trials intended to be included in a marketing application." However, clinical trials, as experiments on human subjects, introduce a heated debate on the ethical concern of randomization. The central question is whether one should use equal randomization (1:1) throughout the recruitment. The proponents of the application of equal randomization in clinical trials maintain that a state of equipoise underlies the very need of conducting a clinical trial and it is retained throughout the trial until the final analysis is conducted and result is known. On the other hand, opponents think that the initial equipoise can be tipped as accrued data point to one treatment better than the other and it is therefore not ethical to use equal randomization throughout. Response-adaptive randomization, in which the randomization probability is changed or updated based on accrued data and is very likely not equal between treatments, is the middle ground where the benefit of randomization is retained while the ethical concern is mitigated when more patients are randomized to the better performing treatment arm. It is this ethical appeal that has motivated the research and application of response-adaptive randomization.

10.1.2 Response-Adaptive Randomization in Clinical Trials

Early response-adaptive allocation methods rooted in the exploration of sequential designs, pioneered by Wald (1947). In Robbins' seminal paper (1952), he not only proposed the famous play-the-winner rule, which assigns the next patient to the same treatment of the current patient or to the other treatment depending on whether the current patient has a success or not, but also declared with amazing prescience that "enough is visible to justify a prediction that future results in the theory of sequential design will be of the greatest importance to mathematical statistics and to science as a whole." The blooming research and application of adaptive designs in clinical trials in the past two to three decades precisely ratified his prediction. The play-the-winner rule is a foundational proposal; however, it is deterministic, in the sense that the next patient is assigned to a treatment with a probability of one or zero. A randomized version was proposed by Wei and Durham (1978), now known as the "randomized play the winner rule," which randomizes the next patient to a winning treatment with a probability between one and zero. We will discuss this procedure in Sect. 10.3. Many different approaches have emerged, including two books (Rosenberger and Lachin 2002; Hu and Rosenberger 2006) with frequentist approaches and a book with Bayesian approaches (Berry et al. 2010) in addition to hundreds of papers in the top statistics and biostatistics journals.

For our purpose we define response-adaptive randomization as any randomization procedure that changes randomization probability between treatment arms based on the accrued data in the course of recruitment. This includes fully adaptive randomization where the randomization probability is updated each time a new patient response is available, group sequential adaptive randomization where randomization probability is updated at an interim analysis of a group sequential design, and anything in between. However, in this paper, our discussion will be focused on fully adaptive randomization.

This chapter is not intended to be a technical survey of statistical methodologies for response-adaptive randomization. Instead we will give a quick scan of different approaches to response-adaptive randomization, and then provide a thorough assessment of practical applicability of such procedures. More specifically, in Sect. 10.2 we will introduce a template that characterizes the relationship between efficiency and degree of skewing to a treatment arm through response-adaptive randomization. Section 10.3 categorizes available randomization procedures into two types, heuristic procedures and optimal procedures, with some typical examples for each type. In Sect. 10.4, we discuss regulatory concerns and most often encountered views against application of response-adaptive randomization procedures. We conclude in Sect. 10.5 with some recommendations for a sensible path forward.

10.2   The Fundamental Question of Response-Adaptive Randomization

Clinical trials are usually multiple objective studies, with some of them competing with each other. For example, cost and ethical concerns demand a trial using as few patients as possible. On the other hand, a large sample size is needed to power a trial to be conclusive. Response-adaptive randomization faces similar challenges to balance different objectives. For instance, through response adaptation, more patients may be randomized to a better performing treatment arm, which is beneficial from ethical point of view. However, this creates an imbalance between treatment arms, and potentially can lead to significant loss of power. To maintain the same power, a larger sample size is called for, which in turn can result in more patients assigned to an inferior treatment arm. Such conflicting objectives require a systematic approach to select the best response-adaptive randomization procedure.

A response-adaptive procedure has two components. The first we call the limiting allocation proportion, which is the proportion of all patients randomized to a treatment arm if N, the total sample size of the trial, tends to infinity. Very often, a limiting allocation proportion depends on parameters that describe treatment endpoints. For example, in case of two treatments A and B with binary responses, a limiting allocation proportion may be $q_B/(q_B + q_A)$, known as urn allocation proportion, where $q_i = 1 - \theta_i, i = A, B$ with θ_i the probability of success for a patient assigned to treatment i. In other words, the number of patients randomized to a treatment is inversely proportional to the failure rate of that treatment, ensuring that more patients will be assigned to the treatment arm with a smaller failure rate. The second component we call the randomization method, which is a process that defines how to update or change randomization probability after new patient response(s) is available. Some randomization methods, for example urn models as described in the next section, always lead to the same limiting allocation proportion; whereas other randomization methods, for example the doubly adaptive biased coin design (DBCD) described in the next section, can target a chosen limiting allocation proportion.

In Hu and Rosenberger (2006), they ask a fundamental question about response-adaptive randomization, *can we develop a response-adaptive randomization procedure that results in fewer failures without loss of power?* Here the power loss is compared to nonadaptive randomization procedure. The question can be addressed using a formal evaluation template by Hu and Rosenberger (2003), which decomposes the expected noncentrality parameter of Z-test for two proportions into three parts, with the first part determined by the limiting allocation proportion of a response-adaptive randomization procedure, the second part determined by the difference between the empirical allocation proportion and limiting allocation proportion, and third part determined by the variance of mean square error of the empirical allocation proportion. Interestingly, the first part is dependent on the limiting allocation proportion only and will be maximized when the limiting allocation proportion is the Neyman allocation proportion, which gives rise to the largest power given the total sample size and is to be derived in Sect. 10.3.2.

The second part vanishes if the empirical allocation proportion approaches to the limiting allocation fast and the third part is a function of the variance of the empirical allocation proportion (we call the variance of the randomization method) and is always negative. For a technical treatment of this template, refer to Hu and Rosenberger (2003). This template therefore presents an explicit link between power of the test, the limiting allocation proportion, and the variance of the randomization method. An ethically desirable response-adaptive randomization procedure should choose an appropriate limiting allocation proportion that reduces the number of failures without much deviation from the Neyman allocation proportion, and should choose an appropriate randomization method leading to the limiting allocation proportion with as small variance as possible.

The same template can be built for other scenarios. For example, Zhang and Rosenberger (2006) gave a similar template for continuous responses. Also note that although the fundamental question by Hu and Rosenberger (2006) is concerned about the ethics and efficiency, it can be generalized as, "Can we develop a response-adaptive randomization procedure that assigns more patients to a treatment arm(s) to achieve a particular objective without loss of power?" The particular objective can be an ethical one, as mentioned above, or quick identification of the best dose in dose finding studies. Then the template can be used to quantify the tradeoff between skewing allocation proportion for a particular objective and efficiency of the statistical test.

10.3 Response-Adaptive Randomization Procedures

Many response-adaptive randomization procedures have been proposed. Some procedures are heuristic while others are based on a formal optimization approach. In this section, we introduce some of these procedures.

10.3.1 Heuristic Procedures

10.3.1.1 Urn Models

The most famous response-adaptive randomization procedure is the aforementioned randomized play-the-winner rule. The rule can be best described as an urn model. An urn contains α balls representing treatment A and α balls representing treatment B. A ball is drawn, say, representing A, and a patient is then assigned to treatment A. If the patient has a success, then add β balls to the urn representing treatment A. Otherwise, if the patient has a failure, then add β balls to the urn representing treatment B. So the urn composition is updated once a patient's response is known, and skewed to the better performing arm at the time. The properties of the randomized play-the-winner rule have been studied intensively (see, for example, Rosenberger 1999).

Other urn models have been proposed, e.g., drop the loser rule (Ivanova 2003) with smallest asymptotic variance among all randomization methods that target the urn limiting allocation proportion (Hu et al. 2007). Interestingly, all these urn models lead to the same limiting allocation proportion, but their variances are different. According to the template, if one wants to choose an urn model, the one with the least variability is desired.

For more details on urn models, readers are referred to Chap. 10 of Rosenberger and Lachin (2002) and Chap. 4 of Hu and Rosenberger (2006).

10.3.1.2   Treatment Effect Mappings

An intuitive method to determine the limiting allocation proportion is to map the treatment effect into a function between 0 and 1. Such a treatment effect mapping method appeared first in Rosenberger (1993). Bandyopadhyay and Biswas (2001) proposed a treatment effect mapping for continuous responses. Consider a trial comparing two treatments with patient responses normally distributed with mean μ_i, $i = A, B$. They defined the limiting allocation proportion as

$$\Phi\left(\frac{\mu_A - \mu_B}{T}\right),$$

where $\Phi(\cdot)$ is the cumulative distribution function of the standard normal distribution and T is a tuning parameter. It has been shown that this allocation proportion leads to significant loss of power due to its significant deviation from Neyman allocation (Zhang and Rosenberger 2006).

10.3.1.3   Bayesian Response-Adaptive Randomization

The Bayesian approach is a natural way to incorporate available data as a prior for decision making and therefore is advocated in response-adaptive randomization for clinical trials (Biswas et al. 2009). However, because of emphasis of regulatory agencies on controlling type I error rate, this method is often discouraged as a decision making tool for confirmatory trials in drug approval applications. In this section, we consider the Bayesian approach for Phase II trials where a better dose of a treatment needs to be identified in dose ranging studies or a treatment is compared to a control in proof of concept studies.

Thall and Wathen (2007) is an excellent introductory reference for why and how the Bayesian approach is used in response-adaptive randomization. We shall proceed with our introduction following their paradigm. The general procedure for Bayesian response-adaptive randomization:

1. Choose a prior distribution for the parameters in the response variables, usually noninformative at the beginning and ideally a conjugate distribution to that of the

response variable. For example, if the response variable has a binomial distribution, a conjugate prior distribution will be a beta distribution.

2. Determine the posterior distribution each time a patient's response becomes available.
3. By comparing posterior distributions or means of different arms, update the randomization probability for each treatment arm.
4. Randomize the next patient and go back to step 2.
5. Repeat steps 2–4 until some stopping rule is satisfied or until the maximum sample size is attained.

In the following, we illustrate this idea by considering a trial comparing two treatments with binary responses and a maximum sample size N. Suppose responses of patients assigned to treatments A and B have a Bernoulli distribution with parameters θ_A and θ_B, respectively. We follow the steps listed above. Step 1 is to choose a prior distribution and a conjugate prior in this situation is a beta distribution. Since we assume there is no information to compare these two treatments at the beginning, a noninformative prior of Beta distribution with parameters 0.5 and 0.5 or Beta(0.5, 0.5) is used for both treatment arms. In step 2, suppose N_A and N_B patients have been assigned to treatments A and B with s_A and s_B successes, respectively. It is straightforward to determine that the posterior distributions for θ_A and θ_B are $Beta(s_A + 0.5, N_A - s_A + 0.5)$ and $Beta(s_B + 0.5, N_B - s_B + 0.5)$. In Step 3, we need to generate a metric representing the treatment difference using the two posterior distributions. An intuitive metric, as in Thall and Wathen (2007) and traced back to Thompson (1933), is $\text{Prob}(\theta_A > \theta_B)$, denoted by $P_{A>B}$. Although this metric is not necessarily the optimal one, as will be commented shortly, we will use it in the following discussion for demonstration. The randomization probability for the next patient to treatment A, ρ_A, is defined by

$$\rho_A = \frac{(P_{A>B})^c}{(P_{A>B})^c + (1 - P_{A>B})^c} \tag{10.1}$$

where c is a tuning constant, with $c=0$ for equal randomization and $c=1$ for $\rho_A = P_{A>B}$. Based on their simulation (Thall and Wathen 2007), $c = (N_A + N_B)/(2N)$ leads to a randomization procedure with the least variability. Again there are many ways to construct randomization probability in (10.1). In Step 5, a stopping rule is implemented in Thall and Wathen (2007) to select treatment A as better if $P_{A>B} > 0.99$ and to select B as better if $P_{A>B} < 0.01$. Otherwise, the trial proceeds until all N patients have been randomized.

Several comments are in order for this Bayesian response-adaptive randomization procedure. Firstly, this procedure can be readily generalized to more than two arms. For example, in the case of three treatments A, B, and C, the metric in Step 2 can be generalized to be $\text{Prob}(P_A > P_B, P_A > P_C)$, denoted by PA. Then Eq. (10.1) can be modified to

$$\rho_A = \frac{PA^c}{PA^c + PB^c + PC^c}.$$

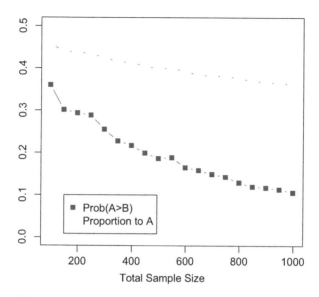

Fig. 10.1 Probability of posterior of A larger than posterior of B and proportion of patients assigned to A

Another way to generalize to more than two treatment arms is to use as a metric $\text{Prob}(P_A > \bar{P})$ where $\bar{P}$ is the average of P_A, P_B and P_C, as in Lee et al. (2012).

Secondly, ρ_A is not stabilized even when N is very large, which results in significant variability of this procedure. Figure 10.1 depicts posterior $\text{Prob}(\theta_A > \theta_B)$ (line with squares) and proportion of patients assigned to treatment A (line with solid circles) when true $\theta_A = 0.25$, $\theta_B = 0.30$ and no stopping rule is included. Note that even when N tends to 1,000, both $P_{A>B}$ and ρ_A remain decreasing, although the latter decreases more slowly since $c = (N_A + N_B)/2/N$ approaches to 1/2 as N gets large. In fact, we can reasonably infer that the limiting allocation proportion of this procedure is zero. In other words, the limiting proportion to treatment A is 0 as long as $\theta_A < \theta_B$, which leads to an undesirable deterministic procedure.

Using the template, it is very easy to understand why this Bayesian response-adaptive randomization procedure will have loss of power. The limiting allocation proportion, 0, deviates significantly from Neyman allocation proportion. This leads to a significant reduction in the first part of the decomposition in the template, therefore a significant loss of power no matter what randomization procedure is used. Response-adaptive randomization procedures based on the frequentist approach will suffer from the same problem if an inappropriate limiting allocation proportion is chosen, as will be seen in the following section.

10.3.2   Optimal Allocation Procedures

Based on the template, a desirable response-adaptive randomization procedure must select an appropriate limiting allocation proportion that balances ethical consideration and preservation of power, and use a randomization method to target this proportion with a small variability. In this section, we describe the optimal allocation approach to derive limiting allocation proportions that can preserve power, and a family of randomization methods targeting the proportions with small variance. In the following we again use a trial comparing two treatments with binary responses to demonstrate the optimal allocation approach.

Suppose we use the following Z-test to compare two treatments.

$$\frac{\hat{\theta}_A - \hat{\theta}_B}{\sqrt{\dfrac{\hat{\theta}_A(1-\hat{\theta}_A)}{n_A} + \dfrac{\hat{\theta}_B(1-\hat{\theta}_B)}{n_B}}},$$

where n_i is the number of patients randomized to treatment i and $n_A + n_B = N$. To derive a limiting allocation proportion that balances ethical consideration and power preservation, we use the following optimal problem,

$$\begin{cases} \min \quad n_A(1-\theta_A) + n_B(1-\theta_B) \\ \text{subject to} \quad \dfrac{\theta_A(1-\theta_A)}{n_A} + \dfrac{\theta_B(1-\theta_B)}{n_B} \equiv constant, \end{cases} \tag{10.2}$$

which minimizes the expected total number of failures with the constraint that the denominator of the test statistic is held constant. Solving this problem, we have

$$\frac{n_A}{n_B} = \frac{\sqrt{\theta_A}}{\sqrt{\theta_B}},$$

or equivalently, the proportion to treatment A, ρ_A, is given by

$$\rho_A = \frac{\sqrt{\theta_A}}{\sqrt{\theta_A} + \sqrt{\theta_B}}.$$

This optimal allocation appeared first in Rosenberger et al. (2001) and has been called RSIHR proportion (acronym of authors' initials). This optimal allocation proportion does not deviate much from Neyman allocation, which is the solution to (10.2) when the objective function is replaced with $n_A + n_B$, and proved to offer a desirable tradeoff between minimization of total failures and preservation of power after extensive comparison to other proportions (Rosenberger and Lachin 2002).

Now since we have an appropriate limiting allocation proportion, next we consider a randomization method that targets this proportion. We recommend two methods, the DBCD method (Hu and Zhang 2004) and the efficient randomized adaptive designs (ERADE) (Hu et al. 2009). We start with the DBCD method, which is defined by the following allocation function.

$$g(x, y) = \frac{y[y(1-x)]^\gamma}{y[y(1-x)]^\gamma + (1-y)[x(1-y)]^\gamma},$$

where γ is a tuning parameter with $\gamma = \infty$ defining a deterministic allocation method and $\gamma = 0$ defining the sequential estimation method (Melfi et al. 2001). Usually $\gamma = 2$ is recommended and is used in the following discussion. During randomization, after j patients have been randomized, x will be replaced with $N_A(j)/j$, the empirical proportion of j patients to treatment A, and y will be replaced with an estimate of ρ_A, $\hat{\rho}_A$, based on responses of j patients. Then $g(N_A(j)/j, \hat{\rho}_A)$ is the randomization probability of the next patient to treatment A.

The ERADE method uses a discrete allocation function, defined by,

$$g(x, y) = \begin{cases} \eta y & \text{if } x > y \\ y & \text{if } x = y \\ 1 - \eta(1 - y) & \text{if } x < y \end{cases}$$

where $0 \leq \eta < 1$ is a tuning parameter reflecting the degree of randomization and a value between 0.4 and 0.7 is recommended. The allocation function was developed based on Efron's biased coin design (Efron 1971), which can be obtained by forcing $y = 1/2$ and $\eta = 2/3$, an adaptive randomization method intended to assign equal number of patients to each treatment. The implementation of the ERADE method is the same as the DBCD method.

Figure 10.2 depicts the allocation functions of both methods when $y = 0.7$ with tuning parameters $\gamma = 2$ and $\eta = 2/3$. Note that for both methods, when $x < 0.7$, then $g(x, 0.7) > 0.7$; when $x > 0.7$, $g(x, 0.7) < 0.7$; when $x = 0.7$, $g(x, 0.7) = 0.7$. In other words, based on j patients' responses, if $N_A(j)/j$ is larger than ρ_A, then next patient will be randomized to treatment A with a probability larger than ρ_A. On the other hand, if $N_A(j)/j$ is smaller than the estimate of ρ_A, then next patient will be randomized to treatment A with a probability smaller than ρ_A. In the long run, both $N_A(j)/j$ and ρ_A will converge to ρ_A, the desired proportion to treatment A. However, these two functions are different in that the function for the DBCD is continuous whereas that of ERADE is discrete. This difference proves to be fundamental. By taking only three different values, the ERADE method is less variable than the DBCD method. In fact, it has been shown that the ERADE method is asymptotically best, which means that the method has the least possible asymptotic variance of all response-adaptive randomization methods that target the same limiting allocation proportion.

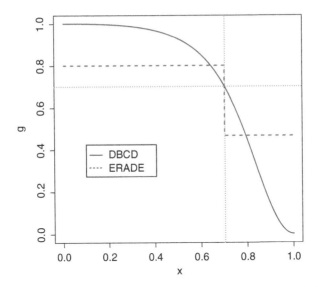

Fig. 10.2 The allocation functions of the DBCD and ERADE methods when $y=0.7$

Extensive simulations have showed that these two randomization methods perform very well with finite sample size (Hu and Rosenberger 2006). They are versatile in that they can target any limiting allocation proportions, for example, the limiting allocation proportion of urn models.

Recently, Flournoy et al. (2013) conducted a comprehensive comparison of different response-adaptive randomization procedures, including the ones we discussed in this section, with recommendations on choice of randomization procedures for binary outcomes and continuous outcomes.

10.4   Benefit–Risk Assessment

The major motivation for using response-adaptive randomization is initially for ethical considerations in that more patients can be randomized to a better performing treatment dictated by accumulated data. The application of such procedures has met significant resistance from major clinical trial stakeholders, such as statisticians, clinicians, and regulators, after the first ECMO trial using randomized play-the-winner rule (Bartlett et al. 1985) that gave rise to a controversial design with ten out of total eleven patients allocated to the winning treatment arm. Although Bayesian response-adaptive randomization procedures have recently gained some momentum, strong opposing voices still are heard frequently to challenge the value of response-adaptive randomization procedures (Chevret 2012; Korn and Freidlin 2011). In this section, we conduct a comprehensive benefit–risk assessment of using response-adaptive randomization and point out situations where such procedures can be applied with the most net benefit.

10.4.1 Regulatory Considerations

In February 2010, the Food and Drug Administration (FDA) released a draft guidance (FDA 2010) on adaptive design clinical trials for drugs and biologics. According to the guidance, trials are categorized into adequate and well-controlled (A&WC) studies (usually Phase III trials) and exploratory studies (usually Phase II trials) and the FDA has different perspectives on adaptive randomization for these two types of studies.

In the guidance, response-adaptive randomization is labeled as "Adaptive study designs whose properties are less well understood," and "should be used cautiously in A&WC studies, as the analysis is not as easily interpretable as when fixed randomization probabilities are used. Particular attention should be paid to avoiding bias and controlling type I error rate." Since response-adaptive randomization aims to assign more patients to a treatment arm, thus creating a possible "poor balance in patient characteristics between the groups at the end of the study," introducing bias into treatment effect estimate, the guidance concludes that "such poor balance in important characteristics could be a very significant problem for an A&WC study." We think that the regulatory concern about potential bias due to imbalance treatment assignment is sensible and we will address this concern later. However, their concern on controlling type I error rate is ungrounded, since there is adequate research by theory or by simulation showing optimal response-adaptive randomization procedure controls type I error rate very well (Hu and Rosenberger 2006). Even for trials using Bayesian response-adaptive randomization, the frequentist framework has been proposed for data analysis that strongly controls type I error rate (Gaydos et al. 2012). Also there is vast literature that analysis of data from trials using response-adaptive randomization is as straightforward as when fixed designs are used, either following the standard methods based on normality or nonparametric methods based on linear rank test (Zhang and Rosenberger 2012). There is no difference in how to interpret the analysis results compared to fixed designs.

For exploratory studies (e.g., Phase II trials), the guidance in fact encourages companies to use adaptive designs, including response-adaptive randomization. According to the guidance, "Outcome dependent adaptive randomization is particularly valuable for exploratory studies because it can make practical an increase in the number of tested treatment options (increased breadth to the range of doses tested/and/or decreased step size between doses) explored for the drug's activity and facilitate estimation of the dose-response relationship, and hypothesis testing is not the objective." The authors agree with the guidance and think that more research is needed for optimal response-adaptive randomization procedures for Phase II trials. As shown in last section, the Bayesian procedure, though being easy to understand, has very large variability compared to the optimal procedure. The optimal procedure proposed in the literature mostly focuses on balancing ethical concerns and preservation of power. In general, regulatory agencies have not emphasized concerns about the ethics of randomization and a scan through the FDA's guidances, EMA's guidances and ICH guidances on clinical trials suggests no texts discussing about allocating more patients to a treatment arm based on ethical consideration. In fact, the regulatory agencies are more concerned about potential bias due to treatment assignment imbalance and in the FDA guidance on adaptive design, "to address the concern regarding patient characteristics, we recommend that sponsors maintain randomization to the placebo group to ensure that sufficient patients are enrolled into the placebo group along the entire duration of the study." Therefore, an optimal procedure for Phase II trials should be using a different objective function instead of one based on ethics. For example, one can minimize the total variances of parameter estimate if a parametric dose response model is specified and to be characterized. Such response-adaptive randomization procedures based on optimal properties should yield smaller variability and therefore either use fewer patients for a particular power or larger power given the number of patients.

In summary, although regulatory agencies labeled response-adaptive randomization as "less well understood" adaptive designs and are cautious of using such procedures in A&WC trials, they are in general open or encourage companies to use response-adaptive randomization in exploratory studies. We also want to emphasize that by "less well understood" adaptive designs, the FDA intends to think these are designs that lack of regulatory experiences, rather than designs that are too biased to be valid, too difficult to understand, or too complex to implement. With accruing knowledge and experiences with response-adaptive randomization, the regulatory agencies may become confident for its use in A&WC trials, in addition to exploratory studies.

10.4.2 Benefit–Risk Assessment of Using Response-Adaptive Randomization Procedures

Response-adaptive randomization was initially proposed to assign more patients to the better performing treatment by changing randomization probability based on accruing data. This ethical orientation has created significant controversies. The central question is, "does the benefit of response-adaptive randomization justifies the associated risk?" In this section, we will review most frequently cited drawbacks of response-adaptive randomization and present situations where such designs can be justifiably applied.

We start with the purpose of response-adaptive randomization. As mentioned above, the initial intention was on ethical considerations. As noted in the FDA guidance, "this randomization method had been used in placebo controlled studies chiefly to place more patients into the group with better outcomes." However, we strongly remind the readers that the ethical appeal is not the only reason for using response-adaptive randomization. Instead, we would point out that *the purpose of response-adaptive randomization is to achieve a particular trial objective by changing randomization probabilities in the middle of patient recruitment*. The ethical consideration is only one of such objectives. Another objective may be, as mentioned in the FDA guidance, "…to suit the objective of dose response evaluation," because "response adaptive randomization appears to have the potential to obtain a more precise description of the dose response relationship by starting with a broader range of doses…" Another objective may be to maximize the power of a statistical test with a given total sample size and response-adaptive randomization with Neyman allocation (Zhang and Rosenberger 2006) can achieve the goal.

With this in mind, next we will examine many views in the literature against using response-adaptive randomization.

Response-adaptive randomization can only assign negligibly more patients to the better performing treatment. A typical example is a recent article (Korn and Freidlin 2011), "Outcome-adaptive randomization: Is it useful?" in which the authors conclude that "Adaptive randomization is inferior to 1:1 randomization in terms of acquiring information for the general clinical community and offers modest-to-no benefits to the patients on the trial, even assuming the best-case scenario of an immediate binary outcome." First, we note that the magnitude of benefit is a judgment call. For example, if a trial using the adaptive randomization with the same number of patients obtains the same analysis conclusion as using the fixed design, but causing five less patient deaths, is this benefit modest or large? Different people may have different opinions. Secondly, usually binary outcomes are used to demonstrate response-adaptive randomization, just as we did in previous sections. However, response-adaptive randomization in trials with other outcomes can produce larger benefits (e.g., continuous outcomes, Zhang and Rosenberger 2006 and survival outcomes, Zhang and Rosenberger 2007). Third, the purpose of response-adaptive randomization is not necessarily ethically oriented, and therefore it can still be used to achieve other objectives.

"…these trials [Bayesian adaptive randomization] are complex to design because there is a lot of flexibility in the selection of data sampling rules, allocation rules, early stopping rules, dose selection rules, models (doseresponse and longitudinal) and prior definitions. These are also among the most difficult approaches to implement well." (Gaydos et al. 2012). First, non-Bayesian adaptive randomization procedures are available which do not require prior definitions. Second, these designs do not necessarily have stopping rules and dose selection rules and if they do, they are no more difficult than other adaptive designs with similar rules. Third, for companies that run such trials the first time, some challenges exist. However, with the advance of technology, for example, the central data monitoring, interactive voice response services (IVRS) and interactive web response service (IWRS), the added complexity in implementation of such trials is eased and becomes manageable, with sufficient blinding like fixed designs. In fact, many clinical research organizations can facilitate such randomization procedures.

Poor balance in patient characteristics can cause significant treatment effect estimate bias. This is also a great regulatory concern, as mentioned in previous sections. One remedy may be to use block adaptive randomization and block adjusted analysis (Korn and Freidlin 2011) for large or long-term trials. Another remedy is to use covariate adjusted response-adaptive randomization (Hu and Rosenberger 2006). We agree that careful consideration should be taken to avoid bias.

"The statistical inference is complicated because the treatment assignments and the responses are correlated; as a consequence, rerandomization tests must be used instead of traditional likelihood-based tests." (Buyse 2012). We agree that the response-adaptive randomization generates correlated patient responses and a re-randomization test can (not must) be used for data analysis. However, it is well established that under moderate regularity conditions (satisfied in most trial settings), traditional likelihood based tests can be used for inference with well-controlled type I error rate (Hu and Rosenberger 2006).

"Adaptive randomization can cause accrual bias (if patients wait for the probability of receiving the better treatment to increase) and/or selection bias (if patients are aware of the emerging difference among the treatment groups)." (Buyse 2012). The accrual bias, coined by Rosenberger (1996), can be avoided by using a double blind strategy and the selection bias mentioned can be avoided under most trials settings where patients are not usually aware of the treatment effect difference.

More simulations are needed to understand the operating characteristics of such trials and more interactions are needed with the regulatory agencies. In general, all adaptive designs, including well-understood adaptations according to the FDA guidance, need more simulations than traditional designs. However, with more experiences gained by all stakeholders, such simulations will help improve clinical trial design and understanding response-adaptive randomization will become a routine.

Of course, we cannot exhaust the list of all objections to response-adaptive randomization, but we want to emphasize that as any type of study design, response-adaptive randomization cannot be applied with significant net benefit in all situations. We believe that a path forward will be to use such procedures in exploratory studies first. As more experiences are gained by industry and regulatory agencies, response-adaptive randomization may become "well understood" and applied in general settings including the A&WC trials.

10.5   Conclusions

In this paper, we introduced response-adaptive randomization procedures that can help achieve a specific objective or balancing conflicting objectives by skewing randomization probability during the course of recruitment. The objective can be a traditional one as assigning more patients to a better performing treatment arm, or to get a more precise estimate of dose response relationship. Although the FDA guidance labels such adaptive randomization procedures as "less well-understood," it in fact means these procedures, like sample size adaptation based on interim effect size, are not widely applied in practice. "This guidance encourages sponsors to gain experience with the less well-understood methods in the exploratory study setting." As more experiences are accumulated, we believe response-adaptive randomization can find its best niche in clinical research.

Many misconceptions about response-adaptive randomization are ungrounded as addressed in the last section. Another misconception we want to address here is concerning the Bayesian procedure and optimal procedure. It seems that the Bayesian procedure has been most applied in Phase II trials and the optimal procedure has been proposed toward A&WC trials. In essence, these two types of procedures can be applied in both scenarios. Which procedure should be used in a particular scenario depends only on which procedure can achieve the desired objective more efficiently. In this regard, more research should be conducted on using optimal response-adaptive randomization procedures in exploratory studies or Phase II trials and on type I error rate control of Bayesian procedures in A&WC trials.

References

Bandyopadhyay U, Biswas A (2001) Adaptive designs for normal responses with prognostic factors. Biometrika 88:409–419

Bartlett RH, Roloff DW, Cornell RG, Andrews AF, Dillon PW, Zwischenberger JB (1985) Extracorporeal circulation in neonatal respiratory failure: a prospective randomized study. Pediatrics 76:479–487

Biswas A, Liu DD, Lee JJ, Berry D (2009) Bayesian clinical trials at the University of Texas M. D. Anderson Cancer Center. Clin Trials 6:205–216

Berry SM, Carlin BP, Lee JJ, Muller P (2010) Bayesian adaptive methods for clinical trials. Chapman & Hall/CRC, Boca Raton, FL

Buyse M (2012) Limitations of adaptive clinical trials. Am Soc Clin Oncol 32:133–137

Chevret S (2012) Bayesian adaptive clinical trials: a dream for statisticians only? Stat Med 31:1002–1013

Efron B (1971) Forcing a sequential experiment to be balanced. Biometrika 58:403–417

FDA (2010) Guidance for Industry: adaptive design clinical trials for drugs and biologics

Fisher R (1935) The design of experiments. Oliver and Boyd, Edinburgh

Flournoy N, Haines LM, Rosenberger WF (2013) A graphical comparison of response-adaptive randomization procedures. Stat Biopharm Res 5:126–141

Gaydos B, Koch A, Miller F, Posch M, Vandemeulebroecke M, Wang SJ (2012) Perspective on adaptive designs: 4 years European Medcines Agency reflection paper, 1 year draft US FDA guidance-where are we now? Future Sci 2:235–240

Hu F, Rosenberger WF (2003) Optimality, variability, power: evaluating response-adaptive randomization procedures for treatment comparisons. J Am Stat Assoc 98:671–678

Hu F, Rosenberger WF (2006) The theory of response-adaptive randomization in clinical trials. Wiley, New York

Hu F, Rosenberger WF, Zhang LX (2007) Asymptotically best response-adaptive randomization procedures. J Stat Plann Infer 136:1911–1922

Hu F, Zhang LX (2004) Asymptotic properties of doubly adaptive biased coin design for multi-treatment clinical trials. Ann Stat 32:268–301

Hu F, Zhang LX, He X (2009) Efficient randomized adaptive designs. Ann Stat 37:2543–2560

ICH (1998) Statistical principles for clinical trials

Ivanova A (2003) A play-the-winner type urn model with reduced variability. Metrika 58:1–13

Korn EL, Freidlin B (2011) Outcome-adaptive randomization: Is it useful? J Clin Oncol 29:771–776

Lee JJ, Chen N, Yin G (2012) Worth adapting? Revisiting the usefulness of outcome-adaptive randomization. Clin Cancer Res 18:4498–4507

Melfi VF, Page C, Geraldes M (2001) An adaptive randomized design with application to estimation. Can J Stat 29:107–116

Robbins H (1952) Some aspects of the sequential design of experiments. Bull Am Math Soc 58:527–535

Rosenberger WF (1993) Asymptotic inference with response-adaptive treatment allocation designs. Ann Stat 21:2098–2107

Rosenberger WF (1996) New directions in adaptive designs. Stat Sci 11:137-149

Rosenberger WF (1999) Randomized play-the-winner clinical trials: review and recommendations. Contr Clin Trials 20:328–342

Rosenberger WF, Lachin JL (2002) Randomization in clinical trials, theory and practice. Wiley, New York

Rosenberger WF, Stallard N, Ivanova A, Harper C, Ricks M (2001) Optimal adaptive designs for binary response trials. Biometrics 57:173–177

Thall PF, Wathen KS (2007) Practical Bayesian adaptive randomization in clinical trials. Eur J Canc 43:859–866

Thompson WR (1933) On the likelihood that one unknown probability exceeds another in view of the evidence of two samples. Biometrika 25:285–294

Wald A (1947) Sequential analysis. Wiley, New York

Wei LJ, Durham S (1978) The randomized play-the-winner rule in medical trials. J Am Stat Assoc 73:840–843

Zhang L, Rosenberger WF (2006) Response-adaptive randomization for clinical trials with continuous outcomes. Biometrics 62:562–569

Zhang L, Rosenberger WF (2007) Response-adaptive randomization for clinical trials with survival outcomes: the parametric approach. J Roy Stat Soc C 53:153–165

Zhang L, Rosenberger WF (2012) Adaptive randomization in clinical trials. In: Hinkelmann KI (ed) Design and analysis of experiments, vol 3: Special designs and applications

Part II
Trial Implementation Considerations

Chapter 11
Implementing Adaptive Designs: Operational Considerations, Putting It All Together

Olga Marchenko and Christy Nolan

Abstract The use of adaptive clinical trial designs for a drug development program has clear advantages over traditional methods, given the ability to identify optimal clinical benefits and make informed decisions regarding safety and efficacy earlier in the clinical trial process. However, operational execution can be challenging due to the added complexities of implementing adaptive designs. These complexities deserve additional attention. Key operational challenges occur in several areas: availability of statistical simulation tools for clinical trial modeling at the planning stage; the use of trial simulation modeling approaches to ensure that the trial is meeting expected outcomes; and challenges regarding rapid data collection, clinical monitoring, resourcing, minimization of data leakage, IVRS, drug supply management, and systems integration. The purpose of this chapter is to highlight several operational challenges that must be taken into consideration in conducting an adaptive clinical trial. Adaptive design implementation strategies are also discussed in this chapter.

Keywords Adaptive design • Trial execution • Operational challenges • Implementation strategy

O. Marchenko (✉)
Quintiles, 352 Arlington Drive, Saline, MI 48176, USA

Quintiles, 4820 Emperor Blvd., Durham, NC 27703, USA
e-mail: Olga.marchenko@quintiles.com

C. Nolan
Quintiles, 5364 Notting Hill Rd, Gurnee, IL 60031, USA

Quintiles, 4820 Emperor Blvd., Durham, NC 27703, USA
e-mail: Christy.nolan@quintiles.com

W. He et al. (eds.), *Practical Considerations for Adaptive Trial Design and Implementation*, Statistics for Biology and Health,
DOI 10.1007/978-1-4939-1100-4_11, © Springer Science+Business Media New York 2014

11.1 Introduction

Execution at the operational level can be challenging given the additional complexities found when implementing adaptive designs; however, there are clear approaches to operational conduct that can be utilized successfully across each unique adaptive design method.

The successful conduct of any clinical trial requires cross-departmental coordination. Implementation of an adaptive design requires far greater integration from all functional teams which include biostatistics, data management, clinical operations, clinical research, regulatory, interactive randomization system (IVR system), and drug supply. Although this level of integration can provide operational complexities, it can also allow for a unique opportunity to optimize the methods for which we work, thereby improving clinical trial execution by requiring highly efficient and fully integrated processes from study design to final project delivery.

The logistical infrastructure required to support the conduct of an adaptive design must reflect the unique elements of the final design. The long and successful tradition of "non-flexible" double-blind randomized parallel group designs has led to the development of our current systems, tools, and processes as they are now established across the industry. Supporting adaptive designs with the currently available infrastructure although not impossible may be viewed as challenging. Adaptive designs stray from the traditional development models as they benefit from building (1) the capability for high-speed data acquisition, analysis, and integrated reporting into the trial supporting infrastructure; (2) focused real-time remote clinical monitoring efforts for specified critical safety and efficacy data elements; and (3) increased flexibility to implement the required adaptation.

Given the unique operational needs for adaptive designs, the implementation of integrated systems and processes with enhanced flexibility and speed will clearly act as enablers for execution of adaptive designs; however, it is not an absolute requirement. This needs to be highlighted, to avoid misperceptions that adaptive design implementation is only possible in an advanced technology environment. Nevertheless, it should be acknowledged that advances in technology will hold the key to realizing transformational change in the clinical development paradigm. It is from within this environment that we anticipate that adaptive designs will move from being a minor player, as they are today, to becoming a major player from exploratory- through confirmatory-phase clinical development programs, ultimately leading to significant advances in drug development.

As technology improves, it is conceivable that informatics platforms will be available that allow for real-time data capture, interoperability with electronic medical records (EMR), reduced dependencies on source verification, and the provision of fully integrated statistical analysis tools that will trigger patient randomization, monitor and dispense drug supplies, and utilize decision support methodologies to facilitate pre-planned adaptations and futility analysis, all of which will be invisible to the investigator, study teams, and sponsor. However, use of existing systems available today, along with integrated process methodologies and approaches, allows for conduct of an adaptive clinical trial.

Given the preceding remarks, the following sections discuss some of the key operational considerations and challenges when implementing an adaptive design. Adaptive design implementation should not be a daunting experience, as there are consistent best practices that can be applied at the operational level regardless of a design method. The key to a successful trial execution will require the application of each of the principles that will be discussed in the following section, along with an in-depth planning stage taken place prior to study initiation. The planning stage is a critical component for adaptive design studies and will set the stage for project success.

11.2 Planning Stage

The planning stages for an adaptive clinical trial must be completed prior to finalizing the decision to proceed. Adaptive designs should be considered only if they add benefit to the overall drug development process, allow for effective operational implementation, and provide efficiency gains, thus ensuring increased probability of success for a given compound. Adaptive designs are not a one-size-fits-all approach and should be carefully considered prior to implementation. Adequate planning can take 3 to 12 months, depending on clinical trial complexities. We recommend that the planning stage consist of three components—statistical design simulations, and operational simulation, followed by systems integration approaches—to ensure that all specified design requirements can be executed at the operational level. The planning and design phase requires cross-functional collaboration and should include areas such as clinical research, biostatistics, pharmacology, regulatory, and clinical operations. Planning and executing an adaptive design study challenges the traditional approach to clinical trial conduct and requires a fully integrated team, nontraditional resourcing, and integrated informatics approaches.

There are common operational approaches that can be applied across all adaptive design methodologies; therefore, the operational teams would benefit from understanding the basic types of adaptive designs that are commonly used today.

11.2.1 Adaptive Designs

An adaptive design is defined as "a multistage study design that uses accumulating data to decide how to modify aspects of the study without undermining the validity and integrity of the trial" (Dragalin 2006). To maintain study validity means providing correct statistical inference and minimizing operational bias, and to maintain study integrity means providing convincing results, pre-planning, and maintaining the blind of interim analysis results.

Flexibility does not mean that the trial can be modified any time. Modification and adaptations must be pre-planned and should be based on data collected during the course of the study. Accordingly, the draft guidance of the US Food and Drug Administration (FDA) for industry on adaptive design clinical trials defines an adaptive design clinical trial as "a study that includes a prospectively planned opportunity for modification of one or more specified aspects of the study design and hypotheses based on analysis of data (usually interim data) from subjects in the study FDA (2010)." Analyses of the accumulating study data are performed at pre-planned time points within the study, with or without formal statistical hypothesis testing. Ad hoc, unplanned adaptations may increase the chance of misuse or abuse of an adaptive design trial and should therefore be avoided FDA (2010, 2012) and EMA.CHMP (2007).

Operational teams must have a general understanding of adaptive design methods to proceed to the planning and design stage. To support this process, we have listed six commonly used adaptive design types:

- *Adaptive randomization designs.* Here, alterations in the randomization schedule are allowed depending upon the varied or the unequal probabilities of treatment assignment. Adaptive randomization categories include restricted randomization, covariate-adaptive randomization, response-adaptive (or outcome-adaptive) randomization, and covariate-adjusted response-adaptive randomization. Restricted randomization procedures are preferred for many clinical trials because it is often desirable to allocate equal number of patients to each treatment. This is usually achieved by changing the probability of randomization to a treatment according to the number of patients that have already been assigned. Covariate-adaptive randomization is used to ensure the balance between treatments with respect to certain known covariates. Response-adaptive randomization is used when ethical considerations make it undesirable to have an equal number of patients assigned to each treatment. Adaptive assessment is made sequentially, updating the randomization for the next single patient or a cohort of patients using treatment estimates calculated from all available patient data received so far. In this situation, it should be feasible to identify the "better" treatment; the "better" treatment should not be associated with any potential severe toxicity; and delay in response should be moderate allowing the adaptation to take place. Covariate-adjusted response-adaptive randomization combines covariate-adaptive and response-adaptive randomization. These randomization categories and methods are reviewed by Rosenberger and Lachin (2002) and by Hu and Rosenberger (2006). Response-adaptive randomization is the most difficult in the execution due to its frequent update and the need of the clean data for the randomization decisions. Chapter 10 of this book provides an overview of the response-adaptive randomization methods and challenges.
- *Adaptive dose-ranging designs.* Insufficient exploration of a dose–response relationship often leads to a poor choice of the optimal dose used in the confirmatory trial, and may subsequently lead to the failure of the trial and the clinical program. Understanding of a dose–response relationship with regard to efficacy and safety prior to entering the confirmatory stage is a necessary step in drug development. During an early development phase, limited knowledge about the compound opens more opportunities for adaptive design consideration.

Adaptive dose-finding designs allow fuller and more efficient characterization of the dose–response by facilitating iterative learning and decision making during the trial. Adaptive dose-ranging designs can have several objectives. For example, they can be used to establish the overall dose–response relationship for an efficacy parameter or efficacy and safety parameters, estimate the therapeutic window, or help with the selection of a single target dose. The allocation of subjects to the dose currently believed to give best results, or to doses close to the best one, has become very popular in clinical dose-finding studies—for example, when the intention is to identify the maximum tolerated dose (MTD), the minimum efficacious dose (MED), or the most efficacious dose. Examples are cited by Lai and Robbins (1978), O'Quigley et al. (1990), and Thall and Cook (2004) and Chevret (2006). More rigorous approaches are based on the introduction of utility functions, which quantify the "effectiveness" of a particular dose, and penalty functions, which quantify potential harm due to exposure to toxic or non-efficacious doses. Examples are provided by Li et al. (1995) and Fedorov and Leonov (2013) and Marchenko et al. (2014). Chapter 7 of this book discusses different statistical approaches for dose selection in adaptive trials.

One of the appeals of early development adaptive designs such as adaptive dose-ranging designs is their greater acceptance by regulatory agencies. In fact, the FDA draft guidance on Adaptive Design Clinical Trials for Drugs and Biologics encourages sponsors to utilize adaptive designs in early development, to improve the efficiency of exploratory studies, as well as to gain experience with the use of adaptive approaches.

- *Adaptive group sequential designs.* Here, a trial can be stopped prematurely due to efficacy or futility at the interim analysis. The total number of stages (the number of interim analyses plus a final analysis) and stopping criterion to reject or accept the null hypothesis at each interim stage is defined, in addition to critical data values and sample size estimates for each planned interim stage of the trial. At each interim stage, all the data are collected up to the interim data cutoff time point. Data are then analyzed to confirm whether the trial should be stopped or continued. Staged interim analyses are pre-planned during the course of the trial and must be carefully managed by the operational teams. The opportunity to stop the trial early and claim efficacy increases the probability of an erroneous conclusion regarding the new treatment (Type I error). For this reason, it is important to choose the significance levels for interim and final analyses carefully so that the overall Type I error rate is controlled at the pre-specified level. The stopping rules can be based on rejection boundaries, a conditional power, or a predictive power/predictive probability in a Bayesian setting. The boundaries determine how conclusions will be drawn following the interim and final analyses, and it is important to pre-specify which type of boundary and spending function (if applicable) will be employed. The conditional power approach is based on an appealing idea of predicting the likelihood of a statistically significant outcome at the end of the trial, given the data observed at the interim and some assumption of the treatment effect. If the conditional power is extremely low, it is wise to stop the trial early for both ethical and financial reasons. While it is possible to stop the trial and claim efficacy if the conditional power is extremely high, the conditional power is mostly used to conclude futility. The choice of statistical approach and the type of boundaries should depend on the objectives of the trial and the role of the trial in a clinical program. The timing and the number of interim analyses should be carefully considered as well. While by increasing the number of analyses, the chance of stopping prior to the end of the trial increases, many analyses during the trial might not be practical or even possible due to the fast enrollment or financial constraints. Chapter 6 of this book gives more detailed description of interim analyses and the suggested timing of analyses. While considering stopping for the overwhelming efficacy, one should keep in mind the implication of stopping early on the safety profile of the drug. More details on sequential designs can be found in Jennison and Turnbull (2000) and Proshan et al. (2006).

- *Sample size re-estimation designs.* These types of designs allow for sample size adjustment or re-estimation based on observed data at an interim time point(s) for which statistical analysis may be conducted in either blinded or unblinded manner, based on the criteria of treatment effect size, conditional power, and/or reproducibility probability. Sample size re-estimation can improve the outcome of the trial if the information used to calculate the original sample size was unreliable; if the change is necessary due to new or additional information from an ongoing or a finished trial; or if recent research in the therapeutic area has led to new requirements or standards. Although the flexibility to adjust the sample size of a trial during an interim analysis is appealing when information is limited at the design stage, it does not come without a price. When the adjustment is made, it is important to take steps to preserve the Type I error rate. Bretz et al. (2009) review the adaptive design methodology including sample size reassessment in confirmatory clinical trials. Sample size re-estimation is an adaptive design feature mostly used in confirmatory trials, and usually it is used to increase the sample size (not to decrease). Implementation of adaptive procedures for confirmatory trials needs to be carefully planned and executed. Similar to adaptive group sequential designs, the number and the timing of sample size re-estimation require additional considerations. While it is possible to perform the sample size re-estimation multiple times, it is not recommended to perform it more than once during the study. Careful consideration must be given to the total sample size utilized for decision making at the planning stage and the processes that minimize potential bias which may result from knowing an interim observed treatment effect. In the case of unblinded sample size re-estimation, special attention should be given to the management of Data Monitoring Committees (DMC) and the control of the result dissemination. Chapter 14 of this book provides more information on consideration for planning interim analyses and DMCs.

- *Biomarker adaptive designs.* This type of design allows for adaptation using biomarker information. Modifications can be made to an ongoing trial based on the response of a biomarker that can predict a primary endpoint outcome, or one that helps select or change a treatment. Biomarkers can be used to select a subpopulation with an enhanced benefit from the study treatment. Wang et al. (2007) describe approaches to evaluation of treatment effect in randomized trials with a genomic subset. Designs that can be used to perform the subgroup search and identifications based on biomarkers are discussed in Lipkovich et al. (2011) and Lipkovich and Dmitrienko (2014). Stallard (2010) describes a seamless phase II/III design based on a selection using a short-term endpoint; Jenkins et al. (2011) present an adaptive seamless phase II/III design with subpopulation selection using correlated endpoints; and Friede et al. (2012) introduce a conditional error function approach for subgroup selection. Statistical designs that are used to screen biomarkers, validate biomarkers, and enrich the study population based on a biomarker or several biomarkers are of great interest to our industry and society. It should be kept in mind that there is still a gap in clinical development between identifying biomarkers associated with clinical outcomes and establishing a predictive model between relevant biomarkers and clinical outcomes.

- *Adaptive seamless phase II/III designs.* Seamless phase II/III designs have become more popular in drug development. Such designs aim to reduce the overall sample size by allowing the data from phase II patients to be used in phase III analysis (inferentially seamless) and/or eliminating the time between phases, which results in a shorter total drug development time (operationally seamless). An adaptive seamless phase II/III design is a two-stage design consisting of the so-called learning stage (phase II) and a confirmatory stage (phase III). Just as there are a number of phase II designs, there are a number of corresponding phase II/III designs. Seamless designs pose a lot of challenges as the time for planning a confirmatory trial is eliminated or rather combined with the planning time of phase II when the information is limited and the uncertainties of the treatment are bigger. A sufficient benefit should be expected from the combined phase II/III trial as compared to the strategy with a phase II trial followed by a separate phase III trial. In order to retain the validity, a Type I error control is important for the inferentially seamless designs. Approaches based on the combination test principle that combines the stagewise p-values using a pre-specified combination function or on the conditional error principle which computes the Type I error under the null hypothesis conditional on the observed data at interim are used to control Type I error rate. Bretz et al. (2009) provide a comprehensive review of the methods and offer practical considerations.

More details and references on types of adaptive designs can be found in Chap. 1 of this book.

11.2.2 Trial Design and Planning

The design planning session is a critical element of the initial planning phase, for which several design sessions may be required until the design is finalized. Design sessions should include representation from key functional areas. The power of visualization tools cannot be underestimated and is strongly recommended during the planning and design stage. Computer-assisted simulation modeling, traditional business process modeling (BPM) techniques, and other software tools should be used during this stage to support the project teams' understanding, development, and optimization of the proposed trial, the critical data elements for collection, and predicted data flow during the course of the trial. Business process modeling is an activity that allows for the representation and documentation of key clinical trial activities, so that proposed operational processes may be analyzed and optimized. In this capacity, business process modeling is a useful tool that allows for the optimization of complex operational processes that are critical to the successful execution of an adaptive design. Simulations and business modeling diagrams should map all operational activities from study start-up, through patient recruitment and corresponding data collection, and to all pre-specified interim time points for data analysis and decision making, allowing the team to assess the impact of the desired design on clinical operations (e.g., drug supply, treatment assignment, sample size re-estimation). Simulations and diagrams will thereby permit optimization of clinical trial operations and finalization of the design. In addition, access to metadata to address many of the design and operational questions will assist in finalizing the clinical development and implementation plan.

The planning team should have an understanding of the drug candidate, mechanism of action, target product profile (TPP), and commercialization requirements in addition to the existing and future competitive landscape. Such understanding facilitates the development of a comprehensive clinical operational strategy.

At a minimum, the following questions should be addressed during the planning stage.

(a) Country Selection Criteria

What is the optimal placement of the study in relation to the proposed protocol, treatment pathways, current standards of care, availability of patients, and ability to gain regulatory approvals and market authorizations for a specific country?

(b) Patient Recruitment Estimates

What is the estimated rate of patient recruitment per country, based on the targeted therapeutic area, drug indication, and prior performance of targeted study sites with drugs of a similar indication? What is the competitive landscape for drugs currently in clinical trials that may compete for patients? What is the investigator's interest in the protocol, treatment regime, drug class, and likelihood that the trial will be recommended?

(c) Critical Data Elements

What are the essential data elements that must be collected and analyzed for interim decision making during the course of the trial? In what time frame will all essential data elements be collected (days, weeks, or months)? What are the primary, secondary, and safety endpoints for the trial and what is the forecasted event rate?

(d) Electronic Case Report Forms (eCRFs) Design

How will the clinical trial case report forms be designed to capture essential data elements across all proposed patient visits during the course of a clinical trial?

(e) Data Cleaning

What data elements must be cleaned and/or source document verified, to meet design requirements and acceptability by the Data Monitoring Committee? What are the best methods for data cleaning to meet planned analysis, decision making, and proposed design adaptations?

(f)' Data Capture

How will the data be collected by investigators, central laboratories, or other external sources? How will these data be integrated and in what time frame will all data be fully integrated (hours, days, months) to meet data transfer and planned statistical analysis requirements?

(g) Study Start-Up

What is the impact of an adaptive design on study start-up and planned regulatory approvals based on the selected design, estimated patient recruitment, and forecasted time frame for which critical data elements and accumulated trial data will be analyzed for planned decision making and adaptation?

(h) Investigational Product

What is the impact of an adaptive design on drug manufacturing, packaging, drug quantities, and supply chain, and how will investigational product be managed during the course of the clinical trial? Careful consideration is required as the impact to drug supply is directly related to the final design (e.g., will the drug be blinded to the investigators and patients, what route of drug administration will be utilized, how will the proposed clinical trial adaptations impact drug supply, and what will be the mode of drug administration that is of ease for usage by the investigator?). Additional considerations should also be given to the potential impact on patient-informed consents and clinical trial agreements.

(i) Systems

What systems will be utilized for clinical study conduct and how will these systems be fully integrated? Systems may include electronic data capture, interactive voice randomization systems, clinical laboratory systems, centralized reading vendors (imaging, etc.), customized statistical programs (drug supply simulations, interim analysis applications, adaptive randomization), and clinical trial management systems.

(j) Agency Approval

What is the final regulatory strategy, based on final protocol and country selections, which will ensure that proposed regulatory submission and approval timelines meet the final project plan for all study deliverables?

(k) Program Timelines

Given a clear understanding of the critical design elements, time frame for data capture and data cleaning, planned interim analysis, country selection, and patient recruitment, what are the key project milestones for the entire clinical program?

At the end of the planning and design sessions, the team should have comprehensive documentation and clear visualizations that describe all operational deliverables, and corresponding time frames for when each deliverable will be achieved to support the final design. The team should develop a baseline integrated project plan, firmly assess time and cost of the clinical study, and identify potential risks and contingencies if required. Given the implementation of BPM techniques during this stage, and the development of clear process maps for all steps across all functions, the implementation team will have a well-documented roadmap that describes how the study will actually be implemented. As an end result, the team will have a comprehensive analysis of what needs to be accomplished, by what time frame, and precisely how the work will be executed. The importance of this level of detail cannot be underestimated given that a percentage of staff on the execution team might not have adaptive clinical trial expertise. A publication by *Clinical News*, May 2013, an article entitled "Tufts Report Sees Growing Use of Adaptive Trial Designs," documents that it is estimated that approximately 20 % of all clinical trials today are adaptive and adoption continues to grow. Therefore, due to the continued and growing adoption of adaptive clinical trials at this time, it is reasonable to anticipate that project teams, including investigative sites that are selected to perform the adaptive trial, will comprise both experienced and non-experienced staffs. Taking the time to clearly document not only timelines and deliverables, but also process maps and project work instructions that define how the work will be completed, will assist greatly in staff education, training, and optimal execution of the trial.

11.2.3   Clinical Trial Modeling and Simulation

Trial simulations that compare different design's options, evaluate a range of assumptions and possible scenarios, and compare operating characteristics of designs are an essential step in a trial design and planning stage. Gaydos et al. (2009) outline points to consider on trial simulation. As mentioned in the paper, no trial design can be globally optimal. Besides statistical considerations and assumptions, operational assumptions should be evaluated and simulated. Each development and operational team needs to define the criteria for a design optimization. There are several software packages available commercially that one can use to design an adaptive trial, but none of the available software has the full range of assumptions and adaptations built in. It is critical for a statistician responsible for the trial design to have a good knowledge of adaptive design methodology and be able to use a commercial software or to write a customized code if necessary. Chapter 8 of this book provides a review of currently available statistical software.

An important aspect of the planning and design process is to complete the appropriate trial simulations to optimize an individual trial and assess relative impact on overall development. Clinical trial simulation is a key step in evaluating potential clinical outcomes using various design scenarios and clinical trial assumptions to validate the design, ensuring effective execution at the operational level. Simulation models are used to predict the relationships between certain inputs such as patient recruitment, dosing arms, clinical outcomes and event rates (such as endpoints, adverse events (AEs), and serious adverse events), sample size, interim analysis time points, and other inputs that must occur within the study domain. Simulation tools can also be used to monitor clinical trial outcomes during the course of the study, within trial simulation, to ensure that the study is meeting expectations. Clinical trial simulations utilize computer programs to mimic actual conduct of the trial in a virtual capacity, and can be used to reforecast predicted outcomes; simulations might also include an analysis of project cost, and cost management.

Prior to study initiation, and as an output of the planning sessions, the team should have an established baseline simulation model, or enrollment model, that forecasts key deliverables and project milestones which comprise the baseline project plan. The project team will utilize the baseline project plan to ensure that operational execution will allow for implementation of key design elements. The baseline project plan should have, at a minimum, the following planned deliverables and/or milestones: (1) country-specific study start-up deliverables which include site identification, site selection, regulatory submission, and approvals; (2) site initiations and timing for initiations; (3) patient recruitment to include screened, randomized, and country-specific recruitment caps when required; (4) dosing arms; (5) patient exposure; (6) clinical endpoints and key data elements; (7) electronic case report from completion and submission milestones; (8) site and external data submission milestones; (9) planned statistical analysis milestones including within trial, interim, and DMC; (10) remote data cleaning, and data lock deliverables throughout the clinical trial; and (11) clinical resource requirements to meet project deliverables.

A well-built baseline project plan that comprehensively forecasts and documents project deliverables and milestones provides a roadmap for clear execution. Further, reforecasting key program deliverables based on actual clinical trial data received during the course of the trial is an essential component for study management. Otherwise, how would one know if planned study objectives can be delivered on schedule after the study has been initiated? The ability to evaluate project variation from the initial baseline plan and predict future outcomes using clinical trial data collected during the course of the study (predictive analytics) will allow the project team to manage the trial using data-driven techniques. This is important, as data-driven trial execution provides objective evidence to determine if study activities are meeting planned expectations, allowing for implementation of early risk mitigation strategies if the project is not on schedule.

Analyzing project variance from baseline and using actual versus planned parameter's values and predicted versus planned outcomes will allow the team to quickly assess clinical trial status. Simulation modeling and reforecasting techniques, when used during the course of the study, are a significant aid to earned value management (EMV), which is a project management technique for measuring project performance and progress. Earned value management methodologies assess measurements of project scope, schedule, and cost which should be implemented in every program. Although the intent of this chapter is not to delve into the essentials of good project management practice, an adaptive clinical trial requires exceptional project management rigor, provided by a highly seasoned, experienced leader who can implement earned value management using clinical trial simulation tools and data-driven analysis to assist with the overall management of the project.

11.3 IVRS and Drug Supply

The interactive voice randomization system (IVRS), used to manage patient randomization and assignment to treatment arms, must be fully integrated into the clinical trial operational processes. Statistical analysis outputs used for an adaptive randomization or dose–response designs are directly integrated into the IVRS ensuring appropriate subject randomization. The IVRS must be tightly integrated with the EDC platform. A typical IVRS data set may contain the following for newly randomized subjects: country, site, subject ID, date of birth (may be age or month and year of birth as per local requirements), gender, randomization code, randomization date, core study or substudy, enrollment status, drug interruption(s), and drug restart. Study coordinators will call the IVRS to notify the system of patient status, allowing data to be tracked in real time. These data are extremely valuable when managing patient enrollment and trial operations.

The IVRS must also integrate directly with the drug supply chain mechanism. Drug supply requirements need to be simulated during the planning stage as a part of the clinical supply optimization process to ensure appropriate production, labeling, and inventory management. Clinical drug supply optimization parameters typically include simulation and demand forecasting, regulatory strategy for submission and approvals, packaging and labeling strategy, distribution strategy, drug supply plan with trigger methodology, GMP/GDP regulatory review, IVRS specification requirements, and systems integration strategy. Chapter 15 gives more information on drug supply strategies and approaches for clinical supply modeling and simulation.

Appropriate drug formulations, dosing regimens, and routes of administration also need to be identified. For example, various dose levels can be produced by combining two or more tablets of specific doses. For intravenous drugs, varying dose levels can be achieved by requiring drug preparation to be conducted on site, using vials of equal volume dispensed in several dose strengths, and providing instructions as to how much should be removed from each vial to prepare a new dose.

11.4 Site Selections

As discussed earlier in this chapter, and as a result of the growing adoption of adaptive clinical trials, not all investigators that may qualify for study participation will have adaptive clinical trial expertise. It is anticipated that an adaptive clinical trial will utilize a blend of experienced and non-experienced clinical investigative sites. Given the complexities of the adaptive design and the need for near-real-time data entry and cleaning for decision making, sites that are selected for study participation must have adequate, experienced staffs to manage the accelerated pace of the adaptive design. Qualified sites must have experience in the specific therapeutic area and indication, have managed regulated clinical studies conducted under an IND, have the necessary infrastructure to support the added complexities of the trial, and have access to the appropriate patients. The demands of an adaptive clinical trial exceed those of the more traditional designs, and site personal and institutional review boards must be willing to accept additional responsibilities to ensure that the trial can meet the intended design requirements. We have observed that given adequate staff, institutional infrastructure, and thorough study training, non-experienced investigative sites have not only been able to effectively manage even the most complex adaptive designs, but also have been extremely supportive of the clinical trial, as they have recognized that adaptive designs may allow for earlier commercialization of a new drug product which would ultimately benefit their patients.

Sites need to be prepared to handle, at a minimum, (1) near-real-time data entry with minimal quality errors, (2) immediate submission of study endpoints including safety and efficacy, (3) effective drug management and accountability, (4) cooperation with clinical research organizations for real-time remote data cleaning, (5) potential changes to patient-informed consents, and (6) exceptional management, and organization of source documents. Sites must be extremely effective in the area of high-quality data management activities to ensure that all pre-planned statistical analyses can be completed on schedule, and that associated DMC decisions as a result of such analysis are immediately implemented should they impact their institution. Investigators need to be fully committed from study initiation to final database lock given the need for continually clean, accumulating data, which must be obtained during the course of the study across all patients, and which directly impact interim decision making.

11.5   Patient Recruitment

Patient recruitment rates are a critical design element, as the rate of randomization will drive the rate at which treatment data can be collected and analyzed, allowing for appropriate decision making. Recruitment rates are specific to the therapeutic area, indication, protocol requirements, and standards of care for the country in which the study is conducted. Initial patient recruitment assumptions could utilize reliable data sources from historical trials, and estimation using data mining techniques. However, final recruitment assessments should utilize data derived from comprehensive feasibility assessment which is conducted for the specific drug candidate. Recruitment assessments that are specifically developed for a drug candidate should be incorporated into final simulation and enrollment models that comprise the final baseline project plan. Given the requirements of the final protocol and study design, a comprehensive feasibility assessment is an important output of the planning and design phase, and should be considered as one of the key deliverables from this phase to give confidence in patient recruitment estimates, along with baseline project planning deliverables and milestones.

The rate at which patients are recruited determines the treatment data capture rates required for statistical analysis and decision making. As a result, the rate at which the trial recruits must complement the desired adaptive design—faster is not necessarily better. Instead, recruitment rates must be optimized to meet the desired pre-planned analysis within the specified time period. As one example, for dose–response designs, slower recruitment is preferable so that a dose adjustment can effectively be implemented for the next patient or the group of patients. Recruiting too quickly may not allow effective dose adjustment to occur during the specified randomization period. Optimizing recruitment rates based on the unique design requirements has a positive impact on the quality, length, and cost of the clinical trial. The speed of randomization also has a direct impact on key operational components—all of which need to be simulated during the planning stages—such as total number of sites required for study conduct, the rate of study start-up, site initiations, drug packaging, and supply chain management. Chapter 16 discusses approaches for patient recruitment modeling and simulation.

11.6 Treatment Data and Data Collection

Careful consideration should be given to the types of data used for an adaptive design and the method for data collection. Pre-planned statistical analysis must include a detailed assessment of all data that are required to perform an adaptation, in addition to when the data will be available and how they will be collected. Adaptive designs are better suited to the use of early outcome measurements as opposed to delayed ones. Early measures of clinical endpoints, biomarkers, or other efficacy endpoints allow for revised dosing allocations (response-adaptive designs), adaptive randomization (based on specific biomarkers), or other forms of design adaptations. Case report forms should focus on collection of key safety and efficacy data, and not on the collection of nonessential data elements, which can significantly increase trial costs and drive operational inefficiencies in an already complex study design.

Consideration must be given to those data elements that require cleaning rather than full source document verification, as source verification impacts the speed at which data can be utilized for decision making and increases operational complexity and cost. EDC systems are widely used today, which speed up the data collection and cleaning process. However, fully integrated clinical trial platforms—allowing for accelerated data capture, remote data monitoring and cleaning, seamless data transfer, and statistical analysis for DMC decision making—are not yet mainstream. As a result, clinical systems need to be tightly integrated to manage the complexities of an adaptive trial, ensuring minimization of data leakage and protection of the data and preserving blinded trial status. As technology improves, it is conceivable that informatics platforms will be available that allow for real-time data capture, interoperability with electronic health records (EHR) systems, e-Source archives, reduced dependencies on clinical monitoring, and the provision of fully integrated statistical analysis tools used for decision making for adaptive trials. However, use of existing systems, along with integrated approaches, allows for conduct of an adaptive clinical trial, but requires additional up-front planning time.

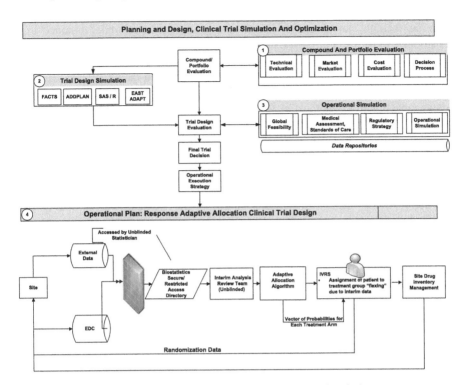

Fig. 11.1 An adaptive design process flow: response-adaptive allocation design

In addition, it is important to develop a comprehensive data management plan that documents all aspects of data handling for adaptive clinical trials. At a minimum, the data management plan should contain the following: (1) data cleaning plan, (2) edit specifications, (3) non-eCRF handling guidelines (include all relevant clinical trial data that are not captured in a traditional electronic case report form), (4) data coding guidelines, (4) SAE reconciliation guidelines, (5) QC plan, (6) data handling guidelines that document deviations from study-specific guidelines and planned procedures, (7) data integration guidelines, (8) local lab guidelines and central lab guidelines, (9) unblinding procedure guidelines, (10) data storage guidelines, (11) DMC guidelines, and (12) study-specific guidelines (e.g., eDC, IVRS).

The intent of the data management guidelines is to ensure proper data handling and data integrity during the course of the study. It is extremely important that rigorous adherence be applied to all data handling rules to ensure that the data are not inappropriately biased in any way. Clinical trial data that are utilized for submission to regulatory authorities and for market authorizations must be protected to ensure that data are of the highest quality. In this capacity, it is important to clearly define roles and responsibilities within the data management and clinical teams, ensuring that appropriate access to data is provided or prohibited to a given party.

As one example, for clinical trials that are conducted in a blinded manner, it is customary to utilize a blinded data management team in addition to an unblinded team. The unblinded team has proprietary access to unblinded clinical trial data, as they will be responsible for data integration of unblinded data and preparation of safety and efficacy reports for the data monitoring committee. However, unblinded data management teams must be firewalled from the clinical team and clinical trial activities, to avoid the introduction of operational bias into the clinical trial, which could potentially reduce the overall integrity of the data and trial.

For individuals that are new or less experienced to the clinical trial arena, we recommend a strong understanding of GCP regulations and best practices in data handling to protect clinical trial data from potential scrutiny by regulators. Data must also reside on secured storage locations, ensuring separation of blinded and unblinded data whether it is data with the actual treatment codes, PK/PD data, or safety information that can unblind treatments. Adherence to good clinical practice (GCP) and data handling procedures is a critical element of adaptive design trials, given the need for more frequent pre-planned statistical analysis and adaptation(s) during the course of the trial, coupled by the need for the operational teams to implement the required adaptation.

11.7 Centralized Remote Clinical Monitoring

A nontraditional clinical monitoring approach should be utilized for adaptive design trials, including a hybrid clinical monitoring approach consisting of centralized remote monitoring in addition to onsite source data verification (SDV). Centralized remote monitoring provides for continuous cleaning across key data elements in near real time, allowing for more immediate data transfers, statistical analysis, and decision making. The onsite clinical monitoring effort should take a risk-based monitoring approach, requiring minimal onsite time and source verification only for key data elements. SDV activities will typically lag behind remote data cleaning, so it is important that decision makers carefully consider those data elements that do not require SDV versus those that do. In general, most planned analyses that result in adaptations rely on data elements that do not require SDV. However, for some design elements, SDV may be required; in these cases, the timing of the data transfer and interim analysis must be carefully planned.

Risk-based monitoring techniques using advanced analytics and signal detection methodologies can also improve data quality by highlighting potential quality issues that need to be addressed during the trial. Some risk-based monitoring analytics utilize statistical analysis and variance around key risk areas that must be mitigated, such as AEs, SAEs, enrollment rates, protocol violations, and missing data.

In conclusion, nontraditional monitoring methods should be employed for adaptive clinical trials, taking account of data flow, timing of data entry, types of data collected, risk, data cleaning requirements, and clinical resource allocations. This will enable study requirements to be met and decision making to be based on the specified design parameters. Remote monitoring efforts must be amplified in addition to advanced analytics methodologies to ensure high-quality clinical trial conduct during the course of the trial.

The last remaining question is that of data cleanliness required for a given analysis. Is 100 % clean truly necessary for a given analysis? The answer to this question will depend upon the total amount of data needed for the analysis, the key data elements that will be used in the analysis, and the degree of risk should a different decision be reached if the data were modified. In general, we believe that more data is usually better than exclusively relying on completely cleaned data. In order to assess true risk of being misled by uncleaned data, one must compare the results of analysis based on:

1. The full dataset (including uncleaned data points)
2. The subset of "completely cleaned" data

The level of data cleanliness and SDV must be established during the design sessions, will be driven by the specific adaptive design that is planned to be implemented, and must take into consideration the key data elements necessary for the analysis, decision making, and subsequent adaptations.

11.8 Data Monitoring Committee (DMC)

DMCs are an important component in adaptive design trials, proactively assessing the risk benefit of the treatment, often at several time points during the trial, and making recommendations for study modifications based on adaptive rules specified in the protocol and/or in the DMC charter. In order to maintain trial integrity and minimize bias, an independent statistical center (ISC) should be utilized to prepare the data for DMC review and decision making. Often, a contract research organization (CRO) or an academic research organization (ARO) plays a role of the ISC. Depending on the design requirements, the ISC may need to comprise an independent unblinded team that has been appropriately firewalled from the rest of the study team to ensure that clinical data is not compromised and data leakage is minimized. The DMC charter outlines roles and responsibilities of DMC and summarizes statistical methods and necessary adaptations; the charter should be prepared at the planning stage and finalized prior to the first look/interim analysis. A DMC is assembled by a sponsor or a CRO/ARO supporting the trial, but free of a sponsor and its designee in terms of financial and professional interests. While there are well-established requirements including the FDA Guidance on Establishment and Operation of Clinical Trial Data Monitoring Committees, adaptive designs present additional challenges for a sponsor, DMC and ISC. It is critical that a CRO/ARO supporting an adaptive trial has extensive experience in performing interim analyses specifically in therapeutic area under study, and have appropriate firewalls established and standard operating procedures (SOP) that guard unblinding processes. Additionally, a CRO/ARO statistician should be knowledgeable in adaptive designs to perform necessary adaptations and analysis, and serve as a link between the sponsor and the DMC by acting as the designated data analysis center biostatistician. Chapter 14 provides more detailed information on this topic.

11.9   Clinical Trial Management and Communication

Given the increased operational complexities of an adaptive design, effective project management and communication is a critical component to success. Adaptive design project teams must work in a nontraditional environment, be tightly integrated, and have the proper resources, instructions, and tools to manage the clinical trial.

Cross-functional collaboration is paramount when designing an adaptive design clinical trial, and the planning and design phase is a critical element that must be implemented to ensure success. How can the success of an adaptive clinical trial be measured? This is an important step because a successful adaptive trial provides benefit to the overall drug development process, allows for effective implementation at the operational level, and provides efficiency gains from the standard model. In addition, we can use existing technologies to develop and operationalize an adaptive design trial, and can leverage common best practices across all unique designs.

11.10   Summary

The number of publications in adaptive designs has increased significantly in recent years, and many of these designs are rapidly growing in use. While adaptive designs add complexity to trials, they allow more efficient use of information for decision making, which ultimately translates into improved probability of success and shorter overall time to market for successful products. Execution of adaptive design trials at the operational level can be challenging, especially in studies involving multiple drugs, doses, biomarkers, and populations, as in the BATTLE (Zhou et al. 2008) and I-SPY2 TRIAL (Barker et al., 2009). The planning stage is a critical component for adaptive design studies. The additional time is necessary for up-front planning and cross-functional coordination. Education should be provided to all key participants to lay out the risks and benefits of applying adaptive designs. Detailed statistical design simulations and operational simulation models are required for studying planning to establish an effective execution. Randomization scheme, recruitment rate, treatment duration, timing of treatment readouts, endpoints, patient and site enrollment, dropouts, study drug formulation, route of drug administration, and drug supply should be considered during the planning stage. Timely data capture is an important enabler for adaptive designs. Electronic data capture should be used for studies with adaptive designs, especially for the trials with decision-critical data. The quality of data, effective data flow, and transfer processes should be discussed and pre-planned prior to interim analyses. Interim analyses have the potential for introducing statistical and operational biases due to the feedback of the information produced by such analyses. To minimize operational bias, interim analyses should be performed and reviewed by an independent statistical center and a data monitoring committee. It is critical that a CRO/ARO playing a role of ISC would have a necessary knowledge in adaptive designs and established processes that support necessary elements of an operational execution of such designs.

In this chapter, we highlighted a few key operational challenges and discussed strategies that must be taken into consideration for conduct of an adaptive clinical trial. Next chapters will provide more details on different aspects of adaptive design implementation such as drug supply, patient recruitment, IVRS, planning of interim analyses and managing DMCs, and available technology to protect trial integrity.

Appendix: Process Flow Example

We previously discussed that business process modeling is an activity that allows for the representation and documentation of key clinical trial activities, so that proposed operational processes may be analyzed and optimized. In this capacity, business process modeling is a useful tool that allows for the optimization of an adaptive clinical trial design. Described below are the essential elements of the trial design planning process, using business process modeling, which can occur in four general stages.

Stage 1: *Compound and portfolio evaluation.* In this stage, the drug manufacturer will proceed with a portfolio management process to make an assessment of which compound will be developed, based on the scientific, technical, medical, and commercial information required to assess the probability of technical success of the molecule. A decision will be made at the end of this evaluation period to either proceed or not proceed with the development of the compound. The information gathered in the stage will be utilized as a part of the adaptive clinical trial development approach.

Stage 2: *Trial design simulation.* In this stage, commercial software or custom software applications will be utilized to simulate key features of the proposed adaptive design and assess operating characteristics of the design. Data from other trials with this compound might be used to understand the uncertainty of treatment effect assumptions. The relative impact of the adaptive design trial on overall development should be considered. Examples of specific adaptive design requirements may include dropping or adding treatment arms; terminating the trial during an interim analysis due to efficacy, futility, or safety; changing patient randomization scheme; re-estimating the sample size; selecting subpopulations; and any combinations of the above.

Stage 3: *Operational simulation.* In this stage, the desired adaptive design is simulated to ensure that the design can actually be executed at the operational level. Simulations will include regulatory submission and approval timelines based on proposed country selections and study protocol, patient recruitment model, data submission timelines (all data elements required for data collection and statistical analysis), pre-planned interim analysis and DMC milestones, drug supply, compliance model, data cleaning activities, resource allocations, and final proposed program timelines. It is important to note that operational simulation efforts may indicate that the proposed study design may not be operationally feasible, which will require modification of the final study design to ensure successful implementation. The process of simulation is a critical element and should not be underestimated.

Stage 4: *Operational execution plan*. In this stage, given finalization of the intended design and appropriate operational simulation to ensure that the trial can be successfully executed, a comprehensive operational plan must be developed to ensure that the appropriate systems are in place and can be fully integrated to meet the final project plan deliverables. Business process flow diagrams are essential to ensure that each operational function understands how the trial will be executed, how the data will flow through the trial, and what key decisions need to be made at specific time points within the trial. This is an essential step in the process when working with multiple business partners, and multiple external vendors. As discussed previously, the planning and design process may take several months to complete, but is well worth the effort (Fig. 11.1).

References

Barker AD, Sigman CC, Kelloff GJ et al (2009) I-SPY 2: an adaptive breast cancer trial design in the setting of neoadjuvant chemotherapy. Clin Pharmacol Ther 86(1):97–100

Bretz F, Koenig F, Brannath W, Glimm E, Posch M (2009) Adaptive designs for confirmatory clinical trials. Stat Med 28:1181–1217

Chevret S (2006) Statistical methods for dose-finding experiments. Wiley, New York

EMA. CHMP 2007. Reflection paper on methodological issues in confirmatory clinical trials planned with an adaptive design. http://www.ema.europa.eu/docs/en_GB/document_library/Scientific_guideline/2009/09/WC500003616.pdf.

Dragalin V (2006) Adaptive designs: terminology and classification. Drug Inf J 40:425–435

FDA (2010) Guidance for industry 2010. Adaptive design clinical trials for drugs and biologics. http://www.fda.gov/downloads/DrugsGuidanceComplianceRegulatoryInformation/Guidances/UCM201790.pdf.

FDA (2012) FDA draft guidance. Enrichment strategies for clinical trials to support approval of human drugs and biological products. http://www.fda.gov/downloads/Drugs/GuidanceComplianceRegulatoryInformation/Guidances/UCM332181.pdf

Fedorov V, Leonov S (2013) Optimal design for nonlinear response models. CRC Press, Boca Raton, FL

Friede T, Parsons N, Stallard N (2012) A conditional error function approach for subgroup selection in adaptive clinical trials. Stat Med 31(30):4309–4320

Gaydos B, Anderson K, Berry D et al (2009) Good practices for adaptive clinical trials in pharmaceutical product development. Drug Inf J 43:539–556

Hu F, Rosenberger W (2006) The theory of response-adaptive randomization in clinical trials. Wiley Inc.

Jenkins M, Stone A, Jennison C (2011) An adaptive seamless phase II/III design for oncology trials with subpopulation selection using correlated survival endpoints. Pharm Stat 10:347–356

Jennison C, Turnbull BW (2000) Group sequential methods with applications to clinical trials. Chapman and Hall/CRC, Boca Raton, FL

Lai TL, Robbins H (1978) Adaptive design in regression and control. Proc Natl Acad Sci USA 75:586–587

Li Z, Durham SD, Flournoy N (1995) An adaptive design for maximization of a contingent binary response. In: Flournoy N, Rosenberger WF (eds) Adaptive designs. Institute of Mathematical Statistics, Beachwood, OH, pp 179–196

Lipkovich I, Dmitrienko A (2014) Strategies for identifying predictive biomarkers and subgroups with enhanced treatment effect in clinical trials using SIDES. J Biopharma Stat 24:130–153

Lipkovich I, Dmitrienko A, Denne J, Enas G (2011) Subgroup identification based on differential effect search (SIDES): a recursive partitioning method for establishing response to treatment in patient subpopulations. Stat Med 30:2601–2621

Marchenko O, Fedorov V, Lee JJ, Nolan C, Piheiro J (2014) Adaptive clinical trials: provides an overview of early-phase designs and their challenges. Ther Innov Regul Sci 48(1):20–30

O'Quigley J, Pepe M, Fisher L (1990) Continual reassessment method: a practical design for phase I clinical trials in cancer". Biometrics 46(1):33–48

Proshan MA, Lan KKG, Wittes JT (2006) Statistical monitoring of clinical trials – a unified approach. Springer, New York

Rosenberger WF, Lachin JM (2002) Randomization in clinical trials, theory and practice. Wiley, New York

Stallard N (2010) A confirmatory seamless phase II/III clinical trial design incorporating short-term endpoint information. Stat Med 29:959–971

Thall PF, Cook JD (2004) Dose-finding based on efficacy-toxicity trade-offs". Biometrics 60:684–693

Wang S, O'Neill R, Hung H (2007) Approaches to evaluation of treatment effect in randomized clinical trials with genomic subset. Pharm Stat 6:227–244

Zhou X, Liu S, Kim ES, Herbst RS, Lee JJ (2008) Bayesian adaptive design for targeted therapy development in lung cancer – a step toward personalized medicine. Clin Trials 5(3):181–193

Chapter 12
Implementation Issues in Adaptive Design Trials

Linda Danielson, Jerome Carlier, Tomasz Burzykowski, and Marc Buyse

Abstract In this chapter we discuss operational challenges that are specific to adaptive trials (as well as complex nonadaptive trials): essentially, the need to validate the design, to control the trial centrally, to collect and analyze key data rapidly, to preserve the trial blinding and integrity, and to document all important adaptive decisions taken. We illustrate these challenges using an actual phase I trial in oncology, and argue that the issues can be addressed through proper planning, choice of experienced vendors and independent groups (coordinating center and DSMB), statistical teams with adequate expertise in the design chosen (randomization and CRM), recourse to efficient computer technology (IWRS, EDC, automated e-mailing), and oversight by a team that must be as flexible as the trial design!

Keywords Operational issues • Phase I • Randomization • Drug supply • CRM (continual reassessment method) • IWRS (interactive web response system) • EDC (electronic data capture) • DSMB (Data and Safety Monitoring Board)

L. Danielson (✉) • J. Carlier
International Drug Development Institute (IDDI),
30 Avenue Provinciale, Louvain-la-Neuve, Belgium
e-mail: linda.danielson@iddi.com; jerome.carlier@iddi.com

T. Burzykowski • M. Buyse
International Drug Development Institute (IDDI),
30 Avenue Provinciale, Louvain-la-Neuve, Belgium

Interuniversity Institute for Biostatistics and statistical Bioinformatics (I-BioStat),
Hasselt University, Agoralaan D, Diepenbeek, Belgium
e-mail: tomasz.burzykowski@uhasselt.be; marc.buyse@iddi.com

W. He et al. (eds.), *Practical Considerations for Adaptive Trial Design and Implementation*, Statistics for Biology and Health,
DOI 10.1007/978-1-4939-1100-4_12, © Springer Science+Business Media New York 2014

12.1   Introduction

The growing enthusiasm for adaptive design trials is sometimes abated by concerns about difficulties with their conduct (Quinlan et al. 2010). While it is undeniable that adaptive design trials are generally less straightforward to implement than classical, fixed sample size designs, potential difficulties can all be addressed prospectively (Krams et al. 2007). Regulatory guidance documents are essential background references (EMA 2007; FDA 2010). Sponsors who choose to conduct adaptive design trials will want to ensure that the providers with whom they partner to conduct the trial have adequate expertise in terms of statistical methodology as well as operational experience in terms of using advanced technology (IWRS, EDC) and dealing with multiple partners (DSMB, drug supply centers, investigational sites).

In this chapter we discuss implementation issues using a phase I clinical trial as a case study. This trial is in many ways more complex than larger scale, later phase adaptive design trials, but it is illustrative of many requirements that are common to all adaptive designs: the need to allow for sufficient planning of the trial design and implementation, to validate the design prior to starting the trial, to oversee the trial progress centrally, to monitor drug supply at all participating sites, to collect patient data in real time, to clean essential data with minimal delays, to analyze the data in a timely fashion for appropriate adaptations to be possible, to revisit some of the design assumptions over the course of the trial if required, to preserve the trial blinding and integrity, and to document all important adaptive decisions taken over the course of the trial for future audits.

12.2   Case Study

The case study used here is based on an actual trial, although details have been modified to preserve anonymity. An experimental drug for supportive therapy of cancer patients had to undergo phase I testing. The goal of the phase I trial was to find the maximum tolerated dose (MTD), defined as the dose of the drug for which the probability of dose-limiting toxicity (DLT) was equal to 33 %. The experimental drug was added (with no expected interactions) to standard anticancer therapy.

12.2.1   Design Constraints

The design of the trial had to fulfill the following requirements specified by the sponsor:

- A continuous dose scale should be used over a pre-specified range of feasible doses.
- About ten patients should be treated at the MTD.
- A placebo group of about ten patients should be included.

- Patients should be randomized in double-blind fashion with less patients randomized to placebo than to the experimental drug.
- The total sample size of the trial should be about 30-40 patients.

These conditions implied that a nonstandard phase I design had to be worked out. It was decided to design the trial using the likelihood-based version of the continual reassessment method (CRM) (O'Quigley and Shen 1996) on a continuous dose scale (Storer 2001). The trial was split into two stages: an initial dose-escalation stage and a model-guided stage. In both stages, patients were randomized to receive placebo or the experimental drug in addition to standard chemotherapy according to a 1:3 randomization ratio. The main reason for including the placebo group was to collect information about the background rate of a particular type of chemotherapy-related toxicity the supportive therapy was aimed at reducing. The information collected was intended to provide some idea about the potential effect of the therapy and could be used by the sponsor for planning (e.g., sample size calculations) of the next trials.

12.2.2 Initial CRM Design

Initially, the design of the trial was specified as follows. In the dose-escalation stage, consecutive patients were assigned to doses equal to multiples of a dose d, i.e., $0.5d$, d, $2d$, $3d$, $4d$, $5d$, $6d$, and $6.7d$. Already at this stage, randomization to placebo (with 25 % probability) was implemented; that is, the assignment of patients to the sequence of the pre-planned active doses was interleaved with a random assignment of placebo.

Upon observing the first instance of dose-limiting toxicity (DLT), the model-guided stage was to be initiated. Note that observing a DLT for placebo did not trigger the stage, nor were placebo-assigned patients used in updating the model.

In the model-guided stage, the hyperbolic-tangent dose-toxicity model was used for selection of the doses for consecutive patients. The model was of the form

$$\pi(x,\beta) = \left\{(\tanh x + 1)/2\right\}^{\beta},$$

where $\pi(x,\beta)$ is the probability of DLT for dose x (Fig. 12.1).

Upon observing the DLT status for a patient, the value of the parameter β would be updated based on all available data. Then, the next patient would be assigned the dose for which the probability of the DLT, based on the updated model, was equal to 33 %. In this stage, doses would be chosen on a continuous scale. That is, the dose with a DLT probability exactly equal to 33 %, according to the updated model, would be selected. Section 12.3.6 describes how these continuous doses were managed. The following stopping rule was used for the model-guided stage: before assigning a dose, the probability of assigning the next four patients to a dose within $\pm(2/15)d$ relative to the last assigned dose was computed.

- If the probability was less than 90 %, then the trial would continue.
- If the probability was equal to at least 90 %, then the number of patients already treated at doses higher or equal to the last assigned dose minus $(2/15)d$ would be determined.

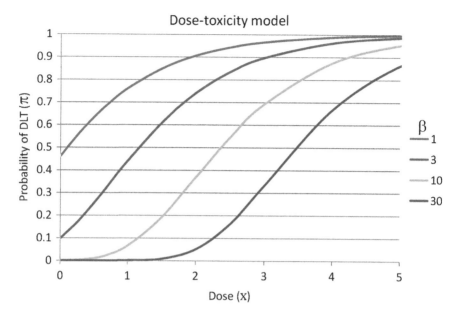

Fig. 12.1 Probability of dose-limiting toxicity (DLT) as a function of dose (x). In the continual reassessment method (CRM), parameter β is re-estimated every time the outcome of a patient (DLT or no DLT) is observed

- If ten or more patients had already been treated at doses higher than or equal to the last assigned dose minus $(2/15)d$, the trial should be stopped.
- If less than ten patients had already been treated at doses higher than or equal to the last assigned dose minus $(2/15)d$, additional patients—maximally four— would be assigned to the last assigned dose in order to reach (if possible) the total of ten patients, after which the trial would stop without reassessing the model.

If, according to the above rules, any additional patients were to be added to the group receiving the experimental drug, and if the placebo group contained less than ten patients, up to two extra placebo patients could be included in the trial, so that the size of the placebo group would get as close as possible to ten patients.

12.2.3 Design Modifications

During the conduct of the trial, several modifications to the design had to be made. In particular:

- After the trial started, it appeared from extensive simulations that the condition used in the stopping rule for the model-guided stage (at least 90 % probability of assigning the next four patients to a dose differing by at most $(2/15)d$ from the last assigned dose) was too stringent and would result in too large a sample size.

Thus, the condition was changed to at least 80 % probability of assigning the next four patients to a dose differing by at most $(3/15)d$ from the last assigned dose. For this condition, the expected number of patients receiving experimental drug would be equal to about 40. The modification was introduced by a formal amendment to the protocol.

- The results observed for an initial sequence of patients included in the initial dose-escalation stage suggested that the drug was safer than assumed and that the MTD could be higher than the initially set maximum of $6.7d$. Hence, the margin of tolerance, used in the condition specified in the stopping rule, was changed from an absolute one to a relative one. In particular, the stopping-rule condition was changed to at least 80 % probability of assigning the next four patients to a dose differing by at most 10 % relative to the last assigned dose.

- Given that the initial results suggested that the drug was safer than assumed, changes to the initial dose-escalation scheme were introduced. First, the escalation of doses beyond the $6.7d$ was formally allowed. To this aim, a second protocol amendment was issued, which also included the change of the margin of tolerance mentioned earlier and an update of the drug preparation and administration procedures implied by the increase of the allowed maximum escalated dose. Next, once the total dose of $10d$ had been reached, the basic increase of dose equal to d, adopted for the initial dose-escalation step, appeared to be much too small. Hence, the increase was changed to 20 % of the last assigned dose. That is, the sequence of doses to be assigned in the initial dose-escalation stage was modified to $10d$, $12d$, $14.4d$, $17.28d$, etc. Moreover, the maximum dose to be used in the trial was reset to $66.7d$. These modifications were introduced by a third protocol amendment, in which additional updates of the drug preparation and administration procedures had to be made.

12.2.4 Trial Conduct

The trial was conducted in five centers. The occurrence of a DLT was assessed during a 5-day period. The DLT status of each patient was reviewed by a Data Safety and Monitoring Board (DSMB), based upon all adverse event data provided by the clinical sites. The DSMB was also charged with the approval of the next dose assignment within the model-guided stage. Hence, the role of the DSMB extended well beyond the traditional role of monitoring safety, adding to it the roles of an adjudication committee and a trial steering committee (Ellenberg et al. 2002; DeMets et al. 2006; Herson 2009; also see Chap. 14 of this book for further discussions).

The study took about 1 year until completion. Eventually, the trial never reached the model-guided stage, as not a single DLT was observed. The assumed level of toxicity of a new drug may in fact be overestimated in phase I trials, which calls for flexibility in the range of doses that are planned to be studied (see, e.g., Paoletti et al. 2006). In this trial, the accrual was stopped with a last assigned dose of the experimental drug equal to $62d$, i.e., close to the (updated) maximum of $66.7d$. The total number of patients included in the trial was equal to 28, with seven patients assigned to placebo.

12.2.5   Challenges

The implementation of this trial raised a number of challenges. These included the need for implementing randomization and blinding, which are not standard practices in a phase I study. The randomization system had to be linked to a drug supply system that monitored the treatment kits available at each of the five sites. The DSMB had to accept or overrule the dose of each patient randomized to receive the experimental drug. The DSMB also had to adjudicate the outcome of each patient, and decide whether a DLT had been observed or not.

The conduct of this trial was further complicated by the additional design modifications made during the conduct of the study, which implied modifications to the system used for randomization and assignment of the doses to the patients. All of these challenges are discussed in more detail in the next sections. Admittedly some of the challenges are peculiar to our case study, such as major design modifications that are typically not permitted in later phase trials but are to be expected in first-in-man trials. However, this case study is of interest because many of the solutions adopted to address the adaptive nature of the trial are generic and can be implemented identically for simpler adaptive designs of later phase trials.

12.3   Implementation

The flow chart of Fig. 12.2 summarizes, in simplified form, the way in which this phase I trial was implemented.

Clearly, implementation of such a design requires integration of several computer systems (Gallo et al. 2006). An interactive web response system (IWRS) was used for patient randomization and for drug supply management and an electronic data capture (EDC) system was used to enter clinical data (case report forms). An automated e-mailing system was used to send messages from the coordinating center to the DSMB and to the five clinical sites where patients were being treated. Documents were stored in, and shared through, a web portal that gave different access privileges to the individuals involved in the trial conduct.

12.3.1   Planning

The planning phase is of key importance to ensure the successful implementation of an adaptive design (Quinlan and Krams 2006). Because the design is nonstandard, custom software must usually be developed, tested, and validated. The various functionalities required for the trial conduct, as outlined in the next sections, usually involve different departments (typically, information technology, data management, biostatistics, and clinical operations). An "adaptive design team" dedicated to the trial should be put in place by the trial sponsor (Fardipour et al. 2009a). This team is responsible for choosing the various technologies required for the trial conduct

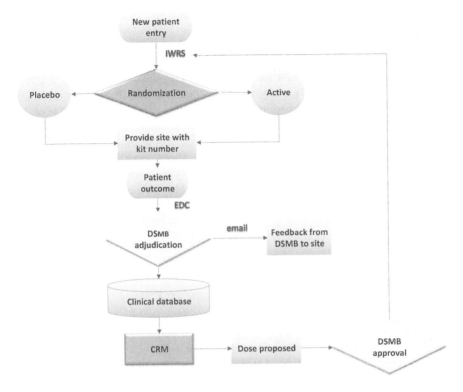

Fig. 12.2 Flow chart showing implementation of phase I design. *IWRS* interactive web response system, *EDC* electronic data capture, *DSMB* Data Safety and Monitoring Board

(IWRS, EDC, CRM or other adaptive statistical module, communication system), as well as any other vendors and the committees involved in the trial (DSMB, drug supply center, independent statistical center). In our example, the adaptive design team was based at the coordinating center of the trial, which also served as the independent statistical center. Adaptive trials have been reported in which two independent statistical centers were put in place in order to fully protect the blinding of interim data (Fardipour et al. 2009a). Generally speaking, blinding is a key consideration in planning adaptive trials (Gallo 2006), especially those in which part of the trial is confirmatory and is intended to be used for registration, such as in seamless II/III designs (Maca et al. 2006).

12.3.2   Randomization

Having a correct and validated randomization system is essential for any randomized trial. A centralized randomization is essential for an adaptive trial where the randomization depends on the totality of the current data. This may sound trivial but a number of trials have failed or have raised serious questions about how patients were randomized. There are several aspects to this issue: First and foremost, does the vendor implementing the randomization system have adequate statistical competence? There exist a number of classical randomization methods (permuted blocks with or without stratification, minimization, etc.), and the choice of a method as well as the details of its implementation are among the most important features of any randomized trial. This is also true when outcome-adaptive randomization is chosen, whereby the probability of treatment allocation varies over the course of the study depending on the observed patient outcomes. Second, is the integrity of treatment allocation ensured, and how? Third, are measures in place to address deviations, such as patients not taking the medication allocated to them? Fourth, is the randomization monitored over time, to ensure that the system does what it is supposed to do? For all these reasons, it may be desirable to choose a vendor that has a proven system and a track record of successful randomization implementations. Chapters 9 and 10 of this book provide details about points to consider regarding randomization in adaptive trials.

12.3.3   Continual Reassessment Method (CRM)

Special-purpose software (a SAS macro) was developed for this trial to implement the CRM method described in Sects. 12.2.2 and 12.2.3. The software was qualified by running extensive simulations aimed at checking the operational characteristics of the design, including the identification of the MTD and the expected sample size. One unusual feature in this trial was the major design changes that occurred during trial conduct, and required software changes and revalidation. The statistician responsible for the trial attended the DSMB meeting during which all relevant data were reviewed. Once the DLT status of a patient was confirmed by the DSMB, the statistician was responsible for including the information into the randomization system. Also, in the model-updating stage, the statistician was responsible for running the CRM module. However, as has already been mentioned, the trial did not reach this design stage.

12.3.4   Interactive Web Response System (IWRS)

The availability of a flexible IWRS was essential to manage the complexity of this adaptive design. The trial was designed to go through two distinct stages, each stage being substantially different from the previous one in terms of the randomization features. The IWRS was also designed to generate information to, and integrate information from, the DSMB, to provide a treatment kit number to the unblinded pharmacist at each site, to control the opening and closure of recruitment at each participating site, and to monitor investigational product needs at each site, taking into account the subjects and site history, as well as the current trial status.

As stated above, the DSMB involvement was continuous in so far as they had to approve the dose to be administered to every patient randomized to the experimental drug. This is unusual and had implications on the choice of DSMB members as well as on the DSMB Charter, which contained clear explanations about the flow of information between the different parties involved in the trial. Every effort was made to keep all processes as simple as possible for DSMB members. They did not have to log into the IWRS; rather, they had stated their preference to send a fax with their decision to the coordinating office which entered the necessary information into the IWRS. All other communications to and from the DSMB were done via e-mailing system, which was largely automated to minimize both the time required and the opportunity for errors.

The sites were informed automatically and in real time of the trial status. This was important since the randomization was stopped and started before and after each DSMB meeting. They needed to know at every moment whether the randomization was open or closed so that they knew when they could randomize patients.

12.3.5 Electronic Data Capture (EDC)

The EDC system in this trial was used to collect key data for the IWRS to act as a central control system. The EDC captured real-time information on the subject treatment and outcome (in this case any dose-limiting toxicity). This information was fed to the clinical database, and was to be used by the CRM for dose selection, and reviewed by the DSMB for dose approval (Fig. 12.2).

12.3.6 Drug Supply Management

The drug supply process can be complex in adaptive trials, especially when the trial proceeds in stages with different types of supplies (product, dose, formulation, etc.) It is important to test the product dosage, packaging, distribution, storage, or usage before trial start, and to monitor these features closely during the early phases of the adaptive design trial. When changes in any of these parameters are mandated by the trial design, all possible scenarios must be simulated to estimate the quantities of the product required, where and when. Further discussions of points to consider for the drug supply process in adaptive trials can be found in Chap. 15 of this book.

An experimental product never comes in unlimited quantities and is often quite expensive; the shipments can have significant costs; storage conditions are not always ideal; product shipments may not arrive immediately. Having these restrictions in mind is key in order to put in place the drug supply process including mechanisms that will help make appropriate real-time decisions in case of unexpected events with drug supply. A challenge that is specific to adaptive trials is to optimize drug supply across all scenarios allowed by the adaptive design.

Whenever possible, the product formulation or packaging should ensure that there will be no need for additional product regardless of the scenario that actually takes place, for example in designing the product kits in such a way that all possible doses can be reconstituted with a given number of kits. This not only reduces the cost of drug supply, but it also ensures the integrity of the trial blind after adaptation.

For the study described above, the treatment was given as an infusion, so there was flexibility in modifying the dose. Since this was a double-blind study, the investigator could not be aware of the treatment being given, so the syringes were prepared by an unblinded pharmacist. The pharmacist prepared two syringes by drawing the appropriate amount of study drug and adding the appropriate amount of sterile water for injection in order to get the final volume needed. The IWRS system provided detailed instructions to the pharmacist on the size of the syringe, and how much active drug and how much saline solution to combine in each syringe. All of this information was dynamic and depended on which dose was to be given. This was defined at the beginning of the study, and then modified and revalidated when the protocol increased the maximum possible dose as the IWRS system had to foresee all possible doses.

12.3.7 Data Safety and Monitoring Board (DSMB)

Adaptive designs, by definition, include interim analyses which may or may not trigger adaptations. Our phase I design is an extreme example in which the outcome of every patient receiving experimental treatment could potentially change the dose for the next patients entered in the trial. In traditional open-label phase I dose-escalation trials, the investigators themselves review the interim data to decide on the next dose to be administered, but in the double-blind trial discussed here the interim analyses were reviewed by an independent DSMB, just as they would be in most other adaptive design trials. The independence of the DSMB was felt essential to maintain the blinding and prevent operational bias from entering the trial post-adaptation, had the investigators and/or the sponsor been aware of interim trial outcomes.

Regulatory guidance documents (EMA 2005; FDA 2006) as well as several books (Ellenberg et al. 2002; DeMets et al. 2006; Herson 2009) discuss requirements for the composition and role of DSMBs, and provide templates for DSMB Charters. The role of DSMBs in adaptive trials is covered in detail in Chap. 14 of this book. The most important role of DSMBs is to ensure the protection of the patients entered in the trial, which entails not only a careful and regular review of safety data, but also a close scrutiny of the trial conduct. As stated above, DSMBs are typically independent from all other parties involved in the trial conduct and the integrity of the trial data is ensured by restricting access to interim trial outcomes to DSMB members only. In our phase I example, the algorithm for dose escalation was fully pre-specified and the DSMB acted mostly as a safeguard against unexpected drug effects. In late-stage adaptive designs used for confirmatory trials, it is also

Table 12.1 Conditions under which sponsor involvement may be considered in adaptive decisions

Condition	Details
Rationale for involvement	There is a strong and documented rationale for a few sponsor representatives to be involved, either to reach the best decision for the trial itself or to secure further funding for the remainder of the trial (e.g., if a sample size increase is considered)
Complete independence from trial conduct	The sponsor representatives are not involved in trial operations, and clearly understand the issues and risks associated with knowledge of interim results (e.g., operational biases)
Minimal data shared	The sponsor representatives receive "minimal" pre-specified interim data, i.e., *only* at the adaptation point, and *only* the data required to reach a decision (unlike a DSMB who has a broader role, and may therefore see more extensive interim data)
Documentation	Any release of information to sponsor representatives is duly documented and tracked using a secure electronic system
Adequate blinding	Adequate firewalls are put in place to guarantee blinding for all individuals other than those involved in adaptive decisions

essential that the DSMB has complete independence. In some situations, however, e.g., in early-stage adaptive design trials, the sponsor may find it difficult to leave important adaptations to a completely independent committee, no matter how carefully chosen. Leaving aside the sponsor's financial interest, it may be the case that the sponsor has access to important information not available to the DSMB, so that it may be in the best interest of the trial that the sponsor be involved in the decision making. If the sponsor needs to be represented at all in the decision making, the PhRMA Working Group on Adaptive Trial Designs (Gallo et al. 2006) recommends that the rationale for this be documented, that the sponsor representatives who receive access to interim results be adequately distanced from the trial conduct, and that their number be limited to the bare minimum. Table 12.1 lists essential conditions under which sponsor involvement may be considered in adaptive decisions.

It should be emphasized that even if all necessary precautions are taken to maintain interim results blinded, adaptations will often convey indirect information on the treatment effects—for instance, when doses are dropped for lack of efficacy. For a detailed discussion of this issue, see Gallo (2006).

One problem that occurred in the trial described above, but also frequently in other trials, is that the DSMB may see data that raise serious questions about the adequacy of the design assumptions. To protect against unwarranted consequences of such problems, it is useful to put in place a trial Steering Committee, involving all parties concerned, and to pre-specify rules for any required interactions between the Steering Committee and the DSMB (Fardipour et al. 2009b). The fact that a trial is planned to be adaptive does not imply that any type of data-derived design changes are feasible; in fact, a well-designed adaptive trial must pre-specify what specific adaptations will be considered, and under what conditions. However, the setup of an adaptive trial ensures that mechanisms are in place to discuss other design changes that might be required, as in our example, whilst preserving the trial integrity.

12.3.8 Communication System

As is clear from Fig. 12.2, the various parties involved in the conduct of the trial (coordinating center, drug supply center, DSMB, participating sites) had to be informed quickly and consistently of new events triggering further actions. This was made possible through implementation of an automated e-mailing system between these parties, which was felt to be more reliable than an e-mailing system triggered by human intervention. Such a system also provided an unalterable record of the sequence of events throughout the course of the trial. In addition to this e-mailing system, a dedicated web portal was built specifically for the trial, with access privileges tailored to each individual involved in the trial conduct.

12.4 Quality Assurance

12.4.1 System Validation

All systems put in place to help conduct a trial (CRM, IWRS, EDC, drug supply) need to be fully validated, whether for an adaptive or a nonadaptive trial. The testing required for system validation is more challenging for an adaptive trial, and can become a hefty mission when the number of potential scenarios is large. However the system validation provides a unique opportunity not just to test the systems, but also to revisit the assumptions underlying the design and the plausible scenarios arising from it. Unsuspected flaws can be uncovered during testing, in which case amendments to the design may prove necessary. Finally, the system validation brings added value because it involves a number of real trial actors and offers an opportunity to identify bottlenecks or obstacles and fine-tune all processes and communication lines.

12.4.2 Simulations

When an adaptive design is implemented, it is essential to investigate the various potential outcomes of the trial under a range of plausible scenarios. From a statistical point of view, the operating characteristics of simple designs can be derived analytically, but for complex designs such as the phase I design discussed here, simulations must be used. If custom-made software is used to implement the design, its validation usually includes simulations aimed at showing that the design and the software deliver the intended outcomes. When we conducted such simulations in our phase I trial, they indicated that the initially proposed stopping rule for the CRM design would result in too large a sample size. Consequently, the stopping rule was modified. For detailed points to consider on trial simulations, see Gaydos et al. (2009).

12.4.3   Documentation

An adaptive design requires more documentation than a traditional design. Unless the design has been described in a peer-reviewed publication, its operating characteristics will need to be documented in detail. The advantages of the chosen design will need to be demonstrated, in comparison to simpler, nonadaptive, designs. The simulation report, in an adaptive design, may be considered a regulatory document alongside the statistical analysis plan. For detailed points to consider on documentation, see Gaydos et al. (2009), and Chap. 14 of this book.

12.5   Other Operational Considerations

12.5.1   Coordinating Center

The coordinating center must have statistical expertise in adaptive designs, as well as relevant experience in managing adaptive trials. Although adaptive designs can have a wide range of purposes (dose finding, seamless transition from phase II to phase III, sample size increase, population enrichment, etc.) with different operational implications, we have tried throughout this chapter to discuss issues that are common to most adaptive trials. As a matter of fact, coordinating centers having experience with sophisticated nonadaptive trials (e.g., trials with complex randomization schemes and trials using sequential or group sequential designs) will already have in place a number of key components discussed above (e.g., IWRS and DSMB experience); hence they will find it easier to extend their capabilities to address specific requirements of adaptive trials. In addition to relevant experience, such a coordinating center needs to have a help desk available to all users at all times. Adaptive designs have more parts that can require assistance for the sites, so it is important for them to be able to call someone to get help whenever needed. Since most trials are now worldwide, this help desk should be reachable 24/7—ideally either by e-mail or by telephone.

12.5.2   Change Management

The sponsor of an adaptive trial, and even more so the coordinating center in charge of the trial conduct, must be prepared to implement change management. In a survey of 13 large- and medium-sized pharmaceutical companies and three statistical consultancy groups, change management was mentioned as a major stumbling block against broader adoption of adaptive designs (Quinlan et al. 2010). Appropriate education and training are both key, but it is equally important for the coordinating center to maintain a spirit of openness, flexibility, and critical thinking rather than over-reliance on a rigid set of standard operating procedures (SOPs). Although project-specific SOPs can be useful in most situations, the personnel involved in the project must be adaptive—i.e., prepared to face unexpected events and changes gracefully and efficiently.

12.5.3 Institutional Review Boards

Because of their inherent complexity, adaptive designs will often need to be explained in detail to Institutional Review Boards (called Ethics Committees in Europe) charged with their approval for local use. Similarly, more time may need to be devoted to develop informed consent forms that are truly informative about the nature of the trial design as well as understandable by patients (and investigators). Although the statistical details of the adaptation can be technically challenging, such details are unnecessary to understand the essence of the design, and in fact are best kept hidden from the trial participants, in order to avoid any operational biases that might arise from such in-depth knowledge. A typical example is the randomization method used to allocate treatments to patients. Although the method must be fully described in the technical documentation of the trial, it should not be described in any detail in the documents that are publicly available (e.g., the trial protocol or the trial summary posted in clinicaltrials.gov).

12.6 Conclusions: Success Factors for Adaptive Trial Implementation

Our example illustrates that implementing an adaptive design does require careful planning and creates an operational overhead which adds to the overall costs of the trial (Quinlan and Krams 2006). We discussed a phase I dose-finding trial in cancer, but many of the operational difficulties would be similar in other adaptive dose-finding trials (Shen et al. 2011). In return for such careful planning of adaptive trials, it is important to emphasize that many of the risks associated with the trial design and execution will have been fully addressed prior to starting patient accrual in an adaptively designed trial, which is fully in line with the recent guidance documents on risk-based quality management from the European Medicines Agency (EMA 2011) and the US Food and Drug Administration (FDA 2013). A dialogue with the agencies is less essential for early phase trials, where there are fewer regulatory concerns about adaptive designs, but for later phase trials an early interaction with the agencies is highly recommended (Chow and Chang 2008).

All in all, the challenges of implementing adaptive designs may be well worth the effort. From an operational point of view the following issues should be considered:

- The vendors in charge of implementing the trial should have knowledge of, and experience with, adaptive and complex designs, which requires both statistical and operational (randomization) expertise.

- The vendors should be involved in the trial as soon as possible, preferably at the design stage.
- The members of the DSMB should have adequate expertise and availability to effectively monitor the trial.
- The key events and transitions between the different stages of the adaptive design should be clearly outlined, all operations (automated/semiautomated/manual) defined, and all actors identified prior to trial start.
- The computerized system (see Fig. 12.2) should be fully implemented, tested and validated, and revalidated in case of major design changes.
- Extensive simulations should be carried out to cover all possible scenarios dictated by the adaptive design, with active involvement of all key actors in "dummy runs".
- Proper documentation must be available to address any question that might be raised during or after the trial.

Acknowledgments   The authors are grateful to Dr. Vlad Dragalin for suggesting useful references, and to the book editors for their careful review of this chapter.

References

Chow SC, Chang M (2008) Adaptive design methods in clinical trials – a review. Orphanet J Rare Dis 3:11

DeMets DL, Furberg CD, Friedman LM (eds) (2006) Data monitoring in clinical trials: a case studies approach. Springer, New York. ISBN 0-387-20330-3

Ellenberg SE, Fleming TR, DeMets DL (2002) Data monitoring committees in clinical trials: a practical perspective. Wiley, Chichester. ISBN 0-471-48986-7

European Medicines Agency. Committee for Medicinal Products for Human Use (CHMP): guideline on data monitoring committees. http://www.ema.europa.eu/docs/en_GB/document_library/Scientific_guideline/2009/09/WC500003635.pdf (July 2005). Accessed 30 Sep 2013

European Medicines Agency. Committee for Medicinal Products for Human Use (CHMP): Reflection paper on methodological issues in confirmatory clinical trials planned with an adaptive design. http://www.ema.europa.eu/docs/en_GB/document_library/Scientific_guideline/2009/09/WC500003616.pdf (October 2007). Accessed 30 Sep 2013

European Medicines Agency. Reflection paper on risk based quality management in clinical trials. EMA/INS/GCP/394194/2011. http://www.ema.europa.eu/docs/en_GB/document_library/Scientific_guideline/2011/08/WC500110059.pdf (February 2011). Accessed 30 Sep 2013

Fardipour P, Littman G, Burns DD et al (2009a) Planning and executing response-adaptive learn-phase clinical trials: 1. The process. Drug Inf J 43:713–724

Fardipour P, Littman G, Burns DD et al (2009b) Planning and executing response-adaptive learn-phase clinical trials: 2. Case studies. Drug Inf J 43:725–734

Food and Drug Administration (FDA) (2006) guidance for industry – establishment and operation of clinical trial data monitoring committees. http://www.fda.gov/downloads/Regulatoryinformation/Guidances/ucm127073.pdf. Accessed 30 Sep 2013

Food and Drug Administration (FDA) (2010) Guidance for clinical trial sponsors – adaptive design clinical trials for drugs and biologics. http://www.fda.gov/downloads/Drugs/.../Guidances/ucm201790.pdf. Accessed 30 Sep 2013

Food and Drug Administration (FDA) (2013) Guidance for industry: oversight of clinical investigations – a risk-based approach to monitoring. http://www.fda.gov/downloads/Drugs/GuidanceComplianceRegulatoryInformation/Guidances/UCM269919.pdf. Accessed 30 Sep2013

Gallo P (2006) Confidentiality and trial integrity issues for adaptive designs. Drug Inf J 40:445–450

Gallo P, Chuang-Stein C, Dragalin V et al (2006) Adaptive designs in clinical drug development – an executive summary of the PhRMA Working Group. J Biopharm Stat 16:275–283

Gaydos B, Anderson KM, Berry D et al (2009) Good practices for adaptive clinical trials in pharmaceutical product development. Drug Inf J 43:539–556

Herson J (2009) Data and safety monitoring committees in clinical trials. Chapman & Hall, Boca Raton, FL. ISBN 978-1-4200-7037-8

Krams M, Burman CF, Dragalin V et al (2007) Adaptive designs in clinical drug development: opportunities, challenges, and scope. Reflections following PhRMA's November 2006 workshop. J Biopharm Stat 17:957–964

Maca J, Bhattacharya S, Dragalin V et al (2006) Adaptive seamless phase II/III designs – background, operational aspects, and examples. Drug Inf J 40:463–473

O'Quigley J, Shen LZ (1996) Continual reassessment method: a likelihood approach. Biometrics 52:673–684

Paoletti X, Baron B, Schöffski P et al (2006) Using the continual reassessment method: lessons learned from an EORTC phase I dose finding study. Eur J Cancer 42:1362–1368

Quinlan JA, Krams M (2006) Implementing adaptive designs: logistical and operational considerations. Drug Inf J 40:437–444

Quinlan J, Gaydos B, Maca J, Krams M (2010) Barriers and opportunities for implementation of adaptive designs in pharmaceutical product development. Clin Trials 7:167–173

Shen J, Preskorn S, Dragalin V et al (2011) How adaptive designs can increase efficiency in psychiatric drug development: a case study. Innov Clin Neurosci 8:26–34

Storer BE (2001) An evaluation of phase I clinical trial designs in the continuous dose–response setting. Stat Med 20:2399–2408

Chapter 13
Implementing Adaptive Designs: Using Technology to Protect Trial Integrity, Reduce Operational Bias, and Build Regulatory Trust

Judith Quinlan and Michael Krams

Abstract Experimental design and the execution environment have to go hand in hand to enable successful implementation of adaptive designs: the more complex, dynamic, and closer to real time the adaptation(s), the greater the demand on the execution environment.

As industry has dipped its toes into the adaptive pond, it has done so cautiously, partly handicapped by a traditional execution environment not designed to entertain real time learning and decision making. Therefore, the majority of adaptive designs currently implemented are of the simpler kind: one or two interim analyses, and limited adaptations: sample size adjustments, possibly dropping a dose, in other words: whatever a traditional and antiquated execution environment can support without requiring more than minor work-around solutions.

The opportunity space for adaptive designs from an experimental design perspective in pharmaceutical drug development is of course much wider (as discussed in other chapters). Here we present a conceptual view of a scalable execution environment, designed to support the full opportunity space of adaptive designs, and highlight the role of enabling technology and integrated processes.

This chapter looks at the role of technology today, but perhaps more importantly, identifies the role and need for technology in providing scalable and more efficient solutions that not only enable larger uptake of the simpler adaptive trials of today, but also support the more operationally demanding of adaptive trials, as well as enabling custom designs to be readily implemented. Systems and processes under

J. Quinlan (✉)
SVP Innovation Center, Aptiv Solutions, 805 Old State Road, Berwyn, PA 19312, USA
e-mail: Judith.Quinlan@AptivSolutions.com

M. Krams
VP Quantitative Sciences, Janssen Pharmaceuticals Inc, 1125 Trenton Harbourton Rd, Titusville, NJ 08560, USA
e-mail: MKrams@ITS.JNJ.com

W. He et al. (eds.), *Practical Considerations for Adaptive Trial Design and Implementation*, Statistics for Biology and Health, DOI 10.1007/978-1-4939-1100-4_13, © Springer Science+Business Media New York 2014

stress introduce an increased risk of mistakes that may threaten trial integrity and introduce operational bias. In this future landscape, technology will play a more significant role not only to increase efficiency, but also to ensure trial integrity is maintained and operational bias is minimized. However technology is only a tool that is managed by humans, and as such, it is critical to remember that technology must go hand in hand with appropriate processes to control human behavior.

Keywords Randomization • Drug supply management • Integrated systems • Scalable solutions

13.1   Introduction: What Do We Mean by Trial Integrity and Operational Bias?

Before we begin a chapter on the role of technology in preserving trial integrity and minimizing operational bias, it is perhaps worthwhile to first ask: What exactly do we mean by "trial integrity" and "operational bias"?

Trial integrity, or more to the point, the potential risk to trial integrity, has been raised as a concern and caused much discussion in relation to adaptive trials for over a decade. The following Wikipedia definition is one of the many definitions available: "Integrity is the concept of consistency of actions, values, methods, measures, principles, expectations, and outcomes." Alternative definitions refer to the concept of incorruptibility, and the quality of soundness and being complete.

Clinical trials in pharmaceutical drug development are prospectively planned studies conducted in humans specifically designed to answer research questions about the benefits of new treatment interventions in terms of safety, efficacy, and effectiveness. We should think of "integrity" as referring to the design and conduct of the trial, but also to the way data are collected, analyzed, and interpreted.

The conduct of the trial must follow the design outlined in the protocol. In addition the data from the trial must be complete, accurate, and reliably collected over the course of the trial, in order for the data to be used to answer the trial's predefined research questions.

Minimizing operational bias and ensuring trial integrity go hand in hand. In their book, Design and Analysis of Clinical Trials by Chow and Liu (2014), the various sources of bias are discussed, referring to the ICH-9 guideline, Statistical Principles for Clinical Trials, that defines bias as the systematic tendency of any factors associated with the design, conduct, and evaluation of the results of clinical trials to make the estimate of a treatment effect value deviate from its true value. They conclude that bias can occur at any stage of the trial. Bias occurring due to the conduct of the trial is referred to as operational bias.

Importantly for results of a trial to be extrapolated and have meaning to the wider scientific community, the trial should be conducted in such a manner as to preserve trial integrity and minimize operational bias.

13.2   What Problem Are We Trying to Solve with Technology?

Now before considering adaptive trials, it is beneficial to consider how traditionally designed trials are conducted.

In general, there is a divide between the planning/designing of a clinical trial and the operationalization of the execution of the trial. Often, the project team designs the trial, which includes determining the size of the trial, the treatments to study, dosing frequency, the data to be collected, and patient population to be studied. The clinical operations' perspective may be nominally represented on the design team, but does the team work in a fully integrated fashion to aligned utilities and incentives? Once the design work is complete and the protocol is signed off, the study gets handed off to an operations team, either internal to the company or from a CRO. The question is: to what degree are the utilities of the design and operations team fully integrated? And to what degree are the milestones and incentives of the different groups driving behaviors towards an integrated goal of wanting to make the correct decision at the earliest time point in the most efficient manner, based on the inferences drawn from the trial?

In preparation for executing the trial, countries, sites, and investigators are selected. The randomization list is predetermined prior to the start of the trial, drug kit numbers are created and linked to the randomization list, and initial drug supply quantities are sent to site. In parallel the database is created to collect clinical and lab data from patients who pass the screening process and are eligible to enter the trial. Within this environment the investigator either logs on via a web system, or calls using Interactive Voice Response System (IVRS) to randomize the patient into the trial, and to identify which treatment kit needs to be administered or provided to the patient. For additional drug supplies, the investigator usually logs onto yet another system to generate a new shipment of supplies that is coordinated by the drug supply management group.

Data is initially recorded on paper at site, and assuming Electronic Data Collection (EDC) later entered into an EDC system. Importantly, data cleaning cannot begin until after data has been entered at site. Oversight and coordination of this whole process is administered by the Project Manager (PM) who works with Clinical Research Associates (CRAs) to monitor the performance of the trial across sites. Ensuring procedures are followed; sites are promptly entering data, completing source data verification (SDV), and investigating the resolution of outstanding data queries issued by data management. The PM is also responsible for managing the budget for the trial which includes investigator payments, and tracking hours spent against the planned budget. For most PMs today this involves the use of a Clinical Trial Management System (CTMS).

With the exception of data safety reviews that may be blinded or unblinded, the data remains blinded throughout the conduct of the trial. At the end of the trial, the database is locked, data unblinded for statistical analysis, and the clinical report written.

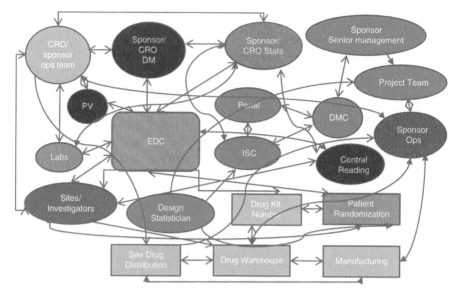

Fig. 13.1 Link between trial design and trial execution

The above is intended only as a top level overview of the process. Nonetheless, even at this level, it is easy to identify that clinical trial execution is complex and involves:

1. Coordination across many functional groups.
2. Many people are involved in the process.
3. The process potentially involves several systems that need to be linked together.
4. "Importantly," clinical trial design and clinical trial execution are primarily operating in siloes.

What may be less obvious by the description above is the issue of data synchronization. This arises as a consequence of multiple systems being in use, often resulting in multiple time views of data. This is generally resolved through data synchronization that is performed periodically, say once a week or some other suitably chosen time period. So understanding what is actually the status of the trial at any particular time point may be far from accurate, creating a challenge when real time learning is the goal.

Therefore even before we consider the impact of what an adaptive trial will have on this process, we already know we are dealing with a complex execution environment, connecting multiple users and multiple systems with multiple and differing demands for information, leading to complex requirements for data flow coordination. This is conceptually depicted in Fig. 13.1.

For now we will ignore what seems an obvious question of whether current practices are actually efficient. What is important for an adaptive trial is that we have been trying to overlay on top of this environment interim decision making that requires the data to be unblinded at least once, or potentially multiple times during the trial in order to make a decision about future trial conduct. Operationally the challenge becomes how to ensure:

- The timely availability of data for the interim analysis.
- Securely control access to unblinded data for interim decision making.
- Speedily and seamlessly implement the interim change without disrupting the conduct of the trial.
- Prevent disclosure of information about the details of the change to those involved in the conduct of the trial.

Within this context we must continue to ensure the data collected from the trial is complete, accurate, and reliable. Importantly, examination of how all these challenges are managed becomes critical for protection of trial integrity and protecting the trial from the introduction of operational bias.

So what does this mean for an adaptive trial? It means we must ensure that the patients entering each stage of the trial are similar so that interim decisions are reflective of whole trial population. All effort must be made during the execution phase of the trial not to disclose the timing of the interim to investigators. Importantly firewalls must be in place to restrict access to unblinded data and any change to trial conduct must be adequately concealed, so as not to influence in any way the type of patients investigators enroll, how future patients in the trial might be treated by the investigator, treatments are administered, how evaluations are made, or how patients may respond.

However given the conceptual diagram above, where there are multiple systems and user requirements for data, it is clear this is by no means a trivial task. Moreover, preservation of trial integrity and minimizing operational bias will depend on how well introducing these new steps required for adaptive trials are executed. In addition, a further requirement for adaptive trials is to be able to demonstrate at the end of the trial that these execution steps were followed, and there was control in terms of data access.

The critical questions to be asked are:

- Who has access; when during the process do they have access; and what information do they have access to. If there is potential for information leakage that would impact the integrity of the trial, or introduce operational bias, have these issues been thought through and what suitable and preventative solutions are implemented? Importantly this needs to be looked at broadly and include both field operations for collecting data as well as the interim analysis workflow process. We refer readers to Chap. 14 for further details about DMCs.
- Following the interim decision what changes need to be implemented:

  - Who will implement these changes.
  - How will these changes be implemented.
  - Again if there is potential to impact the integrity of the trial, or introduce operational bias, what effective and preventative solutions are implemented?

13.3 Building Trust with Regulators

Regulators are mainly focused on trials that are submitted for registration, and so it is important to ensure if adaptive trials are intended as registration quality studies, that all efforts have been made to ensure trial integrity has been preserved, and the possibility of introducing operational bias has been minimized. However these are concepts that are not only applicable to registration studies. These are important concepts that apply to all trials including all adaptive trials. While we may accept differing requirements for the conduct of early phase adaptive trials, where for example the interim analyses are conducted, and the decision body could both be part of the sponsor organization, all efforts should still be made to ensure operation bias is not introduced and trial integrity is not compromised. No matter what the phase of development, we should be confident trial results can be extrapolated and have meaning to the wider scientific community. Otherwise trial results will be misleading, not just to regulators but also to sponsors themselves. Moreover technology and process solutions for adaptive trials should ideally have the flexibility to be applied to all adaptive trials across all phases, including allowance for some aspects to be relaxed for early phase trials. Like the example above where the Independent Statistical Center (ISC) conducting the interim analyses, and possibly the DMC are both internal to the sponsor.

When we think about these issues, we tend to begin by constraining our thoughts to the question of how to achieve this goal for a single trial. While this is definitely important and a good starting place, there is also a broader aspect to consider. For the advancement of adaptive trials we need a framework for execution that includes technology and process that can become an industry standard, uniformly used by industry and CROs alike and accepted by agencies.

What is important to recognize is the interdependency between technology and process in achieving this goal. Technology through the use of role-based access systems can certainly help to facilitate the management of certain aspects, such as controlling who has access to what data from the trial, and in particular who has access to unblinded data. Technology can be used to create audit trails and history logs to provide evidence and assurance following the trial, of who had access to what data and when. Technology can help implement changes to randomization, where treatments need to be dropped or added to the trial, or randomization ratios need to be changed following an interim. Technology can be used to coordinate the accompanying management of drug supplies to sites.

Although technology today can easily control access to unblinded data and interim results, what is needed for the future is for technology to move towards a simplification of the patchwork of systems seen in Fig. 13.1, particularly the integration of EDC, randomization, and drug supply management, as those aspect of clinical trial operationalization are affected the most by requirements for adaptive trials. The integration of these systems will lead to an overall reduction in the number of human touch points involved in the implementation of interim changes to the trial, thereby automating aspects of the workflow process to reduce the number of people who have knowledge that an interim has taken place. While this is a benefit for adaptive trials, the more likely driver to bring about this simplification will be the increased efficiency this brings to trial execution, not just for adaptive trials but for all trials. Moreover integration and simplification will become the cornerstone for creating scalable solutions of the future to manage increased uptake of adaptive trials.

However it cannot be emphasized enough that technology is only part of the solution. Technology is a tool that needs to be managed by humans. Therefore preserving trial integrity and minimizing operational bias will require a combination of technology married together with processes to control human behavior.

An example: a common practice in executing trials with safety interim analyses or group sequential designs is for increased activity by CRAs visiting sites prior to the interim, to encourage the site to enter data because an interim is imminent. Applying the same practice to an adaptive trial, which also includes group sequential trials, becomes a clear announcement to the investigator that an interim is about to occur, and a signal that a possible change to the trial could follow. The reason for this activity is to ensure the maximal amount of clean data is available for the interim, which is directly linked to practices at site for data entry and data management cleaning processes.

If following the interim a treatment is dropped or another added, and the randomization list is not masking the interim, but suddenly displays jumps in numbers, or certain kit numbers are left on the shelf and not used, then an element of disclosure has occurred. This may have no significant consequence at all. However, depending on the design and endpoint, the investigator may be able to make an educated guess or have his own interpretation in regard to the design change, which may impact the type of patients he recruits and how he treats future patients in the trial. This is a potential concern that could introduce operational bias. That being said, this can be rectified at the planning stage, by taking this into consideration when planning the approach to randomization, drug kit numbers, managing CRA visits to sites, and data cleaning processes.

Ideally the timing of the interim should be concealed from investigators, so in their eyes the conduct of the trial appears undisrupted and seamless through the interim process. A possible procedural change to help achieve this would be for all site facing staff such as CRAs not to be told when the interim is due. Information related to the timing of interim analyses could be restricted only to the PM who has oversight of the whole trial, who can continually monitor overall site performance, and ensure site monitoring activity by CRAs is data driven, and does not give away by unusual and increased activity at site the timing of the interim. Additional supportive processes should ensure maximal data is entered and cleaned at all times during the trial, so the data is in a state of interim readiness at all times, negating the need for last minute activity. In many ways the coming of risk-based monitoring algorithms (that include options for adaptive trials to ensure maximal collection of adaptive endpoint (s) data) will help operationally by providing tools for managing CRA activity at site. Depending on the method of randomization, consideration should also be given up front at the planning stages of the trial to the structure of randomization lists and kit numbers in order to mask the timing of the interim from investigators, and minimize the possibility of disclosing information about possible changes to the trial through number configurations. Total concealment is unlikely; however, thoughtful consideration to these aspects is required to reduce the possibility of inadvertently introducing operational bias, an issue that could be resolved through integrated systems that include dynamic randomization.

The timing of site activation is another procedural consideration. For adaptive trials the data collected from each stage of the trial should come from similar patients. If this aspect is overlooked it can adversely impact the results of the trial. This represents a potential change to traditional trial execution, where it is often common practice to regionally stage the startup of sites due to different constraints; for example drug import regulations. If the traditional approach is applied to adaptive trials, this raises the question over the interchangeability between regional and cultural patient populations entering the trial. For example a global trial covering the United States, Western and Eastern Europe, South America, and Japan, a staggered start of regions is likely to occur, and may put into question whether the data used for each interim decision is similar and representative of the whole trial population, or actually different from the data collected from future stages of the trial. This challenge is very much dependent on the number and timing of the interims and the regions covered in the trial. However this is not procedurally impossible and can be managed by trying to ensure at least some representations of sites from all regions are included in each stage of the trial. In an area such as pain for example where it is known that cultural differences can impact patient responses, for a staggered start global trial this would certainly be a concern. However while these issues are highlighted here for adaptive trials, the impact of combining cross-cultural populations in a traditionally designed pain trial should equally be a concern, due to the adverse impact on variability of studying such heterogeneous populations within a single trial.

These examples are used to illustrate that process-driven changes are also used to protect trial integrity and minimize operational bias. Demonstrating that although technology can be used to improve the coordination of changes to randomization and drug supply requirements, and assist with firewalls through role-based access control to unblinded data, technology must also be combined with processes to control human behavior, and procedural changes to traditional approaches to trial conduct.

Like in any trial, traditional or adaptive, it is impossible to provide 100 % assurance. However what can be developed over time are ultimately industry standards in terms of requirements for both IT and processes for the conduct of adaptive trials. This becomes particularly important when considering scalable solutions.

13.4   Different Levels of Risk: Not All Adaptive Trials Are Created Equal

There is a human tendency to try and simplify and categorize in order to manage information. Some may try to simplify trials into a dichotomous classification such as adaptive and nonadaptive. However adaptive trials are not all the same, and present different challenges to existing execution processes and systems. This, in part, is

Fig. 13.2 Link between trial design and trial execution

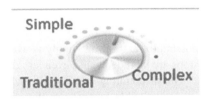

currently driving the uptake of some designs while limiting the uptake of others. It is important this is understood because later we will look at where in the evolution of applying adaptive trials we are today, the limitations of current technology, and look ahead to where we want to be in the future. From this perspective we will begin to see an increasing need for technology solutions.

With this in mind, it is perhaps best to think of trials as belonging to a continuum, as seen in Fig. 13.2. Like a dial that ranges from traditional trials with no interims, through to complex adaptive trials, where in the extreme case we may need data analyzed frequently after every patient, or after small cohorts of patients, and the changes from these interim decisions seamlessly implemented. Moreover as the uptake of adaptive trials increases across industry, this will put pressure on current work-around solutions, creating bottle necks, and technology will become an important and critical player in developing scalable solutions.

So let's first try to identify what is common to "all" adaptive trials and then examine what makes trials simple versus complex. All adaptive trials require work-flow solutions to ensure:

- Timely availability of clean data for interim decision making.
- Appropriate documented processes and a controlled environment in place for conducting the interim decision analyses.
- Identification of the decision body who will make the decision.
- Implementation of the decision.
- *Firewalls* for controlling access to information.

These "must have" elements are not totally new to traditional trials. Producing reports for Data Safety Monitoring Boards (DSMBs) are common place. Group Sequential Designs which are a simple form of adaptive trial, where the decision is only to stop or go, have been in existence for many years. This is not to say that the practices used to execute these trials are perfect, and not in need of improvement. However, processes for their execution do exist and are familiar to operational teams. So in this respect it could be said that the threat to information leakage is not something new. Nevertheless it would be a mistake to say that current practices are equipped to manage all adaptive trials, or to manage a surge in the uptake of adaptive trials where alternative solutions may be required.

To explain, let's first consider an example where current practices need little modification. As long as the important processes mentioned above to ensure consistency of data across stages of the trial, and consideration is given to blinding the timing of the interim, and firewalls are in place for conducting the interim, an adaptive trial where the only adaptation is to increase the sample size causes little other disruption to current practices. The only additional requirement for these trials is to have a longer randomization list produced at the start of the trial, and to ensure potentially extra drug supply is available if needed. Similarly trials where futility stops are included cause even less disruption.

Not discounting that Sample Size Re-estimation (SSR) and early stops for futility are valuable techniques; the opportunity space for adaptive designs is much wider. Unfortunately the execution of some of these other adaptive designs represents greater challenges, because they are considered more operationally complex. All adaptive trials require the must have list above, but the complexity of an adaptive trial is driven by additional factors:

1. How many and how frequently interims need to be conducted?

   (a) Is it just once or required multiple times throughout the trial?

2. How fast is the recruitment speed of the trial?
3. How many treatments are in the trial?

   (a) More treatments mean more options for the following stages of the trial that could include for example adding/dropping treatments, changing the samples size, or changing randomization ratios.

4. How many things are being changed or impacted following the interim decision?

   (a) Is it one or a multiple of the following:
   (b) Changes to sample size.
   (c) Changes to the number of treatments.
   (d) Changes to randomization.

   - Are there only a limited number of treatments and interims during the trial making it possible to predict in advance a finite number of outcomes?
   - Or are there simply so many permutations of what could come next that preplanning in advance to cover all outcomes is impossible?

   (e) Changes to drug supply.

   - Tied to changes in randomization there is a need to coordinate drug supply.

     – Managing the quantities required for adding and/or dropping doses and/or increased amounts due to increases in sample size.
     – Adjusting site floor and ceiling settings that trigger shipments.

   - Managing immediate post-interim quantities:

     – An important time point for drug supply management is preparing for the immediate post-interim decision period.

       How to manage the risk of stock out if an interim decision requires large increases to certain treatments?
       Unavailability of drug at site may result in a pause and interrupt the execution of the trial. This is not desirable because it discloses to the site that an interim has occurred.

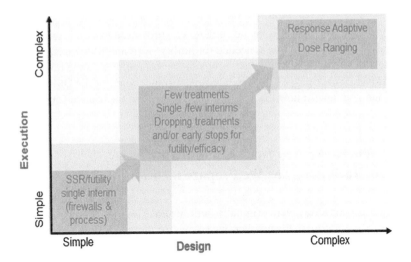

Fig. 13.3 Link between trial design and trial execution

Clearly these are not mutually exclusive factors, and as the combination of adaptation options increases, along with the number of interims required during a trial, so does the executional complexity of the trial increase when trying to use current systems and work practices.

The number of adaptive trials being run at any particular point in time will also give cause for reconsidering how the interim workflow process and execution of the changes may be best implemented. It becomes a very different discussion between how to implement a single adaptive trial, where work-around solutions are plausible solutions versus developing scalable solutions capable of efficiently executing a large number of adaptive trials. Increased uptake of adaptive trials will ultimately impact resources driving the need for alternative solutions. One aspect of this pressure is already being seen today through the impact on the number of DMCs needed, where the shortfall in experienced DMC members has been already identified by many.

Figure 13.3 illustrates the concepts described above, in recognition that both trial design and execution range from the simple to the complex. Simple in the case of execution here indicates little change to the way traditional trials are executed. Along the diagonal are examples of different types of adaptive trials (not meant to be fully inclusive).

Largely today, most adaptive trials being applied belong to trial designs in the bottom left and middle boxes, applying existing firewalls and processes. The pale yellow outer boxes represent the potential overlap in adaptive features. For example a trial that belongs to the center box that has only a few treatment and few interims, which may allow for dropping treatments, and early stopping for futility and efficacy, may also incorporate SSR. While the number of trials falling into the top right hand box remains few by comparison: mainly restricted by lack of expertise and tools for designing these trials, coupled with greater complexity for execution.

While these types of designs are being executed today, they are largely deployed through work-around solutions to utilize existing systems and processes. As described above, little change is needed for futility stops and SSR trials, while those in the middle box largely deploy solutions such as creating separate randomization lists in advance to cover possible interim decision outcomes, or the DMC unblinded statistician generates a new list that is then uploading so the trial can continue.

13.5 Where We Are Today, and the Emerging Role of Technology as We Prepare for the Future

The systems used today were originally built for traditional designs without adaptations, i.e., designs where the number of treatments remains constant, the sample size remains the same, and where data remains blinded throughout the trial. These systems were not built for designs requiring the flexibility to adjust the course of the trial along the way or to support near real time learning. Within this environment the teams and technology used for designing clinical trials, and clinical operations teams and systems for executing trials, were largely able to operate in siloes.

What we have been witnessing over the past decade has been an evolution in innovative change on two fronts. An emerging interest in adaptive trials and the development of adaptive trial design software, paralleled by the development of new technology advances in support systems for clinical trial execution. At the same time industry has come under increasing pressure through patent expirations, driving a need for greater efficiency that we foresee will culminate in a convergence in evolution, merging these two innovative streams together.

Over the past decade the pioneers within industry, who first saw the benefits of adaptive designs, have successfully brought adaptive designs to the forefront of discussion. While 10 years ago we were embroiled in lengthy discussions over the benefits of adaptive trials and there were limited case studies available, and no regulatory guidance, today the situation has changed. The availability of case studies has dramatically increased, as there has been growing acceptance of the methodology, along with the release of draft regulatory guidance on adaptive trials by the FDA in 2010, and the European Medical Agency (EMA) release of their Reflection paper on adaptive designs in 2007. Nevertheless adaptive trials still represent a small fraction of all clinical trials.

Largely the emergence of activity around adaptive designs began as an initiative led by statisticians across the pharmaceutical industry. While knowledge of the methodology and the approach has grown within the statistical community, it is still not applied broadly.

There have been some exceptions; for example one large pharmaceutical company has taken the approach of applying adaptive at the portfolio level, and others appear to soon follow this lead. However largely the adaptive methods applied have been those that can be applied causing limited disruption to current systems and practices. Nonetheless, the success of this approach appears to have gained attention.

We are starting to see evidence that some pharmaceutical companies are also beginning to see adaptive approaches as a means to better manage the risks and costs of clinical development, by identifying failures early and increasing the chances of success for promising compounds. While for these companies the push can be aggressive to apply these methods across their portfolios, they face significant transitional challenges as there needs to be a convergence of education, training, and alignment of technology, both in design and to support execution.

Approaches to building the skills and infrastructure to support the uptake of adaptive designs have been varied across companies. For some adoption has been slow, perhaps not seeing adaptive as a priority. Others have taken the approach to create adaptive internal hubs of expertise to work with project teams on the design of their trials. While for the one pharmaceutical company that stands out from the others and mentioned above, their approach has been to apply adaptive across their portfolio.

There are limitations to both approaches. Small expert hubs can be effective but are unfortunately disconnected from project teams, and often execution teams. Unless these skills are grown at the grass root level of the project team, the growth of adaptive trials will remain limited as specialized hubs will ultimately become a bottleneck. However applying adaptive across the portfolio requires compromise in the types of approaches applied. When widespread application is the goal, consideration has to be given to three important factors:

- First the availability of validated adaptive design software for project statisticians accompanied by training and education.
- Education of clinical functions and operational teams in support of these approaches.
- Consideration to the types of adaptive designs that can be supported by current system infrastructure, and a planned approach for the expansion of uptake, and growth in the methods applied.

However, perhaps the best strategy is recognition that both approaches are essential for triggering change. As shown in Fig. 13.4 below, the availability of validated adaptive software tools in the hands of project statisticians can help facilitate the growth of adaptive designs on a more broad scale. As project statisticians become increasingly more comfortable with the methods we will begin to see an increase in the uptake of the adaptive methods available in the software. In parallel specialized adaptive teams, whether internal or external, provide support for more complex adaptive approaches, developing custom design solutions, and are continually advancing adaptive methods. In addition to the emergence over the past decade of adaptive design software providers, we are also beginning to see the emergence of collaborative efforts across industry and with design software providers to advance adaptive methodology, and transition these new methods into adaptive design software. This in turn will increase the repertoire of designs available to project statisticians. While adaptive statistical methods started in the hands of a few, the increasing availability of technology in the form of statistical design software is now laying the

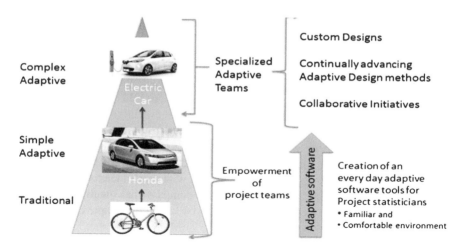

Fig. 13.4 Advancing adaptive trials and the role of adaptive design software

groundwork for more broad scale uptake. However for technology providers in the trial execution space, the challenge or business dilemma is will this increase take place, when will this increased uptake take place, and what do adaptive trials really need that is different from traditional designs. Importantly, and understandably their business question is when should they invest.

In the past trial design and execution have been able to operate mostly in siloes. However what is changing with the coming of adaptive trials is a need for trial design and execution to work together more closely.

Industry has dipped its toes into the adaptive pond cautiously. As mentioned earlier they have largely done so by embracing the simpler types of adaptive trials. Largely trials where only a few treatments are studied and only one or two interim analyses are conducted, and minimal changes following interim decisions are required.

However as advances in adaptive methodology continue, along with the need for custom designs, pressure to push beyond the limitations of the current execution environment and work-around solutions will grow. Pressure will also increase due to the desire to do more of the simpler adaptive trial designs that are done today.

In parallel to the advances in adaptive designs and the development of adaptive design software as an enabler for greater uptake, the past decade has also seen the emergence of technology advances in the field of trial execution: in particular the development of Electronic Data Capture (EDC). As EDC software continues to mature we are beginning to see attempts at the integration of additional capabilities into these systems such as the inclusion of clinical trial management systems and randomization, not necessarily fully integrated or possessing the level of functionality required. However it is a positive signal that the simplification of the patchwork of systems seen in Fig. 13.1 has begun. However as these extra capabilities are added, they are not done so with the execution of adaptive trials in mind. We cannot lose sight of the fact that EDC developers as a business have been naturally and understandably focused on the larger market of traditional designs. When it comes to adaptive trials they have been like outsiders looking in on the growth of adaptive watching to see how it evolves. Unfortunately as observers they are only able to see the tip of the iceberg of adaptive potential, and have lacked the insight to see below the surface, and foresee the user requirements of tomorrow's designs, or the designs of today that are not applied due to being considered too complex for current systems to execute.

However interestingly, some advances have emerged through smaller providers who are involved in the development of adaptive design software, and have taken steps towards developing solutions for executing their own designs, or more generic solutions that could also apply in addition to designs from other software providers. This could perhaps be seen as an analogy to what is occurring in the electric car market. An industry also changing, where electric car manufacturers are not just producing electric cars, but are investing into the infrastructure of battery recharging stations to support and grow the market for their electric cars.

For adaptive designs, one solution is not too dissimilar to work-around solution for other designs of today. Their software is used for designing the trial and a parameter file that individualizes the design is part of the output. The parameter file is then required as input for the corresponding analysis engine to complete the interim analysis. However in terms of process, the response file still needs to be created separately and data is still transferred at the time of the interim, so an analysis can be run and a recommendation returned, sometimes along with a probability vector for the creation of a new randomization.

Another software design provider solution is a standalone solution for managing the interim workflow process. Data, the randomization list, and the code for analysis are all uploaded. The system is able to automatically create the response file, run the analysis, and has the capability to automate a simple report of the recommendation for the DMC. This is all done without unblinding the data used for adaptation to the operator of the system. Access to the system produced reports and information related to input for the interim analyses are all stored within the system, with role base access controlling who has access to unblinded results. A major purpose of the system is to track and provide a history log and audit trail of who had access to what data during the course of the interim analysis workflow process.

A third adaptive software provider has perhaps taken the first step towards a more comprehensive solution by developing an integrated EDC, randomization and drug supply management system, with the beginnings of an embedded adaptive library of designs engines for analysis. This operates similarly to the first option, combining the designs of the first provider with a selection of their own designs to create the library. A parameter file is uploaded, and instead of needing the manual creation of the response file, internal to the system data is extracted from the database, the response file is created, fed to the analysis engine producing a recommendation and a new probability vector for creating the randomization for the next patient(s) into the trial. Importantly there is seamless integration between the EDC system, randomization, and drug supply systems, making the execution of those adaptive designs from the library that require frequent interims and frequent changes to randomization ratios, an easy to implement reality. The system can be operated in both manual and automated mode and is perhaps the framework for a more scalable solution for adaptive trial execution. Moreover by providing a publishable Application Programming Interface (APIs) as an extension to the system, this would provide connectivity for custom designs, allowing them to benefit from the system's seamless execution capabilities, thereby giving rise to an adaptive design execution platform that could cater for a wide range of design types. Flipping the current situation on its head, by providing a system intentionally built with flexibility in mind, where flexibility would be turned off for traditional designs.

However what represents a significant change through the efforts of these smaller adaptive design software providers is recognition that design and execution solutions require integrated thinking and knowledge of adaptive trial design user requirements.

Currently it is too early to know whether any of these solutions will evolve to become the mainstream industry solution of tomorrow. However, perhaps the more likely scenario will be collaboration between design software providers and current IT providers for execution to create a common standard.

The top platform in Fig. 13.5 above represents where we are today with the application of the more operationally simple adaptive approaches that are available in current adaptive design software packages, and can be implemented using current systems and processes. While some more operationally complex trials are being conducted they may require custom design solutions that are executed using the combination of current systems and work-around solutions. However while fit for one off trials and the limited number of adaptive trials of today, these approaches are not an efficient approach for managing greater uptake.

Nevertheless we are already beginning to see some activity on the middle platform, as adaptive design software providers expand their range of design options, from collaborations to further develop methodology, and begin to develop solutions for the execution for some of the more operationally complex designs. In the wake of this advancement, as the repertoire of adaptive trial designs in software expands, we should expect to see a greater range of adaptive trial designs being applied, as project statisticians become more familiar with the methods and some of the barriers to execution begin to disappear.

Importantly we are also beginning to see a signal of what could emerge as the beginnings of a scalable solution for adaptive trial execution, where EDC, randomization, and drug supply management systems are integrated, complete with an embedded library of adaptive trial designs, and the capabilities to provide connectivity for custom designs.

As the transition occurs from the application of the simple adaptive methods of today using current systems and processes, through to scalable solutions, this is not a journey advancing adaptive trial designs alone, but a journey taken together with execution technology. Through this evolution we will also hopefully see that the development of industry standards for adaptive trial execution emerges.

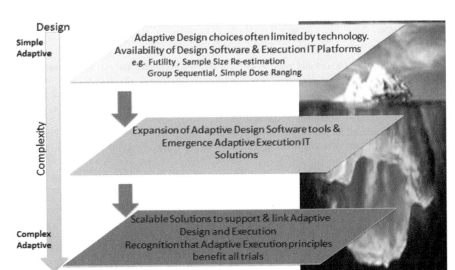

Fig. 13.5 Growth of adaptive designs and the linking of design and execution to create scalable solutions

However it also needs to be recognized that software and technology development is a costly and time-consuming business. How fast this transition occurs, to develop a scalable solution that may appear futuristic to some, could potentially depend on whether collaborations can be forged between adaptive design software providers and current major players in the field of technology for trial execution.

13.6   Conclusion

We believe that the overarching utility of clinical trials in the context of pharmaceutical drug development is to enable making the correct decision at the earliest time point in the most efficient manner. The opportunity space for adaptive designs to contribute to this utility is substantial. To live up to the opportunity there needs to be an integrated effort of clinical trial designers and experts responsible for design execution, which also includes alignment of their incentives and milestones to achieve a common goal. Importantly the message of this chapter is that technology and process go hand in hand to protect trial integrity, minimize operational bias, and build regulatory trust. We argue for designing a simplified execution environment that will ultimately create a common industry standard for integrating design and execution that is scalable, and can accommodate the full spectrum of adaptive and nonadaptive designs. Additionally the execution environment should be able to support designs from multiple adaptive software providers and allow for custom designs to be easily executed.

References

Chow S, Liu J (2014) Design and analysis of clinical trials – concepts and methodologies. Wiley, New York

EMA. CHMP 2007. Reflection paper on methodological issues in confirmatory clinical trials planned with an adaptive design. http://www.ema.europa.eu/docs/en_GB/document_library/Scientific_guideline/2009/09/WC500003616.pdf

FDA (2010) Guidance for industry 2010. Adaptive designs for clinical trials drugs and biologics. http://www.fda.gov/downloads/DrugGuidanceComplianceRegulatoryInformation/Guidances/UCM201790.pdf

Chapter 14
Considerations for Interim Analyses in Adaptive Trials, and Perspectives on the Use of DMCs

Paul Gallo, David DeMets, and Lisa LaVange

Abstract A particularly critical issue for adaptive clinical trials, with potentially great impact on how large a role these trials will come to play in confirmatory stages of clinical development, involves the processes by which accruing data are collected and analyzed, and by which adaptation decisions are made and implemented. The importance of this issue arises from the sensitivity of unblinded interim results and the potential, reflected in current conventions in nonadaptive trials, for access to interim results to introduce biases into the trial conduct and its results. This issue is intertwined with the role of independent Data Monitoring Committees, commonly the only party granted access to interim comparative results in current practice. We discuss the issues of who should be involved in data review for adaptation decisions, how the data flow and access to results is controlled, and the specific role that Data Monitoring Committees might play in this process.

Keywords Interim analysis • Data Monitoring Committee • Operational bias • Group sequential design • Sample size reassessment • Reporting statistician • Seamless design • Firewall • DMC charter • Trial integrity • Confirmatory trial

P. Gallo (✉)
IIS Statistical Methodology, Novartis Pharmaceuticals, East Hanover, NJ, USA
e-mail: paul.gallo@novartis.com

D. DeMets
Department of Biostatistics and Medical Informatics, University of Wisconsin, Madison, WI, USA

L. LaVange
Office of Biostatistics, Office of Translational Sciences, Center for Drug Evaluation and Research, FDA, Rockville, MD, USA

W. He et al. (eds.), *Practical Considerations for Adaptive Trial Design and Implementation*, Statistics for Biology and Health, DOI 10.1007/978-1-4939-1100-4_14, © Springer Science+Business Media New York 2014

14.1 Introduction

Interim analyses of comparative accruing data within ongoing studies are of course a common feature in current clinical trials practice. Major motivations for conducting them include:

- Monitoring data for potential safety concerns that may make it unethical to continue the trial in its current manner.
- Application of formal group sequential methods allowing stopping of the trial with a claim for efficacy if a standard of proof can be met.
- Consideration of stopping a trial for lack of effect, or *futility*, if it seems clear that the study will not achieve its objectives.

These motivations are not mutually exclusive and can overlap. For example, there can be ethical safety implications if an efficacy advantage is demonstrated (or will not be demonstrated) for a treatment for a serious disease condition within an ongoing trial.

Current conventions, especially in trials with registration potential, hold that access to interim results and unblinded data should be carefully restricted, and in particular, not available to trial management personnel, investigators, or other study participants (for the purposes of this chapter, we will view the word "unblinded" as also including *coded*, or semi-blinded, data or results, where treatments are labeled separately but not fully identified, for example, "A," "B," as is sometimes done for interim analysis reports). The rationale behind the regulatory concerns leading to these conventions is thoroughly described in the FDA document *Guidance for Clinical Trial Sponsors on the Establishment and Operation of Clinical Trial Data Monitoring Committees* (US FDA 2006); other relevant references include (CHMP 2005; ICH 1998; Ellenberg et al. 2002; Fleming et al. 2008). The main points of concern can be summarized as follows:

- Trial management personnel can have decisions of various types to make while a trial is ongoing based on objective scientific reasoning, and access to interim results diminishes their ability to manage the trial in a manner which is totally objective, and will be seen to be objective by all interested parties (e.g., regulators and the medical community).
- Knowledge of interim results by trial personnel (e.g., investigators and their staff) could introduce subtle, unknown biases into the conduct of the trial and the study results, perhaps causing slight changes in characteristics of patients recruited, specific details of administration of the intervention, investigator endpoint assessments, etc.

Additionally, interim results may not reliably predict final study results, with different types of serious negative implications if those results are disseminated. As discussed in (Ellenberg et al. 2002), it is important "to minimize the risk of widespread prejudgment of unreliable results based on limited data (that) could adversely impact rates of patient accrual, continued adherence to trial regimens, and ability to obtain unbiased and complete assessment of trial outcome measures. This prejudgment could also result in publications of early results that might be very inconsistent with final study data on the benefit-to-risk profile of the study interventions." The publication issue can take on heightened importance because the general readership may often not adequately understand the limitations of interim results in this regard.

On the basis of such concerns, it has become common practice to address the objectives of interim monitoring through the use of a *Data Monitoring Committee* (DMC), a group of experts possessing all relevant experience and expertise required to perform the necessary monitoring responsibilities. As described in (US FDA 2006), DMC members should be as free as possible of all types of conflict of interest, and should play no role in trial conduct other than to perform their monitoring functions. In pivotal trials, DMC members are typically external to the trial sponsor to maximize their independence and objectivity. Access to unblinded study data and results should be restricted to the DMC and to a small set of individuals providing the necessary statistical and programming support (these support personnel are also independent of other trial activities, and very commonly are external to the sponsor).

Once a DMC has received access to unblinded results, communications between the DMC and other trial entities, such as sponsor trial management personnel or a Steering Committee, would be limited. Communications to the DMC would generally serve to ensure that the DMC remains fully informed in order to most effectively execute its responsibilities, such as in an open session of a DMC meeting. Communications from the DMC should not convey any information about comparative results until such time as there is an ethical issue requiring such communications, or the DMC is prepared to make a major recommendation (e.g., trial termination). Thus, in conventional monitoring practice, access to unblinded interim data and results typically remains restricted to the DMC and its statistical support staff, in order to most effectively achieve the goals of protecting patient safety, maintaining the integrity of the study results, and avoiding the introduction of biases and the potential adverse consequences that can arise from over-interpreting undependable early results.

Recent interest and advances in the area of adaptive trial design suggest opportunities for increased efficiencies in clinical research, in situations where such trials are viewed as appropriate based upon careful consideration and planning. Adaptive design trials allow modification of some aspect of an ongoing trial based on data from within that trial, if this can be done in a manner that maintains the interpretability and statistical validity of the study results, based on implementation of a prespecified plan that achieves these objectives (see US FDA 2010; Gaydos et al. 2009).

There are a number of actions that can be taken within an ongoing trial that fall under the definition of an adaptive design, with which there is a good deal of familiarity and experience, and which can be implemented noncontroversially. These include the application of group sequential designs, blinded sample size reassessment based upon a nuisance parameter, and event-driven designs. These are referred to as "well understood" in the FDA document *Guidance for Industry: Adaptive Clinical Trials for Drugs and Biologics (Draft)* (US FDA 2010), and the roles played by the trial management group and the DMC are generally well established.

Among adaptive designs that are more novel or with which there is less regulatory familiarity, a few particular applications have been considered good candidates for roles in confirmatory trials, including modifying the study sample size, dropping treatment arms, and enriching the study population. In these types of adaptive trials, there is of course an added reason for accessing interim data beyond the more familiar monitoring motivations mentioned earlier, namely, to consider changes to some aspect of the conduct of the trial as it continues. This raises some fairly obvious challenges of several types, due largely to the sensitivity of interim results to which we have already alluded. For example:

- Who are the individuals who will have access to interim results to be used for adaptations?
- What expertise/experience/perspectives should they possess?
- Can processes similar to those used to restrict access within a DMC in conventional monitoring be utilized; or what types of changes or extensions to current practices might be warranted?
- What are the processes by which adaptations, once decided upon, are implemented, and what personnel are involved?
- Is it reasonable or feasible to withhold from trial management personnel or the study sponsor the specific data and analyses which are the basis for modifying a continuing trial?
- What information can observation of adaptations made tell an observer about the nature of the results that led to that adaptation, and does this raise concerns about preserving trial integrity?

In the remainder of this chapter, we discuss such issues in some depth. The major broad topics are: the processes that govern the production and review of interim results and implementation of changes while maintaining the desired degree of confidentiality; and the composition and qualifications of the decision-making bodies (though there is a good deal of overlap between these topics). The specific manner in which these considerations play out will depend on specific details of particular trials, but we will aim to elucidate principles that should be followed in making trial-specific decisions.

14.2 DMCs in Adaptive Trials

14.2.1 The Potential Role of DMCs

Because adaptive trials require access to interim results, there are various reasons why it might seem sensible to consider using a DMC constituted for the more familiar motivations as the party to review data for the purpose of making adaptations.

After all, if a study is already using a DMC for a more conventional purpose (for example, safety monitoring), then the DMC is already allowed access to unblinded interim data. We can expect that the DMC is properly "firewalled," presumably with appropriate confidentiality procedures in place and insulation of trial personnel from access to results. In addition, the same attributes of independence, objectivity, expertise, and experience which would qualify someone for membership on the DMC might suggest that they possess qualifications for advising on adaptations as well.

Questions might arise, however, as to whether this is an optimal role for a DMC. Might there be some type of conflict or mismatch with a DMC's more familiar responsibilities? If so, are these obstacles that can be overcome? And if not, then we still need to address the questions of exactly who will be examining the interim data for adaptation purposes, how the data flow and confidentiality issues will be addressed, and how the changes will be communicated and implemented. Below, we delve further into some of these issues and challenges.

14.2.2 Scope of DMC Decisions in Adaptive Trials

First of all, there sometimes seems to be misunderstanding of the scope that a DMC has in making changes within a trial. For example, because of the independence, objectivity, and expertise that the DMC members possess, it might be perceived that the DMC has wide leeway to potentially pro-actively initiate changes to a trial; that is, in examining the interim data the DMC can choose to modify the study and perhaps steer it in a more favorable direction, even for a trial aspect not originally envisioned as a candidate for modification.

Such a perception reflects a fundamental misunderstanding of adaptive designs. In fact, the DMC is uniquely a party that *cannot* pro-actively modify an ongoing trial, specifically because it has access to unblinded data—this is in fact true for any unblinded monitoring by a DMC for any purpose, regardless of whether the study was designed as an adaptive trial, with an obvious exception of actions arising from a DMC's ethical responsibility to ensure patient safety, which always takes precedence.

If we step back to consider what should be considered a valid adaptive design, we might start with the definition in (US FDA 2010): "an adaptive design clinical study is defined as a study that includes a prospectively planned opportunity for modification of one or more specified aspects of the study design and hypotheses based on analysis of data (usually interim data) from subjects in the study." Also, "the term *prospective* here means that the adaptation was planned (and details specified) before data were examined in an unblinded manner by any personnel involved in planning the revision." The level of detail of prespecification required will depend on the particular trial and type of adaptation, and may or may not follow a rigid numerical algorithm; there just needs to be sufficient specification for the design to be embedded within a valid statistical plan.

In this sense, an adaptation suggested or motivated by unblinded data generally cannot be retrospectively incorporated into a valid adaptive design. Therefore, for a DMC to pro-actively identify an aspect of the trial for potential adaptation based on their review of unblinded data would violate a fundamental tenet of a valid adaptive design. Because it is allowed access to interim results, however, a DMC is a natural party to consider for a main role in the *implementation* of a plan that has been thoroughly developed in advance—they can make recommendations or decisions allowed under that plan. The FDA adaptive design guidance document (US FDA 2010) concisely and elegantly summarizes this, stating that "Because a DMC is unblinded to interim study results, it can help implement the adaptation decision according to the prospective adaptation algorithm, but should not be in a position to otherwise change the study design except for serious safety-related concerns that are the usual responsibility of a DMC."

It is important to keep in mind that the DMC function is to ensure overall patient safety by examining the risk-to-benefit ratio, and also to protect the scientific integrity of the trial to which the patients have contributed their participation. It is *not* to design or redesign the trial—that is the responsibility of a party such as a Steering Committee. An adaptive scheme is an aspect of trial design that similarly falls within the responsibilities of the trial designers, and in fact is generally invalidated if the party designing the adaptive scheme has access to unblinded information. Thus, if a DMC is to play a role in deciding on or recommending a change, it should be on the basis of implementing a plan that has been carefully and thoroughly pre-specified by the trial designers, *not* on the basis of pro-actively identifying candidate aspects for potential adaptation after viewing unblinded results.

14.3 Regulatory Concerns and Viewpoints

Not surprisingly, concerns about access to interim results and the potential for operational bias are featured prominently in the draft FDA adaptive designs guidance document (US FDA 2010). Section IV.A.3, entitled "Operational Bias," addresses these issues in some depth. For example, it is stated that "unblinding of the analysts charged with implementing the planned design revisions… raises concern about the possibility that the analysts might influence investigators in how they manage the trial, manage individual study patients, or make study assessments, bringing into question whether trial personnel have remained unequivocally objective." It is stated further that "knowledge of the interim unblinded data used to make the adaptation decision, or even knowledge only of the specific adaptive choice, has the potential to introduce operational bias into the treatment-effect estimates. This can occur if investigators, because of their knowledge of the specific adaptation decisions, treat, manage, or evaluate patients differently." The section further cites the FDA DMC guidance document (US FDA 2006), which "makes the point strongly that a steering committee or other group that could possibly decide to alter study design (in a partially or fully nonprospectively specified manner) should be blinded to any interim treatment results." Sections IX.B and XI emphasize the need for substantial documentation, including SOPs and DMC charters that are expected to be more detailed and more extensive than is typically the case in nonadaptive settings because of the additional complexities.

An EMEA reflection paper on flexible designs (CHMP 2007) raises similar concerns about the potential for operational bias, pointing out that "interim analyses... always introduce the possibility of damaging the integrity of the trial" and that "a balance has to be struck between the needs for assessing accumulating information and the risk of damaging the integrity of the trial." It is suggested that data before and after an adaptation interim analysis be examined for consistency of within-stage treatment effects. Although acknowledging that discrepancies could be due simply to chance, it states that it would be difficult to convincingly demonstrate that inconsistency was not due to some degree of dissemination of interim results; a similar point is raised in (Koch 2006).

14.4   Who Makes the Adaptation Decision?

14.4.1   Single vs. Separate Decision Boards

A question may arise in adaptive trials as to whether the group evaluating data for adaptations should be different from the group addressing the more familiar interim monitoring types of recommendations—in effect, whether there should be a single DMC, or two separate boards. The FDA adaptive design guidance (US FDA 2010) acknowledges both possibilities, stating that the adaptive decision-making role "could be assigned to an independent DMC when a DMC is established for other study monitoring purposes... Alternatively, a DMC might be delegated only the more standard roles (e.g., ongoing assessment of critical safety information) and a separate adaptation committee established to examine the interim analysis and make adaptation recommendations." Arguments generally favoring the use of a single board are presented in Antonijevic et al. (2013).

A motivation for separating these functions may be that different sets of expertise and experience are necessary to most effectively make the different types of decisions called for in an adaptive design setting. In addition, it might be perceived that the different decision types can most effectively and most objectively be made separately. Perhaps conflicts might arise between decisions of different types; for example, a preplanned sample size reassessment based on the primary endpoint might suggest increasing the number of patients, while an unexpected safety signal might raise concerns about the ethics of such an action, or even whether the study should continue.

Either possible model might be considered, with the specific details of a situation arguing in favor of one over the other. With regard to the relevance of differing expertise, it is only necessary that the decision-making body in aggregate possesses proper perspectives and experience for any actions with which it is charged, a fundamental principle in any DMC setting. Thus, if a single DMC were to be used for both safety monitoring and evaluating a potential adaptation, a board with experienced safety monitoring personnel might be supplemented with individuals having experience in the type of adaptation being made, or more thorough statistical knowledge of the behavior of the adaptation algorithm (this might naturally lead to the presence of more than one statistician on the board). Using separate boards could also raise logistical challenges in terms of what information each receives and when, and under what conditions they might interact with each other.

Regarding the potential for conflict between the types of recommendations to be made, the use of separate boards might not provide an answer, but rather just avoid the question: a conflict will have to be resolved, and some party will need to be defined to do this. Additionally, the potential for such conflict may reflect that the adaptation plan was not adequately developed during trial design. Returning to the illustrative example mentioned above, a sample size modification conflicting with another aspect of the data, perhaps the joint impact of the two aspects could have been taken into account in the development of the adaptation plan. If so, then potential awkwardness in reconciling a conflict after the fact could be avoided. Ideally, the adaptation plan should envision what changes would be appropriate and valid based on the totality of all relevant data and potential outcomes (although with an understanding that some flexibility is often appropriate). Determining the details of the plan should result from extensive advance discussions of hypothetical scenarios that could be envisioned, and what actions seem appropriate in these different scenarios, generally supported by extensive simulations.

The A-Heft trial (Taylor et al. 2004) is a helpful example. Because of uncertainty in the expected treatment benefit for the primary composite endpoint, the A-Heft DMC was charged with the responsibility to authorize a sample size increase based upon interim results, using the method of Cui et al. (1999). This resulted in an enrollment increase of over one-third despite the fact that the DMC viewed that the study was trending towards likely termination on the basis of a mortality benefit for the experimental treatment (and this termination subsequently occurred). Additionally, the sample size increase allowed the possibility that investigators could "reverse engineer" the algorithm and infer the interim treatment effect (see Sect. 14.5). Had the agreed-upon procedures allowed the DMC to overrule the sample size increase algorithm, they may have done so.

This example illustrates a challenge during the current evolution of adaptive designs where actual experience remains limited. Familiar DMC decision making, for example involving whether to terminate a trial, is rarely fully algorithmic, nor does decision making usually depend only on a single parameter. DMCs look at the totality of evidence available to them, and the internal and external consistency of all relevant information, to make the most informed overall risk-benefit decision. On the other hand, novel adaptive statistical procedures might focus solely on results from a single parameter. It may take additional experience to more routinely learn how to effectively integrate these methods with some of the realities and complexities of interim monitoring, allowing the necessary flexibility in DMC decisions while maintaining validity of the study plan and design.

14.4.2   Additional Qualifications

We have referred above to the principle that for any interim monitoring, the DMC membership must include all sets of expertise and perspectives necessary for the types of decisions with which it is charged. More specifically in adaptive trials, the DMC must fully understand the scope of the potential changes, and the implications for the trial and the interpretation of its results. Among the DMC membership there should be individuals experienced in making the types of decisions that might be called for. The DMC must at a minimum include a statistician fully knowledgeable about the statistical methodology and algorithms associated with the adaptation plan. (These conditions hold for the group making the adaptation decision, whether it is an additional responsibility for a DMC constituted for other purposes, or possibly a separate group, as discussed in the previous section.)

In adaptive trials, these added requirements extend to the *reporting statistician*, the individual supporting the DMC who provides the interim reports to the DMC and facilitates their interpretation. As alluded to previously, the group of statistical and programming personnel with access to unblinded data in order to support the DMC possesses all perspectives relevant to its role, is independent of other trial activities, and is "firewalled" similarly as the DMC. In any trial, the reporting statistician must have full understanding of the protocol, trial design and analysis plan, data structures, and monitoring objectives, in order to provide the needed support. In an adaptive trial, the reporting statistician must additionally be fully knowledgeable about the adaptive methodology, adaptation plan, and algorithm, and must be prepared to assist the DMC as needed in monitoring the behavior of the algorithm, including providing additional reports to the DMC upon request.

14.4.3   Sponsor Involvement in Adaptation Decisions

A potentially controversial issue may arise regarding possible involvement of study sponsor personnel in reviewing interim data and making adaptation decisions. In nonadaptive trials with registration potential, it is, as we have described, common practice that the interim data be reviewed by an independent DMC. There would be no access to or knowledge of unblinded interim data by sponsor personnel until such time as a DMC was prepared to make a major recommendation concerning the trial, such as termination. In adaptive trials, it might be suggested that a particular adaptation type is one for which sponsor perspective might be relevant, perhaps to factor in marketing implications associated with different strategies under consideration, or to most fully integrate into the discussion all relevant knowledge about the treatments in question. Also, this may involve decisions that have usually been viewed as a sponsor responsibility in nonadaptive settings, and that have important long-term implications for drug development programs.

Selection of a dose of an investigational treatment for further development comes to mind as an illustrative example. In a traditional development program, doses in a phase III trial are typically chosen by the sponsor based on the results of phase II trials, but this process might be combined into a single adaptive study using what has been referred to as an *adaptive seamless design* (Maca et al. 2006), in which a dose or doses are selected for continuation at an interim analysis. Such a study aims to provide confirmatory evidence for a selected dose, but there might be concern that a DMC entirely independent of the sponsor might not possess all relevant perspectives for a potentially complex decision, and that DMC members experienced in other monitoring contexts might not have experience in this particular type of decision. Thus, it might be viewed that there is a conflict between the familiar desire to insulate the sponsor from access to interim results and the principle of bringing all relevant perspectives to bear in order to make the most fully-informed decision. A question might arise as to whether a sponsor-internal group could be convened to make this type of decision, or whether there should at least be sponsor representation on an otherwise independent DMC for some limited portion of its deliberations.

Once again, planning can play an important role in resolving this conflict. Extensive planning discussions can help mitigate sponsor concerns about allowing an independent DMC to make the adaptation decision without direct sponsor involvement. Prior to a trial's start, or at least prior to any DMC access to unblinded data, it is not controversial for the sponsor and DMC to discuss issues openly. It is important to iron out differing viewpoints at this stage, as this can be very problematic after the DMC has received access to unblinded data. The sponsor can attempt to "educate" the DMC in whatever relevant perspectives it might possess. The planning discussions should include raising varied and complex hypothetical outcome scenarios, and discussing what might seem to be the appropriate recommendations in each; simulation results will often play a large role here. This might then allow the actual data review and recommendations to be performed by the independent DMC without sponsor access to the results, or direct sponsor participation in deliberations.

Though decisions as to how to proceed might depend on situation-specific details, the principles seem fairly straightforward. As described previously, study integrity is best maintained if trial management personnel do not have access to interim results. Sponsor access raises risks by compromising independence, as discussed in (US FDA 2006). Involvement by any sponsor personnel should require clearly-stated and convincing justification, and be *minimal* to meet the needs—including as a desirable special case, *no access*, perhaps achieved through effective planning sessions as mentioned above. As discussed in Gallo (2006), if some sponsor involvement could be convincingly justified:

- The sponsor representatives involved should be the minimum number of individuals possessing the perspectives necessary to assist in arriving at the best decision, probably just one or two sponsor management representatives.
- These individuals should not otherwise be involved in any trial activities, nor contribute to any discussions of trial management issues(noting that identifying personnel with adequate separation of functions may pose logistical challenges for small companies).

- These individuals will have access to results only at the times of adaptation decisions, and they will see only information that is relevant to the decision with which they are assisting (e.g., unlike an independent DMC that may be involved, which may have a broader and ongoing role).
- Appropriate firewalls and process documentation (SOPs, charter) should be in place to ensure that access to results is appropriately restricted, and there should be subsequent documentation that the processes were adhered to; in particular, numerical results remain unknown to other trial participants (trial management team, investigators, Steering Committee, etc.).

There is some similarity here to issues raised in Section 6.5 of the FDA DMC guidance (US FDA 2006), which (in nonadaptive settings) discusses the possibility of sponsor access to interim results for critical business purposes. It is mentioned that such access is "problematic" and introduces risks to trial integrity, and the document cites principles and practices to lessen risks that are quite similar to those we have listed just above. Trial integrity in adaptive trials is most strongly ensured if the adaptation plan can be implemented without sponsor access to interim results, presumably through selection of a qualified independent DMC and sufficient planning.

14.5 "Reverse Engineering"

An issue in adaptive trials with implications for maintaining confidentiality and trial integrity, with some relationship to other DMC-related topics, involves the potential for adaptations to convey information to observers about the interim results that led to those changes. A useful illustrative example would be a sample size reassessment method, such as that of Cui et al. (1999): if the protocol-specified plan is to increase sample size in an algorithmic manner based on the interim treatment effect estimate, then someone who knows the plan and becomes aware of the sample size change can potentially invert the algorithm and "back calculate" or "reverse engineer" to infer what effect estimate led to the change, information that would typically be restricted during an ongoing trial.

It is an unreasonable standard to strictly require that *no* information be conveyed by observation of a mid-trial adaptation. Even in conventional interim analysis settings, this is never the case. All monitoring has potential action thresholds, whether implicit or explicit, and lack of action will generally imply that such thresholds have not been reached. For example, continuation of a trial in which there is safety monitoring usually implies that no large imbalance in serious events exists; continuation of a group sequential trial generally implies that the efficacy results lie within a predefined continuation region (even for some familiar group sequential schemes, this continuation region may be narrower than commonly perceived, especially when an aggressive futility rule is being used). Nevertheless these practices tend not to be questioned, presumably because the information conveyed is judged to be quite limited and with minimal potential for introducing bias, and because the advantages of the interim monitoring with regard to patient welfare and the efficiency of the drug development process outweigh any slight risks. Similar standards should be applied to adaptive designs: steps should be taken where possible to minimize the information that could be inferred by observers, but the amount of such information and its potential for introducing bias should be balanced against advantages that the design offers.

For example, in an adaptive seamless dose selection trial, or in an enrichment design, knowledge of which doses or sets of patients are continuing could be considered to convey *some* information to observers. However, there would usually be little information that could be dependably inferred about the magnitude of treatment effects, and the knowledge available would seem to have minimal potential for introducing biases into the trial. Furthermore, consider as an alternative to the seamless design simply following a conventional separate-trial paradigm; that is, dose selection is performed in a phase IIb study followed by a separate confirmatory trial. In this case, detailed information from the prior trial would be widely available, perhaps impacting equipoise for the subsequent trial in a manner that the seamless approach avoids, which might possibly be considered an advantage for the adaptive approach.

The standard by which adaptive trials should be judged on this issue is thus as follows: is the information conveyed by observing the adaptation limited in regard to discerning the magnitude of interim treatment effects, and with no clear and direct mechanism that can be envisioned for introducing noticeable bias into the eventual trial results? If not, then the risk should be balanced against the perceived advantages that the adaptive design offers.

Beyond the dose selection examples above, other types of adaptations would seem to satisfy this standard if appropriately implemented, for example, sample size reassessment based upon within-trial information on a nuisance parameter. Adaptations which could be more problematic in this regard would include sample size reassessment methods or modification of randomization allocation in a direct algorithmic manner based upon an estimated treatment effect. Open-label trials might be of particular concern, and it may require very careful consideration to decide whether an adaptive design could be implemented appropriately in an open-label setting.

Sample size changes made on the basis of multiple considerations, for example, on both a treatment effect estimate and a nuisance parameter, might mask the interim effect somewhat and thus be less of a problem. "Discretizing" action thresholds might offer an additional possibility for lessening the concern: for example, sample size might be modified not as a continuous function of the treatment effect estimate, but instead might change to one size among a small number of possibilities, corresponding to specified ranges in which the estimate might lie. In general, adaptations that would not be implemented or become apparent until late in a study would be expected to limit the potential for bias.

It is challenging to quantify when a threshold for concern about possible bias will be reached, but the issue should not be overlooked during design of adaptive studies. There should be sensitivity to this possibility and steps should be considered, both during planning and in the process of DMC decision making, to try to limit the information which might be conveyed. It might be considered whether it was acceptable for a trial protocol not to contain full numerical specification of certain action thresholds. For example, if selection of a treatment arm or patient sub-population for continuation is to be made based upon predictive probability criteria, perhaps the general approach might be described in the protocol, with the specific thresholds appearing only in a document of more limited circulation such as the DMC charter and the document relaying the eventual decisions or recommendations. This information could likely not remain unknown to all trial personnel, but at least this approach might limit what other parties (e.g., investigators) could infer from the actions eventually taken.

14.6 Summary and Recommendations

Adaptive designs have potential to bring added benefits and efficiencies to clinical research, when properly planned and utilized in appropriate settings. However, their differences from other more familiar trial settings that involve interim monitoring, and the nature of those differences, raise a number of challenges that must be addressed as we learn how to more effectively utilize them. Some of these challenges involve access to accruing trial results, relative to current conventions aimed at avoiding the introduction of bias. Clearly, in the implementation of confirmatory adaptive trials it will be important to limit or control knowledge of interim results. However, it is not the case that trials must be perceived as compromised if *any* comparative interim information from them becomes available to anyone outside of what we would view as a conventional independent DMC, since that is not the standard even in conventional (nonadaptive) trials with interim monitoring. Current interim monitoring practices have been developed to control information in order to achieve the best balance between the benefits resulting from the monitoring on one hand, and the integrity and interpretability of trial results on the other. For adaptive design implementation, the principle should be much the same. In implementing the interim data review and decision processes, certain critical questions must be carefully addressed: What perspectives and expertise are relevant to the adaptation decision? What is the nature and extent of the information that would become known? Can that information be reasonably considered to have potential to introduce bias into the trial? and What are the specific advantages that the adaptive design offers? General principles and recommendations include the following:

- In line with current conventions, access to unblinded data and knowledge of interim results by trial participants should be restricted, to avoid the potential to compromise trial results. This is particularly important if the trial aims to produce results which are confirmatory or strongly supportive for a potential regulatory submission.
- Review of interim results and decisions regarding adaptations are best made by qualified individuals not otherwise directly participating in the trial. A DMC can play a natural role in implementing an adaptation according to a sound prespecified plan. The membership of the DMC must possess whatever sets of expertise and experience are necessary for the tasks with which they are charged.

- At times sponsor participation in such activities may be considered, but a convincing rationale should be required, there should still be separation of information from trial management personnel, and appropriate firewalls and confidentiality procedures should be in place. Advance planning discussions might avoid the need for sponsor involvement in data review.
- Potential knowledge of interim results by observers or trial participants based on "reverse engineering" is an issue that should be considered in decisions about designing or implementing adaptive trials. In particular, the sensitivity of the specific information that could become known and its potential to introduce bias should be considered, as this might affect the manner in which the adaptive design is implemented. Measures to limit the information that could be inferred should be considered.

References

Antonijevic Z, Gallo P, Chuang-Stein C, Dragalin V, Loewy J, Menon S, Miller ER, Morgan CC, Sanchez M (2013) Views on emerging issues pertaining to data monitoring committees for adaptive trials. Ther Innov Regul Sci 47(4):495–502

Committee for Medicinal Products for Human Use (CHMP) (2005) Guideline on data monitoring committees. EMEA, London

Committee for Medicinal Products for Human Use (CHMP) (2007) Reflection paper on methodological issues in confirmatory clinical trials planned with an adaptive design. EMEA, London

Cui L, Hung HMJ, Wang SJ (1999) Modification of sample size in group sequential trials. Biometrics 55:853–857

Ellenberg SS, Fleming TR, DeMets DL (2002) Data monitoring committees in clinical trials: a practical perspective. Wiley, Chichester

Fleming TR, Sharples K, McCall J, Moore A, Rodgers A, Stewart R (2008) Maintaining confidentiality of interim data to enhance trial integrity and credibility. Clin Trials 5:157–167

Gallo P (2006) Confidentiality and trial integrity issues for adaptive designs. Drug Inf J 40: 445–450

Gaydos B, Anderson K, Berry D, Burnham N, Chuang-Stein C, Dudinak J, Fardipour P, Gallo P, Givens S, Lewis R, Maca J, Pinheiro J, Pritchett Y, Krams M (2009) Good practices for adaptive clinical trials in pharmaceutical product development. Drug Inf J 43:539–556

International Conference on Harmonisation Expert Working Group (1998) ICH harmonised tripartite guideline: statistical principles for clinical trials. Fed Reg 63:49583–49598

Koch A (2006) Confirmatory clinical trials with an adaptive design. Biom J 48:574–585

Maca J, Bhattacharya S, Dragalin V, Gallo P, Krams M (2006) Adaptive seamless phase II/III designs – background, operational aspects, and examples. Drug Inf J 40:463–473

Taylor AL, Ziesche S, Yancy C, Carson P, D'Agostino R, Ferdinand K, Taylor M, Adams K, Sabolinski M, Worcel M, Cohn JN (2004) Combination of isosorbide dinitrate and hydralazine in blacks with heart failure. NEJM 351:2049–2057

US Food and Drug Administration (2006) Guidance for clinical trial sponsors on the establishment and operation of clinical trial data monitoring committees. FDA, Rockville MD

US Food and Drug Administration (2010) Guidance for industry for adaptive clinical trials for drugs and biologics (draft). FDA, Rockville, MD

Chapter 15
Approaches for Clinical Supply Modelling and Simulation

Nitin R. Patel, Suresh Ankolekar, and Pralay Senchaudhuri

Abstract Clinical supply is impacted by decisions and events at every stage of a clinical trial. Protocol design, logistics planning, and operational dynamics pose challenges to the management of clinical supply in terms of complexity and uncertainty. In this chapter, we propose a simulation modelling approach to address these issues and support decision-makers in effectively managing clinical supply. The approach is comprehensively described in terms of underlying structure and process, and is illustrated with adaptive trials involving dropping of arms and a Bayesian responsive-adaptive design for dose finding.

Keywords Adaptive clinical trials • Clinical supply • Simulation modelling • Bayesian response-adaptive design

15.1 Introduction

Clinical supply plays a central role in clinical trials. It is impacted by decisions and events at every stage of a clinical trial. Protocol design determines key drivers of clinical supply such as type of trial, sample size, randomization scheme, treatment regimen, and drug pack-types. Logistics planning defines the supply chain by selecting sites and supply depots in countries and regions, activation schedules for sites, inventory stocking and replenishment policies for sites and depots, and scheduling of packing runs. During the operational stage of a clinical trial, the clinical supply

N.R. Patel (✉) • P. Senchaudhuri
Cytel Inc., 675 Massachusetts Ave., Cambridge, MA 02139, USA
e-mail: nitin@cytel.com

S. Ankolekar
Maastricht School of Management, Endepolsdomein 150, Maastricht, 6229 EP, The Netherlands

W. He et al. (eds.), *Practical Considerations for Adaptive Trial Design
and Implementation*, Statistics for Biology and Health,
DOI 10.1007/978-1-4939-1100-4_15, © Springer Science+Business Media New York 2014

is affected by patient enrolment and randomization, treatment dispensing schedule, inventory and expiry management at sites and depots, clinical events and patient dropouts, and timing of interim looks.

Traditional approaches to estimating drug requirement rely on historical overages and experience with similar trials. The common practice is to use a spreadsheet to perform calculations based on averages. Uncertainty is not modelled in a transparent and explicit manner. The next section of this chapter shows that uncertainty is inherent to medical supply for clinical trials.

The main disadvantages to using such spreadsheet models are:

- There is no quantitative assessment of risk of stock-out (failed randomization).
- Estimates of requirements are not easily defensible because their reliability depends on intuition based on experience. This is especially serious in the case of adaptive designs for which experience is limited.
- There is no systematic way to answer "what-if" questions that help to optimize drug supply (e.g. effect of multi-pack kits, effect of adding more sites).

This chapter focuses on simulating clinical trial supply by explicitly modelling the major sources of uncertainty. The aim of the simulation approach is to support supply related decisions at design, planning, and execution stages of a clinical trial. The chapter is organized in six sections. The next section outlines the key challenges of clinical supply management and motivates the modelling and simulation approach to tackle them. Section 15.3 comprehensively describes simulation modelling of clinical supply for a typical trial. It outlines the simulation process, describes the underlying structure in terms of components, and illustrates the approach through a running illustrative Example 1 of a typical non-adaptive fixed design trial. Section 15.4 extends the clinical supply simulation model to adaptive trials. Two case study examples of an adaptive trial with a single interim look with dropping of arms (Example 2) and a Bayesian response-adaptive design (Example 3) will be used in Sects. 15.4.1 and 15.4.2 respectively to illustrate simulation models for adaptive trials. Section 15.5 discusses strategic issues in medical supply modelling and simulation, computational aspects, re-simulation during the course of trial, and design/medical supply complexity trade-offs. Finally, Sect. 15.6 provides a chapter summary and conclusions.

15.2 Key Challenges

Clinical trials vary widely in complexity in terms of both trial design and global supply chain logistics.

- *Design complexity*: Clinical trial designs are of several types (e.g. traditional having parallel arms with fixed sample size and randomization ratios, crossover, group sequential, adaptive with sample size reassessment, adaptive with dropping of arms, adaptive in randomization ratios). Traditional designs may or may not be stratified, and they can be randomized at the study level or at the site level and can have covariate adaptive randomization. Adaptive designs are even more complex as the adaptations introduce an additional level of uncertainty in the demand patterns for clinical supply at site level. Trials with interim looks involving dropping of arms and/or sample size re-estimation require mid-course reconfiguration of clinical supply system. Trial designs often involve treatment regimens consisting of complex dispensing visit cycles and titration patterns. Double-blinded trial designs can involve preparation of treatment kits from a set of pack-types, offering several choices of combinations of active drugs and placebos.

- *Supply chain complexity*: Clinical trials involve complex global supply chains spanning several regions and countries. Clinical supplies are stocked, shipped, replenished, and eventually dispensed through a multi-echelon structure of central/regional/local depots, and dispensing sites. Expiry of clinical supply has to be managed at all levels of this structure. While clinical supply pack-types are produced at manufacturing facilities in scheduled packing runs, the treatment kits could potentially be prepared at any level of the complex structure. All the links within the structure would have their own lead times between trigger and eventual replenishment of clinical supply stock.

Clinical trials have several sources of uncertainty. The major sources are described below.

- *Enrolment uncertainty*: Prior site enrolment projections are often too optimistic. It is not uncommon to have as many as 30 % of the sites enrolling just one or no patients during the course of entire study. On the other hand, a few sites may contribute most of the patient enrolments. Further, there could be periods of high enrolment at a site followed by a lull period of low or no enrolment.
- *Site activation uncertainty*: Scheduled site activation could face uncertain logistical delays due to local conditions including country-specific regulatory issues. Even after activation, the First Patient First Visit (FPFV) time is often much longer than suggested by the expected enrolment rate.
- *Screening/randomization uncertainty*: Inclusion/exclusion criteria can lead to many screening failures. Randomizations, uncertain by definition, may lead to unbalanced assignments of treatment arms at the site level, even if adequately balanced at the trial level through balancing mechanisms such as permuted blocks and covariate-adaptive minimization algorithms.
- *Dispensing uncertainty*: The first (randomization) visit of a patient is highly uncertain due to enrolment uncertainty described earlier. Subsequent dispensing visits follow specified cycles in terms of periods and frequency and so are relatively predictable, but random delays do occur within specified intervals. A long delay beyond a limit could lead to reverting to a "loading dose" usually associated with the first visit, instead of a "maintenance dose" associated with revisits. The total number of dispensing visits and/or periods as implied by the specified

cycles and frequencies could vary due to random delays and dropouts. Dose levels could also be determined by uncertain clinical or safety events. Trials based on survival endpoints have dispensing uncertainty due to randomness in survival periods.

The challenges posed by complexity and uncertainty in clinical trials can be addressed by using simulation to replicate a given clinical trial several hundred times through a model that captures the inherent complexity and uncertainty of the trial to assess its impact on clinical supply. This approach would enhance efficiency of clinical supply management by minimizing unused supply at the end of the trial while controlling failed randomizations due to supply stock-outs by ensuring availability of the right supply, at the right place, at the right time. Decision-makers at various stages of clinical trial design, planning, and implementation can use simulation to conduct "what-if" analyses of the implications to clinical supply efficiency of decisions and policies and take an integrated view to effectively manage the trial. At the design stage, the simulation model could be used to refine decisions related to various trial parameters such as sample size, number and timing of adaptive interventions, treatment regimen, dispensing cycles, and pack-types. At the planning stage, the model could lead to a better supply chain structure and policies. During trial execution, the model can support effective monitoring and mid-course corrections based on accumulated information.

15.3   Clinical Supply Simulation Model

The clinical supply simulation model embodies key aspects of design, planning, and operations of a clinical trial. Essentially, the model enables virtual replication of a given clinical trial through a simulation procedure to explore various scenarios related to the key aspects. Peterson et al. (2004) and McEntegart and O'Gorman (2005) give detailed descriptions of clinical supply simulation for traditional (non-adaptive) designs.

The simulation procedure consists of three basic steps that are iterated several times to refine and optimize medical supply for a clinical trial. The steps are:

1. Assembling inputs reflecting relevant aspects of a trial scenario. A complete specification of all inputs required to simulate clinical supply for a trial is called a scenario.
2. Running Monte Carlo simulations consisting of several replicates of the trial as defined by the scenario.
3. Analysis of the simulation results database to generate reports.

Iterative cycling through steps 1–3 is used to refine decision and policy parameters that drive supply efficiency. Iteration is performed to answer "what-if" questions aimed at optimizing the drug supply strategy for the trial. This procedure is depicted in Fig. 15.1.

Simulation Overview

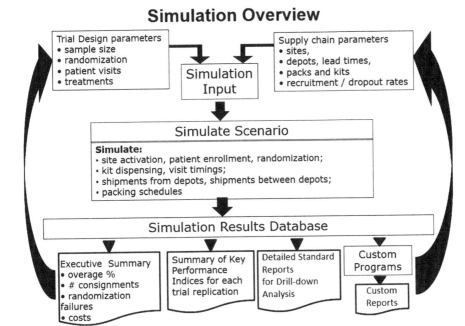

Fig. 15.1 Overview of clinical supply simulation model

15.3.1   Simulation Input

The simulation input consists of trial design and supply chain parameters. The trial design parameters are typically derived from the protocol document. The supply chain parameters are primarily derived from trial planning documents and discussions with supply planners.

The trial design parameters typically include sample size, treatment arms, randomization scheme, treatment regimen, dispensing visit cycles/frequency/dropout assumptions, and clinical supply pack-types. Trials with complex designs may involve additional parameters including number of interim looks, dropping of arms, sample size re-estimation, cross-over schemes, response-adaptive randomization schemes, etc. As a preparatory step before discussing adaptive trials in Sect. 15.4, we will illustrate the various components of a clinical supply simulation model with the simpler case of a typical non-adaptive trial design. Inputs for this non-adaptive trial are described in Table 15.1.

The supply chain parameters typically include depot/site structure, lead times, enrolment rates, and activation plan as described in Table 15.2. The sites are categorized as High, Medium, and Low in terms of the range of enrolment rates. Additional supply chain input parameters for inventory control will be described in Sect. 15.3.2.

Table 15.1 Trial design parameters for Example 1

Sample size	480 patients
Treatment	2 Capsules per day for 6 weeks
Treatment arms	0 (Placebo), 20, 40, 60 mg
Dose pack-types	0 (Placebo), 20, 40, 60 mg
Treatment ratio	1:1:1:1
Randomization method	Permuted block (size=4)
Number of dispensing visits	1
Treatment duration (weeks)	6
Interim looks	0

Table 15.2 Basic supply chain parameters for Example 1

Site categories >	High	Medium	Low
Number of sites			
Country 1	1	1	1
Country 2	3	5	3
Country 3	2	2	2
Enrolment rates (patients/week)			
Country 1	0.86	0.57	0.29
Country 2	1.21	0.80	0.40
Country 3	1.46	0.97	0.49
Range of activation delay (weeks from start of trial)			
Country 1	0–4	0–4	0–4
Country 2	0–9	0–9	0–9
Country 3	9–13	9–13	9–13

15.3.2 Components of Clinical Supply Simulation Model

The clinical supply simulation model consists of the following sub-models that simulate specific aspects of a clinical trial.

- Packing/distribution model
- Site activation model.
- Enrolment model
- Randomization model
- Site inventory model
- Treatment dispensing model
- Treatment kits model

15.3.2.1 Packing and Distribution Model

The packing and distribution model addresses lot scheduling, order fulfilment, and expiry management at central and local depots. Lot schedules specify delivery of lots to the central depot. The quantity, in multiples of the lot-size specified by the

Table 15.3 Supply chain parameters for packing and distribution model

Parameter	Value		
Lot quantity per pack-type	10		
Packing runs schedule	Auto		
Packing expiry time (weeks)	60		
Do not ship time prior to expiry (weeks)	7		
Do not dispense time prior to expiry (weeks)	5		
Cost of drug for 6 week treatment kit	$1,000		
Depot shipment parameters			
Depots >	1	2 (Central)	3
Lead time to country depots from the central depot (days)	10	–	10
Manufacturing and delivery lead time to central depot (days)	–	20	–
Depot to site lead time (days)	3	3	3
Cost per shipment from central or manufacturing to depots	$2,000	$10,000	$2,000
Cost per shipment form depot to site	$500	$500	$500

Table 15.4 Depot stocks required at start of trial

Week	A0	B20	B40	B60
Country 1 (local)				
0	50	50	50	50
Country 2 (central)				
0	290	290	290	290
Country 3 (local)				
0	90	90	90	90

user, should be adequate to take care of required shipments from central depot to local depots and sites, while controlling wastage due to expiry and unused stock. Orders are fulfilled using depot stock on first-in-first-out basis to minimize the wastage due to expiry. The lot schedules can be fully or partially specified (Manual mode) or can be determined by the model automatically for a given lot size (Auto mode). In both cases, the model optimizes the lot delivery schedule to minimize wastage due to expiry and unshipped stock. The delivery of lots and order fulfilment involves lead times and costs. The supply chain parameters related to the packing and distribution model for the Example 1 are given in Table 15.3.

The simulation run control parameters for this example require that the total requirement for each pack-type be manufactured and shipped to the central depot (located in Country 2) at the start of the trial. The quantity to be packed at the central depot was automatically computed to be 1,160 packs (packing overage of 142 %), evenly distributed amongst pack-types, as given in Table 15.4. The central depot in turn would ship 200 packs to the Country 1 local depot and 360 packs to the Country 3 local depot.

The depot stocks required at start of the trial are determined on the basis of time-series of simulated cumulative demand at sites supplied by the depot. These time-series are aggregated per simulation and envelopes across simulations are computed to determine the maximum cumulative demand schedule for the depot.

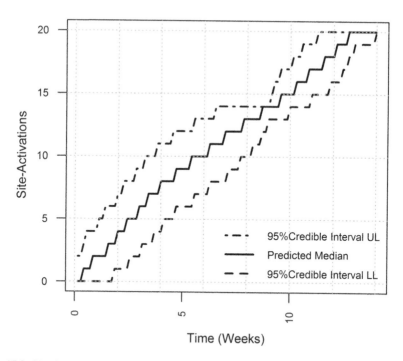

Fig. 15.2 Simulated cumulative site activations for Example 1

The depot stock required at start of the trial is then determined by a simple lookup of the maximum demand schedule at expiry date. The central depot stock is augmented with the stocks of other local depots supplied by it.

15.3.2.2 Site Activation Model

The site model simulates site activation times by random sampling from a probability distribution for activation periods for each country and site category specified by the user. We use a uniform distribution with earliest and latest activation times. A triangular distribution with an additional mode parameter is also popular. Figure 15.2 shows profiles over time of the median and 95 % credible intervals for the cumulative number of activated sites generated by 1,000 simulations for the Example 1.

15.3.2.3 Enrolment Model

The enrolment model generates patient enrolments, screening failures, and patient attributes. A Poisson process is used to generate enrolments, where rates are generated randomly using a uniform distribution within a range around specified enrolment rates. Several papers have proposed Poisson models. In Chap. 16 of this book,

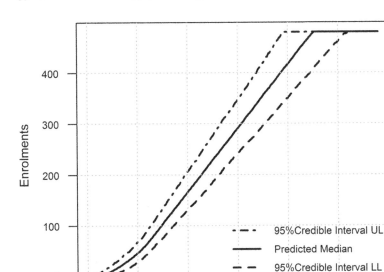

Fig. 15.3 Simulated cumulative enrolments for Example 1

Weili and Xiting describe approaches for patient recruitment modelling and simulation. Anisimov and Fedorov (2007) suggest using a Gamma distribution instead of a uniform distribution for enrolment rates. We have used such distributions in some assignments. However, we have found that drug supply experts find it easier to specify a range of likely rates within which any value is as likely as any other. Screening failure for enrolled patients can be generated through a Bernoulli process. Patient attributes (e.g. Body Mass Index, covariate values) for the screened patients are randomly generated using specified probability distributions and related parameters. Figure 15.3 shows cumulative profiles of enrolled patients at the study level in terms of median and 95 % credible intervals for Example 1.

15.3.2.4 Randomization Model

The randomization model implements the randomization method specified in the protocol. A permuted block randomization is used for most designs. Other methods like stratified permuted blocks, cross-over and covariate-adaptive minimization can be easily simulated with minor modifications to the simulation logic. This is also the case for simpler response adaptive designs such as dropping and adding arms and sample size re-estimation. We will illustrate this approach in the Sect. 15.4.1 where we describe a dropping arms design.

However, for more complex adaptations like Bayesian adaptive randomization it is preferable to leverage outputs from simulations that are routinely carried out to determine operating characteristics of such adaptive designs. This can be done by reading output files with patient randomization sequences from the design simulations as input files for the medical supply simulation. We illustrate this approach in Sect. 15.4.2 where we describe a Bayesian adaptive randomization design for dose finding.

Most randomization methods result in significant imbalance in demand among treatment arms at the site level. Site-level imbalance causes inefficiency in clinical supply, and may result in stock-out in some treatment arms and surplus in others. McEntegart (2003) has proposed a "forced randomization" approach, whereby the randomized subject facing a stock-out is "forced" to be allocated to the next free treatment arm in the randomization list corresponding to available treatment at the site. This approach is motivated by efficiency considerations of clinical supply. This could encounter difficulties with regulators, especially if there are several instances of "forced" allocation.

15.3.2.5 Site Inventory Model

The Initial/Trigger/Resupply (ITR) model is the almost universally used method for controlling supply to sites in trials that use an IVRS system to control randomization and medical supply. Excellent descriptions of how IVRS systems enable implementation of ITR models are given by Byrom (2002) and Waters et al. (2010). Under ITR an initial level of stock is delivered to each site when it is activated. Subsequent orders are triggered to replenish any shortfall below the resupply level set for the site, if the inventory position (stock on hand + on order) for a pack-type falls to its trigger level (or below). The order is placed at the end of the day and a shipment is scheduled at the depot that will be received at the ordering site after a delay known as the lead time. Typically, to reduce the number of consignments, when an order is triggered all pack-types (not just the one that fell below the trigger level) are ordered up to their resupply levels. This practice is known in the inventory control literature as "joint replenishment".

Initial/Trigger/Resupply levels can be either explicitly specified by the user or could be generated by the clinical supply simulator in "Auto mode". The auto mode uses a heuristic algorithm that iteratively computes ITR levels aiming to keep the number of shipments near a target level specified by the user, while ensuring that there are no stock-outs. The trigger level critically influences the probability of a stock-out; higher the trigger level, lower would be the probability of stock-out and vice versa. Basically, the trigger level should be just about adequate to meet the lead time demand between trigger and resupply at a site. Such demand is determined by the rate of enrolment, randomization, and the time points of trigger. Of these, the latter is jointly determined by the initial, trigger, and resupply levels for the site. In other words, the auto mode heuristic algorithm has to co-determine the three levels together, and they in turn determine the number of triggers or shipments.

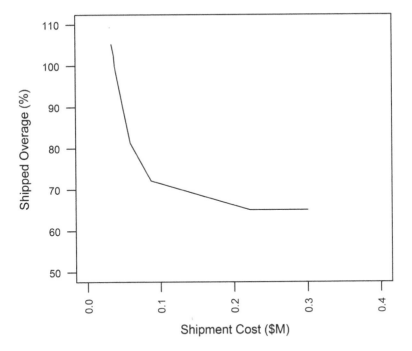

Fig. 15.4 Shipment cost vs. overage trade-off

For a tutorial on heuristic algorithms for optimal inventory policies in supply chains, see Shang (2011). Specifically, the number of shipments is influenced by the initial level and the gap between trigger and resupply level; higher the initial level and/or the gap, lower would be the number of shipments, and vice versa. On the other hand, higher initial, trigger, and resupply levels would increase the shipment overage defined as the fraction of excess site inventory at the end of the trial over total clinical supply dispensed to the patients. The shipment overage should be distinguished from the packing overage defined in Sect. 15.3.2.1, the latter accounting for the excess inventory including at central and local depots. The site inventory policy primarily impacts the shipment overage component of the overall packing overage.

The above discussion implies that setting ITR levels involves a trade-off between the number of shipments and the shipment overage. The auto mode heuristic algorithm generates this trade-off curve for the user to resolve the trade-off by considering the constraints on total availability and cost of clinical supply as well as shipping costs. For Example 1, Fig. 15.4 displays the trade-off curve between average shipment costs and shipped overage, and Table 15.5 gives the trigger and resupply levels for a median shipped overage of about 75 % (corresponding to packing overage of about 142 %) and a total shipment cost of around $80,000 when the initial level is set to be equal to the resupply level.

The trigger/resupply levels discussed so far relate to the first (randomization) dispensing visit of the patient involving uncertain enrolment time at a site and random treatment arm. In the case of trials with multiple dispensing visits, the corresponding

Table 15.5 Inventory policy generated by clinical supply simulator in "Auto" mode

Country	Category	Trigger_A0	Trigger_B20	Trigger_B40	Trigger_B60	Resupply_A0	Resupply_B20	Resupply_B40	Resupply_B60
1	High	2	2	2	2	5	5	5	5
1	Medium	2	2	2	2	5	5	5	5
1	Low	1	1	1	1	4	4	4	4
2	High	3	3	3	3	5	5	5	5
2	Medium	3	3	3	3	6	6	6	6
2	Low	2	2	2	2	5	5	5	5
3	High	3	3	3	3	5	5	5	5
3	Medium	3	3	3	3	5	5	5	5
3	Low	2	2	2	2	4	4	4	4

schedules and treatments are known with certainty for subsequent re-visits, except possibly for a small variation around planned scheduled visit and a chance of drop-out. Therefore, it should be possible to effectively manage the clinical supply for dispensing re-visits with a nearly deterministic process. However, dividing clinical supply between first visit and later re-visits into independent subsystems, each with its own independent set of ITR levels, would lead to sub-optimal control of total inventory. On the other hand, integrating the two subsystems resulting in pooling of clinical supply inventory across the re-visits could potentially increase inventory position at the trigger point. The two subsystems can be integrated through dynamically augmented trigger/resupply levels on the basis of number of patients predicted to report for dispensing re-visit within a prediction window. Byrom (2002) describes setting trigger and re-ordering levels for multiple visit protocols. In addition to the augmented trigger/resupply levels for re-visits, the levels could also be boosted to account for imminent expiry of pack-types in stock as determined by the drug expiry-related parameters. The auto mode heuristic algorithm strives to avoid stock-outs, to the extent possible, by setting optimal inventory policy for augmented dynamic levels, and pre-emptive replenishment of stocks due to expire. If appropriate, for failed randomization due to stock-outs, the user can choose to model dispensing of the required kit at a later date. The ITR mechanism could also be used for replenishment of local depot stocks from central depots. Given the higher depot shipping costs and lead times, however, the ITR mechanism is typically dominated by high initial levels determined as described in Sect. 15.3.2.1 with no further replenishment.

15.3.2.6 Treatment Kits Model

Treatment arms are specified in terms of dose level of active pharmaceutical ingredient (API). For example, the four treatment arms in Example 1 have dose levels of 0 mg (Placebo), 20, 40, and 60 mg, each with its own pack-type. It is possible to improve clinical supply efficiency by restricting pack-types to a subset of dose levels and combining these pack-types for dispensation to all treatment arms. The combinations have to ensure that treatment arms are double-blinded, if required, and the number of packs needed for each treatment arm is minimized to avoid requiring patients to handle too many medications at each administration. Also feasibility in terms of manufacturing/packaging as well as treatment compliance by patients has to be confirmed before considering this option.

Let us now modify Example 1 to a scenario where there is no pack-type of 60 mg. Instead pack-types of 0, 20, and 40 mg are used to dispense all four treatments. Table 15.6 shows how this can be done, while preserving blinding, by dispensing two packs to each patient.

Running 1,000 simulations of this scenario in Auto mode shows that the packing overage comes down very substantially to 85 % compared to the base case overage of 142 %. (Both cases had no stock-out in 1,000 simulations.)

Table 15.6 Dispensing two pack-types for each treatment

	0 mg pack	20 mg pack	40 mg pack
0 mg treatment	2		
20 mg treatment	1	1	
40 mg treatment	1		1
60 mg treatment		1	1

15.3.2.7 Treatment Dispensing Model

The dispensing model reflects the protocol information associated with the treatment regimen (e.g. dispensing cycles, schedule, frequency, treatment kits, permissible delays). The treatment period is often divided into one or more dispensing cycles. If dropout rates are not negligible, the simulation model needs to be provided user inputs on dropouts at each dispensing visit. The treatment kits may be specified to be dependent on patient attributes (e.g. weight). The dispensing model simulates visit times and dropouts, until the specified maximum number of visits or total dispensing duration or dropout, whichever occurs first. Multiple dispensing visits can significantly improve clinical supply efficiency due to "predictive resupply" described earlier in Sect. 15.3.2.5, as the schedule of subsequent revisits is known with greater degree of certainty compared to the randomization visit. This can reduce overage substantially when the proportion of the drug required for subsequent visits is large compared to the first randomization visit. Extending the two pack-types scenario described in Sect. 15.3.2.6 to two dispensing visits for Example 1, the packing overage is reduced further to 75 % compared to the base case overage of 142 %. (Both cases had no stock-out in 1,000 simulations.)

15.3.3 Simulation Results and Database

The model simulates relevant aspects of the clinical trial using sub-models described in Sect. 15.3.2 and stores the results in a database. The database is accessed to produce reports at different levels of granularity to support decisions related to clinical supply. Typically, following standard reports are produced by analysing the simulation database:

- Executive summary reports.

  - Study level Key Performance Indicators (KPI) of clinical supply.
  - KPI report at the pack-type level.
  - Inventory policy in terms of trigger/resupply levels.
  - Inventory policy in terms of packing runs.

- Summary reports for each simulation (trial replication) in a run.

  - Study level KPI per simulation.
  - KPI per simulation at pack-type level.

Table 15.7 Executive summary of clinical supply simulation results for Example 1

	Mean	Std dev.	Min	prct_01	Median	prct_99	Max
Patients randomized	480	0	480	480	480	480	480
Dropout rate (%)	0	0	0	0	0	0	0
FPFV to LPLV (weeks)	43.5	3.3	34	37	43	51	57
Start to LPLV (weeks)	45.1	3.3	35	38	45	53	58
Packs dispensed	480	0	480	480	480	480	480
Packs shipped to sites	842.0	7.3	811	824	842	858	862
Packs expired at sites	0.0	0.0	0	0	0	0	0
Overage on shipped (%)	75.4	1.5	69	72	75	79	80
Packs packed	1,160	0.0	1,160	1,160	1,160	1,160	1,160
Overage on packed (%)	141.7	0.0	142	142	142	142	142
Consignments	125.5	4.2	112	115	125	135	139
Packs per consignment	6.7	0.2	6.1	6.2	6.7	7.3	7.5
Drug cost ($M)	1.2	0.000	1.16	1.16	1.16	1.16	1.16
Shipment cost ($M)	0.1	0.002	0.07	0.07	0.08	0.08	0.08
Total cost ($M)	1.2	0.002	1.23	1.23	1.24	1.24	1.24
% Runs with failed randomization	0	0	0	0	0	0	0
% Runs with failed revisits	0	0	0	0	0	0	0
% Runs with stock-out	0	0	0	0	0	0	0

- "Drill down" reports into selected trial simulations.
    - Patient dispensing details for simulations with stock-outs.
    - Shipment details for simulations with stock-outs.
    - Frequency distribution of stock-outs, if any.
    - Patient dispensing details for a user-specified set of simulations.
    - Shipment details for a user-specified set of simulations.

A typical executive summary report indicating study level KPI for Example 1 with a single dispensing visit and a single pack-type per treatment is given in Table 15.7. The report was generated by performing a run consisting of 1,000 clinical trial simulations using the "Auto mode" ITR levels in Table 15.5. Each row provides a summary of simulation results on a KPI of the trial and the supply strategy. The mean, standard deviation, minimum and maximum values, median, and 1st and 99th percentiles of the KPI are displayed. There were no dropouts specified for this example so the number of patients randomized is equal to the sample size for each clinical trial simulation. FPFV and LPLV are abbreviations for the time of the first visit of the first patient and the last visit of the last patient in the trial. On the average 842 packs were shipped to sites from depots, leaving on average 362 packs at sites at the end of the trial. Thus the shipping overage was 75 % (=362/480). Similarly, the packing overage is 142 % = $100 \times (1,160 - 480)/480$, being almost twice as large due to depot level uncertainty and complexity discussed in Sect. 15.3.2.1. Since the expiry time for lots was long relative to the trial duration no packs were lost due to the expiry date being exceeded. It is common practice to destroy the packs left over at sites at the end of a trial. This can be a significant cost element in the trial because disposal has to be documented carefully in case there is an audit by the regulatory authorities (see Dowlman et al. 2006 for details).

Notice that the number of stock-outs is zero indicating that the Auto mode performed as expected and there were no stock-outs in the 1,000 simulations—all the 480,000 patients simulated in the run were randomized as planned.

The "Consignments" row shows the number of shipments made from depots to sites during the trial. The number varied between 112 and 139. The "Packs per consignment" row shows how many packs were in a shipment. This is useful to know because too high a value could lead to storage difficulties at sites. A low value signals that the number of shipments may be excessive and need to be reduced. The cost rows indicate the components of cost of supply for the trial.

15.4 Clinical Supply Simulation for Adaptive Trial Designs

The cost and feasibility of drug supply required for adaptive clinical trials is often a concern. The adaptive aspect of the design increases uncertainty in the demand for clinical supply. For example, in an adaptive phase 2 dose finding study the demand for a particular dose is not known in advance but evolves dynamically as the trial progresses and randomization to doses is modified by observed responses of subjects to various doses. This is in contrast to non-adaptive designs where the total number of subjects to be allocated to each dose is fixed and known before the trial begins. A simple approach for the adaptive design would be to plan for each dose at the maximum possible level of demand. In an adaptive trial with seven doses where each dose is administered as a single tablet this would lead to increasing the amount of drug overage by a factor of 7 over a fixed allocation non-adaptive design with the same sample size. By exploring options such as multi-pack kits, multiple dispensing visits, and multiple packing campaigns we can reduce drug overage while ensuring an acceptable risk of stock-out. Nicholls et al. (2009) describe the use of simulation to reduce drug overage in an adaptive trial using multi-pack kits.

Adaptive trial designs come in varying degrees of complexity. At the simplest level are designs involving interim looks with dropping of arms. Such designs would have randomization schemes specified for each look. A probability model for dropping of arms can be added to a clinical supply simulator and also modifications may need to be made if the patient enrolment plan calls for slowing down enrolment around interim looks. Such modifications of the clinical supply simulator are feasible for designs involving interim looks with dropping and/or adding arms and sample size re-assessment.

Modifying a clinical supply simulator to handle more complex adaptive trial designs like Bayesian adaptive randomization requires considerable effort and is generally not feasible. Fortunately in such cases, we can leverage the simulation effort that is almost always needed to determine the statistical operating characteristics of complex adaptive designs. In Chap. 9 of this book, Kyle discusses simulation modelling approaches for different types of adaptive trials. Our approach is to save randomization sequences generated by the adaptive design simulator in a file. The clinical supply simulator can be modified to read this file to generate randomization sequences instead of using built-in randomization logic as is the case for simpler designs.

15.4.1 Two-Stage Adaptive Design with Dropping of Arms and Early Stopping

Example 2 is a modification of the fixed sample size design of Example 1 to a two-stage adaptive design with a single interim analysis after 240 patients. Design simulations of the most likely scenario show that there is a 0.8 probability of dropping two of the three arms with active doses, and a 0.2 probability of stopping the trial for futility or efficacy. The enrolment would be halted for 4 weeks at the interim look. While the placebo arm is never dropped, the dropping of any arm with an active dose is equally likely. Also, the design remains balanced after the dropping of arms with block size remaining equal to 4 and treatment ratios of the continued arms are 2:2. If there is just one packing campaign at the start of the trial, the overage is 252 %. If it is possible to schedule a second campaign during the 4 weeks after the interim analysis we can make the second campaign only for the placebo and selected arm if the trial is continued to the second stage. Table 15.8 gives the executive summary for the base case of a single dispensing visit and single pack-type per treatment.

The simulation results indicate higher overage for the single interim analysis design with dropping of arms (159 %), compared to the base case of the traditional fixed sample design (142 %). This is because of uncertainty in the outcome of the interim look in terms of early termination of the trial or which arms are dropped.

The first packing campaign is for 210 packs of each pack-type at the start of the trial. The second campaign is after the arm to be continued is known and is for 170 packs of this arm and 170 packs of placebo.

Table 15.8 Clinical supply simulation results single interim look design: base case

	Mean	Std dev.	Min	prct_01	Median	prct_99	Max
Patients randomized	427.92	98.9	240	240	480	480	480
Dropout rate (%)	0	0	0	0	0	0	0
FPFV to LPLV (weeks)	42.5	10.0	19	21	46	55	59
Start to LPLV (weeks)	44.0	10.0	21	23	48	57	61
Packs dispensed	427.9	99.0	240.0	240.0	480.0	480.0	480.0
Packs shipped to sites	839.9	78.9	669	681	878	898	905
Packs expired at sites	0.0	0.0	0	0	0	0	0
Overage on shipped (%)	96.3	5.1	88	90	94	107	109
Packs packed	1,106.2	140.2	840	840	1,180	1,180	1,180
Overage on packed (%)	158.5	9.6	140	140	164	164	164
Consignments	122.6	23.3	71	75	134	142	145
Packs per consignment	7.0	0.9	6.2	6.3	6.6	9.2	9.5
Drug cost ($M)	1.1	0.140	0.84	0.84	1.18	1.18	1.18
Shipment cost ($M)	0.1	0.012	0.06	0.07	0.10	0.10	0.10
Total cost ($M)	1.2	0.152	0.90	0.91	1.28	1.28	1.28
% Runs with stock-out	0	0	0	0	0	0	0

If we use two pack-types per dispensation as we did in Example 1, the overage goes down to 104 % from 159 %. There is a further reduction to 86 % if we also have two dispensation visits instead of one.

In practice we recommend running simulations for additional likely scenarios to verify robustness of the settings suggested by the above simulations.

15.4.2 Bayesian Response-Adaptive Randomization Design

Our next example, Example 3, illustrates use of simulation to plan medical supplies for an adaptive randomization design. This type of adaptive design is popular for Phase 2 dose finding trials. Example 3 is a study for treatment of dental pain and has eight treatment arms including a placebo and seven doses. For our base case simulations we assume that, in addition to a placebo pack-type, there are seven pack-types, with doses of 1, 2, 3, 4, 5, 6, and 7 units on the log scale. The sample size is 120 (40 placebo and 80 drug) with 10 cohorts of 12 patients each. Subjects in the first cohort are randomized as follows: 4 to placebo, 2 to dose 4, and one each to the remaining six doses. The endpoint is measured 24 h after administration and each subsequent cohort is assigned doses by calculating the Bayesian posterior distribution by updating a weakly informative prior using pain score observations for all subjects in previous cohorts. The allocation ratios to doses are chosen to minimize the variance of the Bayesian estimate of dose response at the target dose. The target dose is the lowest dose with an expected pain score improvement of 15 units in the pain score from placebo. The three likely dose–response scenarios are depicted in Fig. 15.5. The operating characteristics for the design selected for implementation were estimated using simulation. There were 500 trial replications for each dose–response scenario which simulated subject responses for the subjects in cohorts and used the Bayesian calculations described above to allocate subjects to doses for each cohort in each replicated trial. There are five sites each expected to enrol one subject/week. The sites are supplied by a single central depot with a lead time of 1 day. The plan is to have a single packing campaign at the start of the trial to supply all the drug requirements for the trial.

From the point of view of drug supply Example 3 differs from Example 2 in two important respects. First, there are three likely scenarios instead of a single likely scenario. Second, the randomization sequences of subjects depend on the statistical responses of subjects in complex ways (e.g. Markov Chain Monte Carlo calculations for allocation of doses) that are not easy to embed in the drug supply software. Figure 15.6 illustrates how allocation varies for a typical trial replication.

There are two approaches we have used to combine scenarios. The first approach is to assess prior probabilities that reflect the likelihood of each scenario being the true scenario applicable to the trial. The second approach which is more conservative is to ensure that our supply plan is robust under any of the three possible scenarios. We have found that in practice it is not easy to obtain prior probabilities of likely scenarios. We have, therefore, most often used the robust approach that ensures good performance of the supply strategy irrespective of which dose–response scenario holds.

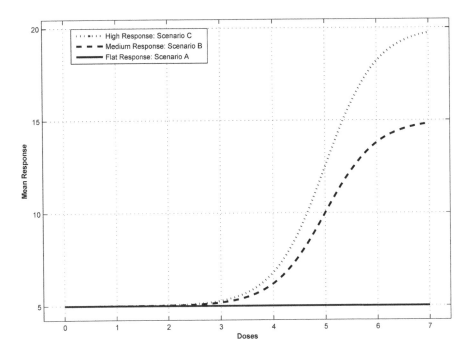

Fig. 15.5 Likely dose–response scenarios for the adaptive design

We first use the simulator to run 500 simulations in Auto mode, one simulation for each of the 500 sequences of subject randomizations generated by the statistical design trial replications executed previously by the Compass software package for dose–response scenario A. These are read by CytelSupply, a clinical supply simulator, from a file that is written by Compass. We repeat the procedure with scenarios B and C to obtain overages of 152, 171 and 165 % respectively. After examining the different sets of trigger and resupply levels we obtained under the three different scenarios we run the manual option in the simulator to investigate overage using a *common set of trigger and resupply levels*. We try several different common sets of levels to determine the lowest overage that gives no stock-out. The set that minimizes the overage is shown in Table 15.9 and the corresponding executive summaries of simulation results for Scenarios A, B, and C are shown in Table 15.10. For all scenarios the overage is the same, 192 %, since the amount packed and dispensed is the same for each scenario.

For benchmarking it is interesting to note that for a non-adaptive traditional trial the simulations with equal randomization ratios for all arms, the overage is 100 %. However the drug supply increase in cost has to be weighed against the improved efficiency of the trial.

The adaptive trial in Example 3 was designed for both Proof-of Concept (PoC) and dose finding. A traditional approach would require a smaller single-dose trial for PoC followed by a dose finding trial with fixed randomization ratios.

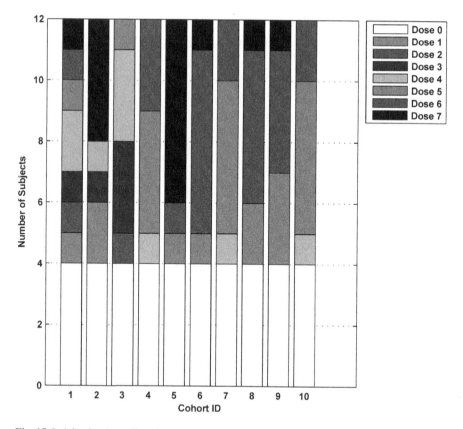

Fig. 15.6 Adaptive dose allocations over cohorts

Table 15.9 Inventory policy for adaptive design

	A0	B1	B2	B3	B4	B5	B6	B7
Trigger	3	2	1	1	1	2	1	3
Resupply	5	4	3	3	3	4	3	5

The accuracy of estimation of the dose–response curve is much better than for a traditional design. Under Scenarios B and C the variance of dose–response estimates at all doses is approximately half that of the traditional design, so that to obtain comparable accuracy the traditional design would need to have twice the sample size (see Orloff et al. 2009 for details). This would increase the cost of traditional design substantially besides increasing the time to market by about 6 months for an efficacious drug.

It is possible to use three pack-types for each dispensation by using combinations of pack-types for each dose as shown in Table 15.11 with inventory policy of Table 15.12. The effect is to reduce overage considerably: from 192 to 74 % as shown in Table 15.13.

Table 15.10 Simulation results for Example 3

	Mean	Std dev.	Min	prct_01	Median	prct_99	Max
Drug-supply Scenario A (base case)							
Patients randomized	120	0.0	120	120	120	120	120
Dropout rate (%)	0	0	0	0	0	0	0
FPFV to LPLV (weeks)	24.2	3.9	15	17	24	35	37
Start to LPLV (weeks)	24.5	3.9	15	17	24	35	38
Packs dispensed	120	0.0	120	120	120	120	120
Packs shipped to sites	257.6	3.1	248	249	258	263	264
Packs expired at sites	0.0	0.0	0	0	0	0	0
Overage on shipped (%)	114.7	2.6	107	108	115	119	120
Packs packed	350.0	0.0	350	350	350	350	350
Overage on packed (%)	191.7	0.0	192	192	192	192	192
Consignments	32.6	1.9	28	29	33	37	39
Packs per consignment	7.9	0.4	6.6	7.0	7.9	8.9	9.1
Drug cost ($M)	0.4	0.000	0.35	0.35	0.35	0.35	0.35
Shipment cost ($M)	0.02	0.001	0.02	0.02	0.02	0.02	0.02
Total cost ($M)	0.4	0.001	0.37	0.37	0.37	0.37	0.37
% Runs with stock-out	0	0.0	0	0	0	0	0
Scenario B (base case)							
Patients randomized	120	0.0	120	120	120	120	120
Dropout rate (%)	0	0	0	0	0	0	0
FPFV to LPLV (weeks)	24.3	3.9	15	17	24	35	39
Start to LPLV (weeks)	24.6	4.0	15	17	24	35	40
Packs dispensed	120	0.0	120	120	120	120	120
Packs shipped to sites	257.5	3.2	246	250	258	264	264
Packs expired at sites	0.0	0.0	0	0	0	0	0
Overage on shipped (%)	114.6	2.7	105	108	115	120	120
Packs packed	350.0	0.0	350	350	350	350	350
Overage on packed (%)	191.7	0.0	192	192	192	192	192
Consignments	31.8	1.8	26	28	32	36	37
Packs per consignment	8.1	0.4	7.0	7.2	8.1	9.3	9.7
Drug cost ($M)	0.4	0.000	0.35	0.35	0.35	0.35	0.35
Shipment cost ($M)	0.02	0.001	0.02	0.02	0.02	0.02	0.02
Total cost ($M)	0.4	0.001	0.37	0.37	0.37	0.37	0.37
% Runs with stock-out	0	0.0	0	0	0	0	0
Scenario C (base case)							
Patients randomized	120	0.0	120	120	120	120	120
Dropout rate (%)	0	0	0	0	0	0	0
FPFV to LPLV (weeks)	24.1	3.7	14	17	24	34	37
Start to LPLV (weeks)	24.4	3.7	14	18	24	34	38
Packs dispensed	120	0.0	120	120	120	120	120
Packs shipped to sites	258.0	3.1	247	250	258	264	265
Packs expired at sites	0.0	0.0	0	0	0	0	0
Overage on shipped (%)	115.0	2.6	106	108	115	120	121
Packs packed	350.0	0.0	350	350	350	350	350
Overage on packed (%)	191.7	0.0	192	192	192	192	192
Consignments	32.5	2.1	26	28	33	37	39
Packs per consignment	8.0	0.5	6.6	7.0	7.9	9.1	9.8
Drug cost ($M)	0.4	0.000	0.35	0.35	0.35	0.35	0.35
Shipment cost ($M)	0.02	0.001	0.02	0.02	0.02	0.02	0.02
Total cost ($M)	0.4	0.001	0.37	0.37	0.37	0.37	0.37
% Runs with stock-out	0	0.0	0	0	0	0	0

Table 15.11 Dispensing three pack-types for each dose

	0 mg pack	1 mg pack	3 mg pack
0 mg dose	3		
1 mg dose	2	1	
2 mg dose	1	2	
3 mg dose	2		1
4 mg dose	1	1	1
5 mg dose		2	1
6 mg dose	1		2
7 mg dose		1	2

Table 15.12 Inventory policy for adaptive design with three pack-types

	A0	B1	B3
Trigger	10	7	7
Resupply	22	12	12

Table 15.13 Clinical supply simulation results for adaptive design with three pack-types

	Mean	Std dev.	Min	prct_01	Median	prct_99	Max
Patients randomized	120	0.0	120	120	120	120	120
Dropout rate (%)	0	0	0	0	0	0	0
FPFV to LPLV (weeks)	24.2	3.9	14	17	24	34	39
Start to LPLV (weeks)	24.5	3.9	14	17	24	35	40
Packs dispensed	360	0.0	360	360	360	360	360
Packs shipped to sites	550.1	11.0	515	525	551	573	579
Packs expired at sites	0.0	0.0	0	0	0	0	0
Overage on shipped (%)	52.8	3.1	43	46	53	59	61
Packs packed	625.0	0.0	625	625	625	625	625
Overage on packed (%)	73.6	0.0	74	74	74	74	74
Consignments	25.3	1.2	21	23	25	28	30
Packs per consignment	21.8	0.9	19.2	19.8	21.7	23.8	25.0
Drug cost ($M)	0.2	0.000	0.21	0.21	0.21	0.21	0.21
Shipment cost ($M)	0.01	0.001	0.01	0.01	0.01	0.02	0.02
Total cost ($M)	0.2	0.001	0.22	0.22	0.22	0.22	0.23
% Runs with stock-out	0	0.0	0	0	0	0	0

15.5 Discussion

15.5.1 Computational Aspects

The Auto mode is important to obtain quick assessments of various strategies for
drug supply. Otherwise we would have to specify a large number of parameters for
the base case and reset them for what-if analyses. In Example 1, not having Auto
mode would require several trial and error runs in Manual mode, each of which

involves specifying 12 trigger/resupply levels. If the randomization was not balanced there could be as many as 48 levels to be set. Although Auto mode does not guarantee minimum overage, we have found the heuristics it employs are effective in giving overages that are close to optimal if not optimal.

The Manual mode is also important. Example 3 illustrates one use of this mode. It can also be used to fine-tune supply chain parameter settings. Since Auto mode uses the same simulations to set supply chain parameters and to compute overage it introduces bias into estimation of stock-outs. The Manual mode offers a straightforward way to estimate this bias by using values of supply chain parameters (such as trigger and resupply levels) calculated in Auto mode in a new set of simulations run in Manual mode using a different random seed. This implements the core idea in data mining and forecasting of using independent "training" and "test" data sets. We have found that with 1,000 simulations the impact is typically small. We tested the inventory and packing runs policies for the Example 1 base case generated in Auto mode for the first 1,000 trial simulations, with 50,000 independent simulations in Manual mode involving a total of 24 million virtual patients. We found that in 48 out of those 50,000 simulated trials, one patient encountered a stock-out. In other words, the probability of a trial with at least one stock-out is less than 0.001, and the probability of a patient experiencing a randomization failure is a negligible 0.000002.

Note that this method of using the Auto and Manual modes in tandem can be used to explore the impact of permitting a small number of stock-outs as may be acceptable in the case of Phase 2 dose finding studies where the API may be in short supply. For example, we could run the Auto mode for 500 simulations with no stock-out. Using the inventory and packing policies from Auto mode we could then run a larger number of simulations (say, 10,000). This would lead to more stock-outs than Auto mode policies computed from 1,000 simulations. If the stock-outs are too high we could repeat the process with, say, 700 simulations in Auto mode. If they are too low, we would repeat the process with, say, 300 simulations. This process can be continued until we have found a suitable range of trade-offs between overage and stock-out risk.

Computational performance of a simulator can be a bottleneck if supply chain policies are to be generated and tested on a large number of simulations for a large multi-site, multi-country, multi-depot, multi-dispensing trial. The simulator used for illustrative examples, CytelSupply, has been enabled for high performance parallel computing to benefit from modern multiprocessor computers. It is able to run 1,000 simulations in Auto mode of our Example 1 base case in less than 5 min on a standard quad-processor PC. Manual mode is slightly faster.

15.5.2   Re-simulation During Execution of the Trial

Re-simulation can lead to substantial efficiencies if we use accumulated data from the IVRS to update parameters that are major drivers of overage such as enrolment, screening failure, and dropout rates. We can subjectively do the updating or use a

Bayesian model to compute posterior distributions from prior values of these parameters. Abdelkafi et al. (2009) describe deployment of a Bayesian model to re-evaluation of the supply strategy using accumulating data that becomes available as a clinical trial progresses. In Chap. 12 of this book, Danielson et. al. describe considerations of IVRS vendor capabilities for AD trial implementation.

Re-simulation is also very useful when new sites are added or protocol amendments such as inclusion–exclusion criteria changes are made.

15.5.3 Evaluating Design and Implementation Complexity Trade-Off

Ideally simulation of supply strategy and adaptive design should be performed hand in hand with simulation of the statistical design performed to obtain statistical operating characteristics. Designs such as Example 3 involve increased complexity in managing medical supplies and the increase in cost and risk due to this complexity has to be weighed against superior statistical performance. We have had experience with a consulting assignment where an adaptive design such as Example 3 was superior in terms of statistical operating characteristics to a design similar to Example 2. However, the latter design was preferred because of less complex supply management.

15.6 Summary and Conclusions

In this chapter we have described how modelling and simulation can help in developing efficient supply strategies for adaptive clinical trials while ensuring acceptable performance in terms of meeting demand at study sites. Traditional approaches that involve use of thumb rules from past experiences combined with spreadsheet models are inadequate as they do not quantitatively evaluate the impact of the various uncertainties inherent in adaptive trials. Since trial designs vary over a wide range of adaptive complexity we have used two case examples of adaptive trials. Both designs are among the most popular adaptive designs used in practice. The first design uses the simple adaptive method of dropping arms. The second design employs the substantially more complex adaptive method of modifying randomization ratios adaptively depending on observed responses.

Since our focus has been on modelling and simulation we have not discussed important broader considerations to effectively supply adaptive trials. An excellent paper by the Drug Supply Subteam of the DIA Adaptive Design Scientific Working Group (Burnham et al. 2014) covers these aspects in detail with valuable checklists and suggestions on the processes, systems, and technologies for managing drug supply. Amongst their most important suggestions are:

- Establish a formal study team for joint strategy development and decision making for drug supply to enable cross departmental collaboration between Supply Chain, Data Management, Clinical Science, Operations, Data Monitoring, Statistics and Programming functions.
- Determine requirement of the Active Pharmaceutical Ingredient (API) well in advance of the start of the trial since lead times for manufacture and release of API can be long (4–12 months).
- Consider using just-in-time packaging and labelling strategies instead of traditional approaches.
- To avoid the risk of unblinding, "scramble" packing lists so that packs are assigned in random order to avoid the risk of a pattern in the sequence of dispensed pack numbers revealing the randomization arm being dispensed.

References

Abdelkafi C, Beck B, David B, Druck C, Horoho M (2009) Balancing risk and costs to optimize the clinical supply chain – a step beyond simulation. J Pharm Innov. doi:10.1007/s12247-009-9063-5

Anisimov V, Fedorov V (2007) Modelling, prediction and adaptive adjustment of recruitment in multicentre trials. Stat Med 26:4958–4975

Burnham N. Quinlan J, He W, Marshall M, Nichols N, Patel N, Parke T, Wong LB (2014) Effective drug supply for adaptive clinical trials: Recommendations by the DIA adaptive design scientific working group drug supply subteam, Therapeutic Innovation & Regulatory Science, published online 22 May 2014, doi:10.1177/2168479014530968

Byrom B (2002) Managing the medication supply chain using interactive voice response systems. Life Sci Today 3:16–18

Dowlman N, Kwak M, Wood R, Nicholls G (2006) Managing the drug supply chain with e-processes. Appl Clin Trials 15(7):40–45

McEntegart D (2003) Forced randomization: When using interactive voice response systems. Appl Clin Trials 12(10):50–58

McEntegart D, O'Gorman B (2005) The impact on supply logistics of different randomization and medication management strategies using interactive voice response systems. Pharm Eng 25(5):36–46

Nicholls G, Patel N, Byrom B (2009) Simulation: A critical tool in adaptive clinical trials. Appl Clin Trials 18(6):76–82

Orloff J, Douglas F, Pinheiro J, Levinson S, Branson M, Chaturvedi P, Ette E, Gallo P, Hisrsch G, Mehta C, Patel N, Sabir S, Springs S, Stanski D, Evers M, Fleming E, Singh N, Tramontin T, Golub H (2009) The future of drug development: advancing clinical trial design. Nat Rev Drug Discov 8(12):949–957 doi:10.1038/nrd3025

Peterson M, Byrom B, Dowlman N, McEntegart D (2004) Optimizing clinical trial supply requirements: simulation of computer-controlled supply chain management. J Soc Clin Trials 1(4): 399–412

Shang K (2011) Simple heuristics for optimal inventory policies in supply chains. Chapter 7 in Tutorials in Operations Research, INFORMS, pp 106–127, doi:10.1287/educ.1110.0086

Waters S, Dowlman I, Drake K, Gamble L, Lang M, McEntegart D (2010) Enhancing control of the medication supply chain in clinical trials managed by interactive voice response systems. Drug Inf J 44(6):727–740

Chapter 16
Approaches for Patient Recruitment Modeling and Simulation

Weili He and Xiting Cao

Abstract Accurate enrollment information is critical for timely decision-making and execution for clinical trials. Enrollment must be carefully planned and monitored in order to maximize business benefit and to achieve study objectives. This is particularly true in adaptive designs (AD) trials, where too slow or too fast patient enrollment along with inaccurate enrollment prediction will imperil the timing of and/or invalidate the planned adaptations in AD trials. This chapter will discuss the key considerations for patient enrollment management and present and discuss different patient recruitment models.

Keywords Bayesian hierarchical models • Adaptive designs • Recruitment modeling • Poisson-gamma model • Enrollment time prediction • Unconditional model • Conditional model • Monte Carlo Markov chain • Poisson-gamma model • Site initiation model • Patient enrollment model • Individual model • Structure model • Transition model • Shrinkage factor • Dynamic site ready time • Monte Carlo simulation

16.1 Introduction

Clinical demonstration of the safety and efficacy of new medicines is the most complex and expensive step in the development of new human therapeutics. While many steps of clinical trial execution can be readily managed or predicted by trial

W. He (✉)
Clinical Biostatistics, Merck & Co., Inc., Rahway, NJ, USA
e-mail: Weili_he@merck.com

X. Cao
Outcomes Research, Medical Data Analytics, Merck & Co., Inc., White House Station, NJ, USA
e-mail: xiting.cao@merck.com

W. He et al. (eds.), *Practical Considerations for Adaptive Trial Design and Implementation*, Statistics for Biology and Health, DOI 10.1007/978-1-4939-1100-4_16, © Springer Science+Business Media New York 2014

sponsors, the time taken to enroll the required patients remains the most variable and least predictable activity (Drennan 2002). Clinical trial enrollment is dependent on multiple, highly variable parameters, from country regulatory approval, to site ethical IRB review, to competitive enrollment at a specific region and study site, and to patient availability and willingness to participate. Ethical drivers also dictate that clinical studies are carried out with minimum numbers of subjects, to maximize knowledge gain while minimizing patient risk. The concept of adaptive design trials is in alignment with the ethical drivers to minimize number of patients in a study and to maximize clinical knowledge (Dragalin 2006; Gallo et al. 2006; PhRMA Working Group on Adaptive Designs 2006). However, adaptive design trials often place added complexity to enrollment.

As mentioned in Chap. 15 on clinical supply, from implementation point of view adaptation schemes that may have impact on the logistics planning include sample size adjustments, changes to the randomization algorithm based on interim analyses, such as dropping/adding of treatment arms/doses, changes to the allocation ratio/treatment assignment probabilities, or re-randomization of the same patients, as well as trials stopping early for either efficacy or futility. Accurate enrollment information is critical for timely decision-making and execution in AD studies. Enrollment must be carefully planned and monitored in order to maximize business benefit and to achieve study objectives. Slower or faster than the expected enrollment rates along with inaccurate enrollment predictions will imperil the timing of and/or invalidate the planned adaptations in AD trials. Therefore, for adaptive design trials patient recruitment forecast is a critical piece in the clinical development and affects clinical trial planning and execution on several levels. On the overall trial level, an imprecise enrollment forecast for the trial may lead to inaccurate or incorrect estimates of timeline projections for interim and final analyses. Each clinical trial serves certain purposes in the overall clinical development paradigm. Inaccurate timeline projection for one trial may also necessitate the adjustment of timeline and/or resource for other clinical studies, which may eventually translate into impact on the filing date and/or Net Present Value (NPV) projection for the entire clinical development program. At country and study site level, clinical supply chain process relies heavily on recruitment and randomization processes, and imprecise enrollment forecast may result in drug supply wastage and/or stock out at study site level (He et al. 2012). As a result, patient recruitment management and forecast has become a well-recognized bottleneck for new drug development as randomness or uncertainty in recruitment process substantially affects all stages of study execution.

Efficient enrollment management requires cross-functional collaborations and should focus on three key areas: process, Infrastructure capability, and education (He et al. 2012). A process is required and critical for a cross-functional team to follow in setting up an enrollment plan with the study sites, in getting real time enrollment data and tracking enrollment progress throughout a trial, and in making adjustment to enrollment projections as needed. Infrastructure capability speaks to the need for system and technology support to capture enrollment information and monitor enrollment status. For adaptive design trials, it is often important to capture and track multi-stage enrollment information and be able to drill down the information at the trial, country, and site levels, so that study teams can project the approximate timing for interim analyses. This can be accomplished by a combination of study track systems, such as SPECTRUM and customized IVRS web reports. Education is another important aspect of enrollment management. For efficient implementation of enrollment plan and enrollment management, it is crucial that study team members know the specific AD features of the trial to ensure optimal site selections and performance. Furthermore, educating site personnel the specific AD features of a trial and how that may relate to the study design and enrollment management requirement will go a long way to ensure good relations, understanding, and a sustained interest in AD trials (He et al. 2012).

Another critical aspect of patient enrollment is enrollment forecast and prediction. As is well known, Modeling and Simulation (M&S) is essential to determine statistical operating characteristics of adaptive trial designs. However, these operating characteristics typically depend on the rate of patient enrollment. As such M&S can be extended to include support of patient enrollment planning decisions. This chapter will focus on patient enrollment M&S, and where appropriate, discuss the relevant applications to AD trials.

16.2 Literature Review of Existing Modeling Methods

Barnard et al. (2010) undertook a comprehensive search and review of literature pertaining to patient enrollment. Based on their review, they summarized the existing proposed models into five categories: the unconditional model, the conditional model, the Poisson model, Bayesian models, and Monte Carlo simulation of Markov models. In their review, Barnard et al. found that one of the common means of estimating trial enrollment time is simple linear models which assume constant enrollment rates over the life of the trial ("unconditional" models), and that while simple and readily evaluated, they ignore center recruitment and other factors that may have impact on enrollment speed. A second class, "conditional" models (Carter et al. 2005), allows enrollment rate to vary over the course of trial enrollment dependent on multiple factors, such as number of sites recruiting, time of year, exhaustion of patient pools, etc. However, such models are simple to construct but difficult to verify: they vary in structure according to trial design and thus must be constructed anew for each trial. Several authors have modeled patient accrual as a Poisson process (Carter et al. 2005; Anisimov and Fedorov 2007; Williford et al. 1987), where individual site enrollment events can be simulated as rates from a Poisson distribution with λ equal to the average enrollment rate. Notably Anisimov and Fedorov (2007) derived a closed form solution for a model in which individual site enrollment averages follow a gamma distribution, while enrollment at the sites within a given time interval follows a Poisson process (Poisson-Gamma). Two additional classes of models described in Barnard et al. (2010) include the Markov chains and Bayesian models (Gajewski et al. 2008; Abbas et al. 2007; Haidich and Ioannidis

2001). Markov chain Monte Carlo systems model a process as a series of mutually exclusive and exhaustive states and the transition probabilities between states. Abbas et al. (2007) demonstrated a sophisticated application of this approach to patient enrollment modeling. However, while they demonstrated that such a model could readily handle such process complexities as variable length screening periods, the model was both complex and computationally intensive, even without incorporating center recruitment. Bayesian models start with a "prior" probability distribution for the value of interest based on previous knowledge and use new evidence as data accumulates to produce a "posterior" probability distribution. Bayesian models rely on data being available to establish prior probabilities of recruitment, which can be updated over the course of the study. This can limit precision at study onset and make them challenging to use for decision making during planning. Their strength is the ability to incorporate information as it accumulates, so recruitment projections become more accurate as more trial data becomes available.

As is clear to anyone who has examined trial enrollment data, the two primary drivers of patient accrual are the rate of clinical center activation, and the rate of patient enrollment per active center. Based on the review of existing methods, it becomes apparent that a recruitment model needs to possess one or more of the following features. First, it should be simple to use and understand. This was also a required criterion described in Barnard et al. (2010) for model evaluation. Next, it should be able to accommodate different starting times for various centers as the time for country specific regulatory rules and IRB approval process may be different for different regions, countries, and study sites. In addition, as most trials nowadays are multi-center global trials, enrollment rates can be different from center to center. Moreover, within each center the enrollment rates may also vary over time. Recruitment models that can allow such flexibility in recruitment rates would be more desirable than the ones that can't. Another important factor to consider in recruitment models is the local factors that influence a model's parameters. Examples would include delays in center start times caused by variations in local ethics and local governance approvals or the existence of trials competing for the same patient pool. Delays caused by governance processes could be estimated from the previous experience. Patient competition must be estimated from knowledge of ongoing or planned trials, potentially run or funded by other groups and estimates of those factors could be used to adjust the parameters used in the recruitment model—for example by reducing the expected number of patients recruited while a competitive trial is underway. Specifically to local factors, it may be important to establish a set of important factors that have major impacts on recruitment, such as time from protocol approval to site readiness, time from site readiness to first patient enrolled, adaptation schemes for adaptive design trials, past performance of the sites, disease being investigated, and inclusion/exclusion criteria, to name a few. For adaptive design trials, it may not be a stretch to establish base case scenarios for enrollment patterns for different AD trial types in different disease areas by building a database to capture past AD trial enrollment patterns and exploring and discerning important factors that impact enrollment. Having outlined a few important factors to consider for recruitment models, trialists need to be cautioned that the flexibility of a recruitment model that is able to accommodate various and many aspects of enrollment regional variability needs to be balanced with the principle of simplicity and understandability of the model, as the applicability of a recruitment model may be rapidly decreased with increased complexity of the model.

The Poisson-gamma model Anisimov and Fedorov (2007) introduced took into account the variability in the recruitment rates across regions or study centers by considering the rates as Gamma random variables. In addition, their model also allows for the incorporation of different sites initiation times. Zhang and Long (2010) proposed a nonhomogeneous Poisson process and modeled the underlying time-dependent accrual rate using cubic B-splines. Their intent was to propose a flexible model that handles recruitment rates that may not be constant over time within study centers. Mijoule et al. (2012) investigated a Poisson-Pareto model for recruitment. They defined the model in the same way as the Poisson-Gamma model (Anisimov and Fedorov 2007; Anisimov 2011), but with a Pareto distribution of the rate instead of a Gamma one. These recruitment models (Anisimov and Fedorov 2007; Zhang and Long 2010; Mijoule et al. 2012) possess many essential features we consider important and yet are practical to use in real applications.

When considering the applications of such recruitment models, at trial level, the chief interest is to obtain estimate of timeline of when a desired enrollment goal can be reached for a particular trial. This is especially important for adaptive design trials, where interim analysis timelines may be achieved when a prespecified number of patients were enrolled or treated for a period of time, and can be predicted based on recruitment models. At program level, it would be of interest to obtain the timeline estimates of when all planned trials can reach enrollment goals. At specific study site level for a particular trial, it is of interest to the clinical operation team and clinical supply personnel to know the projected patient enrollment and timeframe at the specific study site to facilitate clinical supply roll out and site preparation activities, although it is well recognized that site performance varies not only between trials but also within trials, making accurate enrollment prediction at site level extremely difficult.

For the rest of the chapter, we describe a recruitment modeling framework via Bayesian Hierarchical Models. The framework consists of two interconnecting parts. The first part is to model the recruitment process and estimate model parameters based on historical clinical trial data. Once we obtain the estimates of the model parameters, we utilize the information to model and predict the enrollment time for a new clinical trial. We use the similar Poisson-Gamma model that was first introduced by Anisimov and Fedorov (2007). Where appropriate, we make certain extensions of Anisimov and Fedorov's approach to incorporate key factors that are considered important features of recruitment models, while keeping in mind simplicity and understandability of these models. To assist trialists with enrollment planning and projection, we also derive a few important statistics for timeline projections. Applicability of the models to adaptive design trials is also discussed, where applicable.

16.3   Recruitment Model Framework

Enrollment experience from past clinical trials reveals that enrollment time varies
across different regions, especially the interval from protocol approval to site ready,
due partly to country specific regulatory rules and IRB approval process. In addition, patient enrollment rate may differ among different study sites, countries, or
regions. We define enrollment time T_i for site i into two time periods, $T_i = T_{0i} + T_{1i}$.

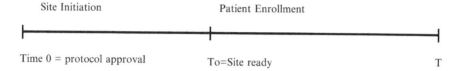

Site Initiation   Patient Enrollment

Time 0 = protocol approval   To=Site ready   T

T_{0i} is the time from protocol approval to site ready and we model it with a Gamma
distribution based on historic information. If such historic information is missing
for a specific region, a uniform random site initiation time can be assumed, as
described in Anisimov (2011). T_{1i} is the patient enrollment time from site ready to
the last screened patient. We model the patients' accrual as a Poisson process whose
rate for site i follows a Gamma distribution, following Anisimov and Fedorov
(2007). Since the enrollment rates rely largely on the geographic region of the site,
we allow a more flexible setting of Poisson-Gamma (P-G) model which takes into
account the sites' characteristics. The parameters in both site initiation model and
patient enrollment model are estimated through Bayesian framework conditional on
the historical data.

16.3.1   Site Initiation Model

Consider a multicenter clinical trial which recruits a total number of M patients
from L sites spreading in J regions. Let T_{0i} denotes the time from protocol approval
to site ready for site i, then we assume the following Gamma model for T_{0i}:

$$T_{0i} \sim \Gamma(\tau, \tau / \lambda_i),$$
$$\log(\lambda_i) = \alpha_1 + \sum_{j=2}^{J} \alpha_j I(site\ i\ is\ in\ region\ j) + \sum_{p=1}^{v-1} \varphi_p V_p,\ i = 1, \ldots, L,$$

Here, $\Gamma(a, b)$ denotes the gamma distribution with shape a and rate b, with expectation a / b and variance a / b^2. In the above Gamma model, we assume that the time
to site ready for each site follows Gamma distribution with mean initiation time λ_i.
A covariate structure, including geographic region and any other possible covariates, is further imposed on the mean parameter through a log link function. In the
above log-linear model, $V_1, \ldots, V_{v-1}$ are additional covariates besides region that
may have impact on site ready time. When $v = 1$ in the proposed model above, the

log-linear model only includes the region factor. Notice that if $\tau = 1$, then T_{0i} is an exponentially distributed random variable. In the above setting when $v = 1$, the mean initiation time for sites in the same region will be the same:

$$\lambda_{\text{region1}} = \exp(\alpha_1),$$

$$\lambda_{\text{region}j} = \exp(\alpha_1 + \alpha_j), j = 2, \cdots, J.$$

The above provides a generic form of site initiation model with the flexibility of incorporating any important local factors as covariates as needed. However, as mentioned in Sect. 16.2, any local factors that may have impact on recruitment need to be weighed in with model simplicity.

We adopt a Bayesian approach for estimating the parameters α_j, $j = 1, \ldots, J$, ϕ_p, $p = 1, \ldots v - 1$ and τ. Choosing a noninformative prior for the parameters, $\alpha_j \sim N(0, 100)$, $\phi_p \sim N(0, 100)$ and $\tau \sim \Gamma(0.001, 0.001)$, the posterior samples can be drawn with Markov chain Monte Carlo (MCMC) approach using BRugs, an R package calling OpenBUGS from R, whose current version (0.2–5) is only available for Windows (Thomas et al. 2006). Details of the MCMC procedure are reported elsewhere (Gelman et al. 1995; Gilks et al. 1995; Robert and Casella 1999).

16.3.2 Patient Enrollment Model

When study sites are ready to enroll, patients coming to the sites who pass the screening criteria will be enrolled into the study. Denote $M_i(t)$ as the total number of subjects screened at site i from site ready up to time t and μ_i as the rate of subjects coming to site i for screening. Similar to Anisimov and Fedorov (2007), we assume that μ_i can be viewed as a sample from a gamma-distributed population and consider a competitive recruitment policy with no restrictions on the number of subjects being recruited to be screened by study centers. Since not all patients screened at the site can be randomized into the study, let $N_i(t)$ denote the number of subjects that are actually randomized into the treatment groups at site i at time t. We assume subjects come to each site as a Poisson process but with some probability $1 - p_0$ of being not randomized (screen failure) and suppose t_i is the site specific enrollment time. We adopt a hierarchical model similar to the one proposed by Christiansen and Morris (1997). Although we include the number of subjects who were screened in addition to the number of subject who were randomized, to allow for differential screen failure rates across different application settings, the model process can be easily simplified to use directly the number of subjects who were randomized.

Similar to Christiansen and Morris (1997), the proposed hierarchical model, Level 1 "Individual Model," assumes that the number of subjects coming to each site follows a Poisson process with different rates μ_i which is then modeled to follow a conjugate gamma distribution. At Level 2 "Structure Model," the individual site's mean rate is modeled as a linear combination of region and other factors, possibly different across sites, through a log link function. It should be cautioned, similar to

Sect. 16.3.1, additional parameters may add extra errors in estimation and may reduce the quality of global prediction compared to simpler models with only a few parameters. Therefore, balance between the number of local factors to include and model simplicity must be considered. At Level 3 "Transition Model," the number of patients successfully randomized follows a binomial distribution.

Level 1: Individual Model:

$$M_i(t_i) \mid \mu_i \sim Poisson(\mu_i t_i),$$

where

$$\mu_i \sim \Gamma(\theta, \theta / \eta_i),$$

Level 2: Structure Model:

$$\log(\eta_i) = \beta_1 + \sum_{j=2}^{J} \beta_j I(site\ i\ is\ in\ region\ j) + \sum_{k=1}^{r-1} \gamma_k X_k,$$

Level 3: Transition Model

$$N_i(t_i) \mid M_i(t_i) \sim Binomial(M_i(t_i), p_0).$$

In the above hierarchical model framework, $\eta_i = E(\mu_i)$ is the expected rate for each site and is a linear function of region and/or any other possible factors through a log link function. The rates $\mu_1, \ldots, \mu_L$ are called the "individual parameters" by Christiansen and Morris (1997). The approximate distributions of these individual parameters must be estimated to make inferences about rate of enrollment. Often the individual parameters are predicted by $r-1$ additional number of study site level covariates $X_1, \ldots, X_{r-1}$ (e.g., time from site readiness to first patient enrolled, past performance of the sites, disease being investigated, and inclusion/exclusion criteria) along with region factor through a log-linear model involving regression coefficients, $\beta_1 \ldots \beta_j, \gamma_1, \ldots, \gamma_{r-1}$. When $r=1$ in our proposed model above, the log-linear model only includes the region factor.

To make inference of the model parameters, we note that the marginal distribution of $M_i(t_i)$ has a negative binomial distribution,

$$P(M_i(t_i) = m_i) = \frac{\Gamma(m_i + \theta)}{\Gamma(\theta) m_i!} \left(\frac{\theta}{\eta_i t_i + \theta} \right)^{\theta} \left(\frac{\eta_i t_i}{\eta_i t_i + \theta} \right)^{m_i}.$$

$M_i(t_i) \sim NB(\theta, 1 - B_i)$, where $B_i = \dfrac{\theta}{\eta_i t_i + \theta}$ is called the "shrinkage factor" and when θ is large, the negative binomial distribution is approximately Poisson distribution. Choosing a small value of θ allows for extra variance beyond the Poisson variation and could account for the over-dispersion problem.

To construct posterior distributions to make inference on model parameters, we note the following:

Level 4: Distributions on the model parameters. We consider the following prior distributions for the parameters $\beta_0, \beta_1, \ldots, \beta_J, \gamma_1, \ldots, \gamma_J, \theta$ and p_0, assuming prior independence of the parameters:

$$\beta_j \sim N(0,100), j = 0, \ldots, J,$$
$$\gamma_k \sim N(0,100), k = 0, \ldots, r-1,$$
$$\theta \sim \Gamma(0.001, 0.001),$$
$$p_0 \sim Unif(0,1).$$

To obtain inference from the hierarchical model, we employ MCMC to draw samples from the posterior distribution. Once the posterior inference on the model parameters can be drawn using the available historical data for a specific disease category, we could make predictions on the site ready time and enrollment prediction time for a new study at the planning stage with the obtained parameters' posterior distribution in the next section.

16.4 Site Ready Time and Enrollment Time Prediction

As mentioned in Sect. 16.2, the utility of recruitment models lies with the interest of trialists in obtaining estimates of timeline for reaching various desired enrollment milestones. Specifically, it is of great interest to assess the following quantities to assist with the planning and execution of a clinical study: (a) dynamic site ready time, measured as the time when a certain percent of the total sites are ready, (b) the length of time to enroll certain number of patients for interim analysis or the total length of enrollment time for a clinical trial, at study planning stage, and (c) the remaining enrollment time, both for a targeted number of patients for an interim analysis or for the entire study, while a study is ongoing. For any new studies, at the planning stage, information from historic trials of similar clinical setting, or planned recruitment data provided by study center coordinators, or information about patients' availability from medical databases can be used as the starting point. This point will be further discussed in the last section of the chapter. Using the hierarchical model described in Sect. 16.3, we obtain the posterior distributions of the model parameters. The following sub-sections provide derivations for site ready time and enrollment time prediction based on the posterior estimates of model parameters.

16.4.1 Site Ready Time Prediction

When planning and executing a clinical study, the primary interest of the study team is to obtain an early projection on site ready time, e.g. the time when 25 %, 50 %, or 80 % of the sites are ready. This will allow study teams plan timelines as well as clinical operations and clinical supply activities ahead of time to meet the study start-up as well as study conduct needs. This is also important for adaptive design trials with regard to projecting the timeline for interim analysis, as site ready time is directly linked to total enrollment time.

Denote SRp as the time when $\frac{p}{100} \times 100\%$ sites are ready. We derive the following:

$$\Pr\left(SRp < t\right) = \Pr\left(\sum_{i=1}^{L} I\left(T_{0i} < t\right) > pL\right),$$

where $I(T_{0i} < t)$ indicates whether or not site i is ready and $\sum_{i=1}^{L} I\left(T_{0i} < t\right)$ is the total number of sites that are ready by time point t. The above equation denotes that if $SRp < t$, then at time point t, at least pL sites are ready.

To calculate the probability of $\Pr\left(\sum_{i=1}^{L} I\left(T_{0i} < t\right) > pL\right)$, we need to first derive the distribution of $\sum_{i=1}^{L} I\left(T_{0i} < t\right)$. Since $I(T_{0i} < t), i = 1, \ldots, L$ are independent Bernoulli random variables with success probability $p_i = \Pr(T_{0i} < t)$, we can easily show that the random variables $I(T_{0i} < t), i = 1, \ldots, L$ satisfy the Lyapunov condition (Ash and Doléans-Dade 1999) and by central limit theorem,

$$\frac{\sum_{i=1}^{L} I\left(T_{0i} < t\right) - \sum_{i=1}^{L} p_i}{\sqrt{\sum_{i=1}^{L} p_i\left(1 - p_i\right)}} \sim N\left(0,1\right).$$

Therefore, we establish the distribution function of SRp as,

$$\Pr\left(SRp < t\right) = \Pr\left(\sum_{i=1}^{L} I\left(T_{0i} < t\right) > pL\right)$$

$$= \Pr\left(\frac{\sum_{i=1}^{L} I\left(T_{0i} < t\right) - \sum_{i=1}^{L} p_i}{\sqrt{\sum_{i=1}^{L} p_i\left(1 - p_i\right)}} > \frac{pL - \sum_{i=1}^{L} p_i}{\sqrt{\sum_{i=1}^{L} p_i\left(1 - p_i\right)}}\right)$$

$$= 1 - \Phi\left(\frac{pL - \sum_{i=1}^{L} p_i}{\sqrt{\sum_{i=1}^{L} p_i\left(1 - p_i\right)}}\right).$$

By utilizing historic information on site ready time, p_i can be estimated through the cumulative distribution of $\Gamma(\hat{\tau}, \hat{\tau}/\hat{\lambda}_i)$ up to time t. By plugging in $p=0.25, 0.5, 0.8$ or 1.00 (100 %) or any percentage of interest, we can obtain the median time along with the 95 % credible interval for the above site ready time.

16.4.2 Enrollment Time Prediction at Study Planning Stage

When planning and executing a clinical study, another indicator on enrollment time that study teams would be greatly interested in is the length of enrollment time for a planned clinical study or for a prespecified number of patients for planned interim analyses. Based on previous clinical study enrollment data, we can obtain the parameter estimates for the hierarchical models in Sect. 16.3.

To make a projection of the enrollment time for a new clinical trial, assuming that we need to recruit N patients from L sites, we denote the quantity as $T(L, N)$. Suppose for any future time point t, the number of patients screened at each individual site up to time t, $M_i(t)$, follows a Poisson distribution with parameter $\mu_i(t - T_{0i})I(t > T_{0i})$. Here $I(\cdot)$ is the indicator function, T_{0i} is the random variable of the individual site ready time and μ_i is the individual site screen rate as defined in Sect. 16.3. If the time point t is later than the site starting date T_{0i}, the site has a screen rate of μ_i, otherwise the site has screen rate 0. Denote the total number of patients screened up to time t by all sites as $\sum_{i=1}^{L} M_i(t)$. The feature of Poisson distribution guarantees that the sum of independent Poisson random variables also follows a Poisson distribution. Hence

$$\sum_{i=1}^{L} M_i(t) \mid \mu_i, T_{0i} \sim Poisson(\Lambda(t)) \text{ where } \Lambda(t) = \sum_{i=1}^{L} \mu_i(t - T_{0i})I(t > T_{0i}).$$

Note that not all patients screened can be successfully randomized in the clinical trial due to screen failures, and we assume for each site, $N_i(t)$ is the actual number of patients who were randomized in the clinical trial and

$$N_i(t) \mid M_i(t) \sim Binomial(M_i(t), p_0).$$

Since the sum of binomial random variables with the same success probability is also a binomial random variable, we have

$$\sum_{i=1}^{L} N_i(t) \mid \sum_{i=1}^{L} M_i(t) \sim Binomial\left(\sum_{i=1}^{L} M_i(t), p_0\right),$$

assuming that the screen failure rate being the same across study sites for a single study.

We derive the distribution function of the enrollment time $T(L,N)$ as follows:

$$\Pr(T(L,N) \leq t) = \Pr\left(\sum_{i=1}^{L} N_i(t) \geq N\right)$$

$$= 1 - \sum_{n=0}^{N-1} \Pr\left(\sum_{i=1}^{L} N_i(t) = n\right)$$

$$= 1 - \sum_{n=1}^{N-1} \sum_{m=n}^{\infty} \Pr\left(\sum_{i=1}^{L} N_i(t) = n \mid \sum_{i=1}^{L} M_i(t) = m\right) \Pr\left(\sum_{i=1}^{L} M_i(t) = m\right)$$

$$- \sum_{m=1}^{\infty} \Pr\left(\sum_{i=1}^{L} N_i(t) = 0 \mid \sum_{i=1}^{L} M_i(t) = m\right) \Pr\left(\sum_{i=1}^{L} M_i(t) = m\right)$$

(16.1)

The marginal distribution of $\sum_{i=1}^{I} M_i(t)$ is calculated as

$$\Pr\left(\sum_{i=1}^{L} M_i(t) = m\right) = \int \Pr\left(\sum_{i=1}^{L} M_i(t) = m \mid \mu_i, T_{0i}\right) f(\mu_i) f(T_{0i}) d\mu_i dT_{0i},$$

and can be approximated by Monte Carlo simulation. For a given time point t, we first simulate T_{0i} and μ_i from the previous model with the posterior samples of the parameters, then calculate the conditional probability $\Pr\left(\sum_{i=1}^{L} M_i(t) = m \mid \mu_i, T_{0i}\right)$ for any given integer m. Repeat the above procedure for a total of B iterations, we get,

$$\Pr\left(\sum_{i=1}^{L} M_i(t) = m\right) \approx \frac{1}{B} \sum_{b=1}^{B} \Pr\left(\sum_{i=1}^{L} M_i(t) = m \mid \mu_i^b, T_{0i}^b\right).$$

To calculate the probability in Eq. (16.1), some approximations are needed. As m increases and n fixed, $\Pr\left(\sum_{i=1}^{L} N_i(t) = n \mid \sum_{i=1}^{L} M_i(t) = m\right)$ decreases rapidly. Thus finite sums can be used as a good approximation to the infinite sum. In addition, by using a large B in the Monte Carlo simulation, the error can be reduced significantly.

For application of the above enrollment time estimate to an adaptive design trial with a prespecified number of patients for interim analyses, similar derivations can be used, where the total number of patients N for the trial is replaced with the number of patients prespecified for the interim analyses. Other relevant parameters, such as the number of study sites L, can also be replaced with any appropriate number of study sites for an interim analysis, if not all study sites were up and running at the point of interim analysis.

16.4.3 Enrollment Time Prediction for an Ongoing Study

Sections 16.4.1 and 16.4.2 describe the prediction of site readiness and enrollment time at study planning stage of a new trial. It is often of equal importance to make prediction of the remaining enrollment time at the interim stage of a trial, based on more updated and realistic site ready, recruitment, and screen failure information. The approach we employ here is similar to Anisimov and Fedorov (2007) but with extension to more a general setting. Specifically, we estimate screening failure rate and provide detailed solution to obtain the predicted enrollment time when incorporating different site initiation time. In addition, we predict the remaining enrollment data of a study with the use of all available information, combining both historic study data and current study information.

Suppose t_0 is the time of an interim study time where at least one site has started recruiting patients. Denote $M_i(t_0)$ as the number of patients screened at site i up to time t_0 and $N_i(t_0)$ as the number of patients randomized in the study at site i up to time t_0. Then the total number of patients screened and randomized at time t_0 by all sites are $M(t_0)$ and $N(t_0)$ respectively. Bayesian framework is utilized in the derivation. Suppose

$$M_i(t_0) \sim Poisson\left(\mu_i(t_0 - T_{0i})I(t_0 - T_{0i} > 0)\right)$$

and the enrollment rate μ_i follows a Gamma distribution $\Gamma(\hat{\theta}, \hat{\theta}/\hat{\eta}_i)$, where $\hat{\theta}$ and $\hat{\eta}_i$ are the posterior estimates based on historical data. To incorporate not only the historic information but also the information accumulated in the current study at the interim, it can be easily implemented by using the same approach as described in Sect. 16.3.2 by treating the partial current study data as part of the historic information in order to obtain an updated estimates of $\hat{\theta}$ and $\hat{\eta}_i$.

To update the enrollment rate of the sites which had started screening patients, we calculate its posterior distribution as

$$f\left(\mu_i \mid M_i(t_0)\right) \propto f\left(M_i(t_0) \mid \mu_i\right)\pi(\mu_i) \propto \mu_i^{K_i(t_0)+\hat{\theta}-1} \exp(-\mu_i(t_0 - T_{0i} + \hat{\theta}/\hat{\eta}_i))$$

Thus $\mu_i \mid M_i(t_0) \sim \Gamma(M_i(t_0) + \hat{\theta}, t_0 - T_{0i} + \hat{\theta}/\hat{\eta}_i)$.

The actual randomization rate can also be updated using Bayesian framework as follows:

$$N(t_0) \mid M(t_0) \sim Binomial\left(M(t_0), p_0\right),$$

where the posterior distribution of p_0 based on historical data can be used as a prior distribution:

$$\pi(p_0) \sim Beta\left(\sum_{i=1}^{L} N_i + 1, \sum_{i=1}^{L} M_i - \sum_{i=1}^{L} N_i + 1\right).$$

Thus the posterior distribution of p_0 is calculated by combining the updated data as

$$f\left(p_0 \mid N(t_0), M(t_0)\right) \propto p_0^{\sum_{i=1}^{L} N_i + N(t_0)} \left(1 - p_0\right)^{\sum_{i=1}^{L} M_i - \sum_{i=1}^{L} N_i + M(t_0) - N(t_0)},$$

i.e., $p_0 \mid N(t_0), M(t_0) \sim Beta\left(\sum_{i=1}^{L} N_i + N(t_0) + 1, \sum_{i=1}^{L} M_i - \sum_{i=1}^{L} N_i + M(t_0) - N(t_0) + 1\right).$

To predict the remaining enrollment time, we follow the same procedure as described in Sect. 16.4.2. At an interim time point of a study, we have already randomized $N(t_0)$ patients in the study. We want to obtain an estimate of the remaining time that $N - N(t_0)$ patients will be randomized from L sites. Thus the cumulative distribution of $T(L, N - N(t_0))$ is,

$$\Pr\left(T\left(L, N - N\left(t_0\right)\right) \leq t\right) = \Pr\left(\sum_{i=1}^{L} N_i\left(t\right) \geq N - N\left(t_0\right)\right)$$

$$= 1 - \sum_{n=1}^{N-N(t_0)-1} \sum_{m=n}^{\infty} \Pr\left(\sum_{i=1}^{L} N_i\left(t\right) = n \mid \sum_{i=1}^{L} M_i\left(t\right) = m\right) \Pr\left(\sum_{i=1}^{L} M_i\left(t\right) = m\right)$$

$$- \sum_{m=1}^{\infty} \Pr\left(\sum_{i=1}^{L} N_i\left(t\right) = 0 \mid \sum_{i=1}^{L} M_i\left(t\right) = m\right) \Pr\left(\sum_{i=1}^{L} M_i\left(t\right) = m\right)$$

Calculating the marginal distribution of $\Pr\left(\sum_{i=1}^{L} M_i\left(t\right) = m\right)$ is similar and Monte Carlo simulation is used. The difference is that we only need to generate T_{0i} for the sites which are not ready yet, and generate μ_i for the sites that have started recruiting patients using the updated posterior distribution.

Similarly as in the discussion in Sect. 16.4.2, the application of the above enrollment time estimate to an adaptive design trial with planned interim analyses is straightforward by using similar derivations with the use of prespecified number of subjects for the interim analyses, where the total number of patients N for the trial is replaced with the number of patients prespecified for the interim analyses. Other relevant parameters, such as the number of study sites L, can also be replaced with any appropriate number of study sites for an interim analysis, if not all study sites were up and running at the point of interim analyses.

16.5 Application

In this section, we apply the proposed hierarchical models and enrollment time prediction to historic study data to obtain site ready and enrollment time prediction at study planning stage and while a study is ongoing. The historical data contains the site initiation and enrollment information for multicenter studies in 15 therapeutic areas conducted in the company since 2006. Within each therapeutic area, we could fit the hierarchical model with the pooled data from all the studies under the same therapeutic area to get the posterior estimates of the parameters.

16.5.1 Model Fitting

Based on historic study site ready and enrollment data, we fit the Gamma model and the hierarchical Poisson-Gamma model for the site initiation and enrollment process respectively. The data includes 11 multicenter studies within a total of 14

Table 16.1 Posterior estimates of parameters in the site initiation model

	Mean	Median	SD	2.5 % percentile	97.5 % percentile	Notes
Alpha[1]	5.339	5.341	0.0565	5.228	5.441	Americas (baseline)
Alpha[2]	−0.394	−0.393	0.0731	−0.533	−0.251	Region effect of Asia
Alpha[3]	−0.213	−0.213	0.103	−0.409	0.00625	Australia/New Zealand
Alpha[4]	−0.288	−0.290	0.0766	−0.434	−0.131	Big Six
Alpha[5]	0.0907	0.0913	0.0883	−0.0840	0.268	Central/Eastern Europe
Alpha[6]	−0.115	−0.116	0.183	−0.451	0.278	India
Alpha[7]	−0.0885	−0.0952	0.119	−0.312	0.144	Mid Europe
Alpha[8]	−0.217	−0.218	0.0854	−0.379	−0.0487	Scandinavia
Alpha[9]	−0.603	−0.604	0.105	−0.801	−0.389	US
Alpha[10]	−0.705	−0.704	0.0923	−0.878	−0.509	US (Area)
Alpha[11]	−0.360	−0.362	0.0805	−0.513	−0.201	US (Central)
Alpha[12]	−0.546	−0.547	0.0859	−0.718	−0.379	US (Eastern)
Alpha[13]	−0.429	−0.431	0.0986	−0.615	−0.230	US (K-Force)
Alpha[14]	−0.326	−0.329	0.0756	−0.472	−0.166	US (Western)
Lambda[1]	208.6	208.7	11.75	186.5	230.7	Americas
Lambda[2]	140.5	140.2	6.523	128.1	154.2	Asia
Lambda[3]	168.9	168.2	14.81	143.1	202.2	Australia/New Zealand
Lambda[4]	156.3	156.1	8.342	140.9	174.2	Big Six
Lambda[5]	228.6	228.4	16.25	199.3	260.3	Central/Eastern Europe
Lambda[6]	188.4	185.5	32.97	135.6	261.7	India
Lambda[7]	191.7	189.7	20.73	156	236.7	Mid Europe
Lambda[8]	168.0	167.8	10.81	148.3	190.6	Scandinavia
Lambda[9]	114.4	113.9	10.46	95.44	136.3	US
Lambda[10]	103.1	102.6	7.421	89.62	118.2	US (Area)
Lambda[11]	145.6	145.3	8.608	129.9	163.9	US (Central)
Lambda[12]	120.9	120.5	7.685	106.8	136.8	US (Eastern)
Lambda[13]	136.1	135.4	10.96	116.7	158.7	US (K-Force)
Lambda[14]	150.5	150.4	7.308	136.9	165.3	US (Western)
Tau	6.036	6.026	0.366	5.348	6.786	Shape parameter

regions, which include Americas, Asia, Austrailia/Newzealand, Big Six (Germany, Italy, Spain, United Kingdom, France, Canada), Central/Eastern Europe, India, Mid Europe, Scandinavia, US, US (Area), US (Central), US (Eastern), US (K-Force), and US (Western). Only region and therapeutic area were included as covariates in the model because more variables may compromise the accuracy of the parameter estimates given the small number of studies available for this application. Regions with similar characteristics can be pooled together to reduce the number of parameters. Table 16.1 presents the posterior estimates of the parameters in site initiation model and Table 16.2 shows the posterior estimates of the parameters in the enrollment model. To check the fit of the model, we created a Quantile-Quantile (Q-Q) plot of the true quantile of the data and model-generated quantile using the data generated from the model based on the posterior samples. Figure 16.1 shows the Q-Q plot. The proposed model shows good fit of the data.

Table 16.2 Posterior estimates of parameters in the enrollment model

	Mean	Median	SD	val2.5pc	val97.5pc	Notes
Beta[1]	−1.563	−1.568	0.104	−1.756	−1.355	Americas (baseline)
Beta[2]	−0.0393	−0.0393	0.137	−0.310	0.247	Region effect of Asia
Beta[3]	−0.288	−0.285	0.189	−0.657	0.0916	Australia/New Zealand
Beta[4]	−0.0483	−0.0470	0.141	−0.321	0.224	Big Six
Beta[5]	0.247	0.252	0.158	−0.0659	0.537	Central/Eastern Europe
Beta[6]	0.1004	0.101	0.326	−0.514	0.757	India
Beta[7]	−0.201	−0.208	0.218	−0.617	0.250	Mid Europe
Beta[8]	−0.306	−0.305	0.168	−0.615	0.0355	Scandinavia
Beta[9]	−0.317	−0.316	0.199	−0.722	0.0709	US
Beta[10]	−0.308	−0.315	0.179	−0.662	0.0395	US (Area)
Beta[11]	−0.316	−0.312	0.151	−0.626	−0.0273	US (Central)
Beta[12]	−0.332	−0.330	0.159	−0.647	−0.0234	US (Eastern)
Beta[13]	−0.126	−0.129	0.174	−0.460	0.216	US (K-Force)
Beta[14]	−0.346	−0.342	0.136	−0.618	−0.0844	US (Western)
Eta[1]	0.210	0.208	0.0221	0.172	0.258	Americas
Eta[2]	0.202	0.201	0.0177	0.171	0.240	Asia
Eta[3]	0.159	0.157	0.0254	0.116	0.217	Australia/New Zealand
Eta[4]	0.200	0.199	0.0187	0.167	0.240	Big Six
Eta[5]	0.270	0.267	0.0324	0.213	0.345	Central/Eastern Europe
Eta[6]	0.243	0.231	0.0776	0.129	0.430	India
Eta[7]	0.174	0.170	0.0346	0.118	0.256	Mid Europe
Eta[8]	0.155	0.153	0.0203	0.121	0.198	Scandinavia
Eta[9]	0.154	0.150	0.0273	0.108	0.216	US
Eta[10]	0.155	0.153	0.0226	0.115	0.204	US (Area)
Eta[11]	0.153	0.152	0.0171	0.122	0.189	US (Central)
Eta[12]	0.151	0.150	0.0186	0.120	0.192	US (Eastern)
Eta[13]	0.186	0.184	0.0272	0.141	0.244	US (K-Force)
Eta[14]	0.148	0.147	0.0135	0.124	0.177	US (Western)
Theta	2.169	2.161	0.154	1.873	2.483	Shape parameter

16.5.2 Site Ready Time Estimation

For a particular clinical study where the study team has a concrete plan for targeted regions for recruitment, the models as described in Sect. 16.3 can be fitted including only targeted regions based on historic data.

Based on the posterior samples from the site initiation model, we can obtain the estimates of time when a certain percent of sites are ready, e.g. SR80, measured by the time when 80 % of the sites are ready. Figure 16.2 shows the estimated SR80 time along with a 95 % creditable interval with the true SR80 time for each therapeutic area. As can be seen, large variations exist in site ready time in different therapeutic areas. Since local factors may differ in different regions, we also obtained estimates of SR80 for each region. Figure 16.3 shows the true SR80 time in each region and the estimated SR80 with a 95 % creditable interval. When fitting

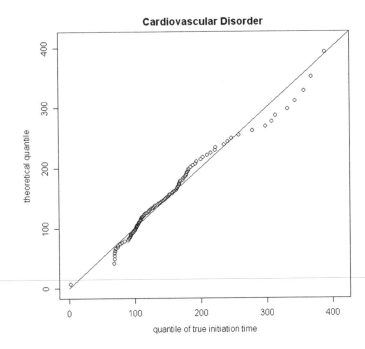

Fig. 16.1 QQ plot of the true quartile of the site initiation time vs. the quartile of the generated site initiation time from the model

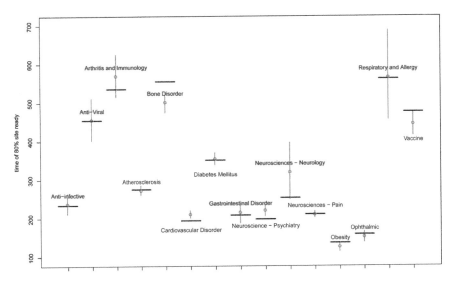

Fig. 16.2 True SR80 time with the estimated SR80 time and a 95 % creditable interval. *Black bar* is the true SR80 time, and *red circle* with a *vertical line* is the estimated SR80 with 95 % creditable interval

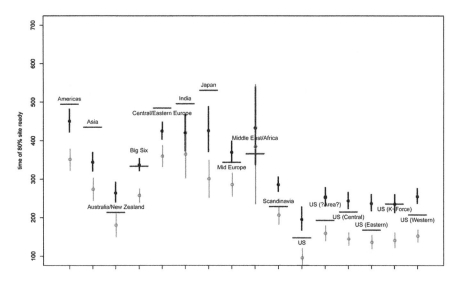

Fig. 16.3 True SR80 time with the estimated SR80 time and a 95 % creditable interval. *Black bar* is the true SR80 time, *circle* with a *thin vertical line* is the estimated SR80 with 95 % creditable interval without justifying therapeutic area and *black dot* with a *thick vertical line* is the estimated SR80 with 95 % confidence interval justifying the therapeutic area

the model, we first obtained the site ready time estimates by region without adjusting for disease area. However, as evidenced by Fig. 16.2, large variations exist in site ready time in different therapeutic areas. As a result, the site ready time was under-estimated in most regions. We then included the disease area as a covariate, shown as black dot and thick line. It appears that this model fits the data well. This better fit can also be reflected by the DIC value, where the preferred model including disease area as covariates yield a DIC value of 72070 while the model pooling all disease area together has a larger DIC value of 73660.

16.5.3   Total Enrollment Time Estimation

We applied the enrollment model to one study in the area of Cardiovascular Disease. The study enrolled 2,430 patients from 183 sites across 14 regions. Using the enrollment model with parameters estimated from the historic study data, our estimated median enrollment time, T(183, 2,430), for this study was 274 days with the 95 % confidence interval of (262, 284) days. The true enrollment time was 279 days. It should be noted that due to the limited availability of historic data for this application in cardiovascular disease area (only two historic studies were available), the 95 % confidence interval for the above point estimate is artificially narrow. Additional discussions related to the importance of building an recruitment database can be found in the last section.

16.6 Discussion

In this chapter, we described a recruitment modeling framework via Bayesian hierarchical models to predict site ready time and patient enrollment time. In building our models, to the extent possible we proposed a general framework that is sufficiently flexible to account for a number of factors that may have impact on enrollment. By modeling two interconnecting parts of the total enrollment time separately, the proposed models are intuitive and easy to use. The general model framework accounts for different enrollment rate in different sites or regions and allows for inclusion in the models of extrinsic epidemiological and environmental factors that have impact on enrollment. Such modeling framework is easily applicable to adaptive design settings, where the number of subjects needed for a prespecified interim analysis is described in study protocols, and hence the same model framework and derivations can be used to project interim analysis timeline.

Regarding the extrinsic epidemiological and local environmental factors, we provided a general framework to incorporate these factors in the recruitment model. It is important to establish a set of important variables or factors that have major impacts on recruitment, such as time from protocol approval to site readiness, time from site readiness to first patient enrolled, adaptation schemes for adaptive design trials, past performance of the sites, disease being investigated, and inclusion/exclusion criteria, to name a few. For adaptive design trials, it is not a stretch to establish base case scenarios for enrollment patterns for different AD trial types in different disease areas by building a database to capture past AD trial enrollment patterns and exploring and discerning important factors that impact enrollment. During this research, we found that such database is lacking, and research is limited in discerning important epidemiological and/or local environmental factors that have impact on recruitment. This may in large part account for the deviations we observed between our projected site ready times versus the observed ones. Concerted efforts with cross-functional contributions will be needed. It should also be noted that with the increase in the number of epidemiological and/or local environmental factors in the model, the errors in estimation may increase. It is critical to evaluate the need and importance of these factors versus the simplicity of the model. If warranted, sensitivity analyses may be carried out to evaluate and discern the importance of these factors.

We described the use of historic information for the estimation of model parameters. Based on our experience in real clinical trials, regional or global patient recruitment specialists generally have recruitment planned data in specific disease areas and regions to guide the selection of appropriate historic trials for a new clinical trial in a specific disease area and potential regions. This again speaks to a concerted effort with cross-functional contributions to enrollment planning and prediction. We suggest that a set of criteria for the selection of relevant historic trials be put in place prior to the actual selection by a cross-function team, not unlike the selection criteria put together prior to a meta-analysis.

Our proposed framework via Bayesian hierarchical models can be easily extended to allow for time-variant recruitment rates within a study site, following the approach for a nonhomogeneous Poisson process as proposed by Zhang and Long (2010). Additionally, future research may include adding site capacity in the models. If data are available from historic trials, it would be of great interest to assess and make inference on extrinsic epidemiological and/or environmental factors that have impact on recruitment in various regions. The information can then be used by trialists in their planning for clinical trial start-up activities.

References

Adaptive designs in clinical trials (2006) special issue. Biom J 4:491–737

Abbas I, Rovira J, Casanovas J (2007) Clinical trial optimization: Monte Carlo simulation Markov model for planning clinical trials recruitment. Contemp Clin Trials 28:220–231

Anisimov V (2011) Statistical modeling of clinical trials (recruitment and randomization). Comm Stat Theor Meth 40:19–20, 3684–3699

Anisimov V, Fedorov V (2007) Modelling, prediction, and adaptive adjustment of recruitment in multicenter trials. Stat Med 26:4958–4975

Ash RB, Doléans-Dade CA (1999) Probability and measure theory, 2nd edn. Academic, New York, NY, p 307

Barnard K, Dent L, Cook A (2010) A systematic review of models to predict recruitment to multicentre clinical trials. BMC Med Res Methodol 10:63

Carter RE, Sonne SC, Brady KT (2005) Practical considerations for estimating clinical trial accrual periods: application to a multi-center effectiveness study. BMC Med Res Methodol 5:11

Christiansen CL, Morris CN (1997) Hierarchical poisson regression modeling. J Am Stat Assoc 92:438, 618–632

Dragalin V (2006) Adaptive designs: terminology and classification. Drug Inf J 40:425–435

Drennan KB (2002) Patient recruitment: the costly and growing bottleneck in drug development. Drug Discov Today 7(3):167–170

Gajewski BJ, Simon SD, Carlson SE (2008) Predicting accrual in clinical trials with Bayesian posterior predictive distributions. Stat Med 27:2328–2340

Gallo P, Chuang-Stein C, Dragalin V, Gaydos B, Krams M, Pinheiro J (2006) Executive summary of the PhRMA working group on adaptive designs in clinical drug development. J Biopharm Stat 16:275–283

Gelman A, Carlin J, Stern H, Rubin D (1995) Bayesian data analysis. Chapman & Hall/CRC, New York

Gilks W, Richardson S, Spiegelhalter D (1995) Introducing Markov chain Monte Carlo. In Markov Chain Monte Carlo in practice. Chapman & Hall/CRC, New York, pp. 1–17

Haidich AB, Ioannidis JP (2001) Determinants of patient recruitment in a multicenter clinical trials group: trends, seasonality and the effect of large studies. BMC Med Res Methodol 1:4

He W, Kuznetsova K, Harmer M, Leahy C, Anderson K, Dossin N, Tymofyeyev Y, Li L, Bolognese J, Schindler J (2012) Practical considerations and strategies for executing adaptive design trials. Drug Inf J 46(2):160–174

Mijoule G, Savy S, Savy N (2012) Models for patients' recruitment in clinical trials and sensitivity analysis. Stat Med 31(16):1655–1674

PhRMA Working Group on Adaptive Designs (2006) Full white paper. Drug Inf J 40:421–484

Robert C, Casella G (1999) Monte Carlo statistical methods. Springer, New York, NY

Thomas A, O'Hara B, Ligges U, Sturtz S (2006) Making BUGS open. R News 6:12–17

Williford WO, Bingham SF, Weiss DG, Collins JF, Rains KT, Krol WF (1987) The "constant intake rate" assumption in interim recruitment goal methodology for multicenter clinical trials. J Chronic Dis 40:297–307

Zhang X, Long Q (2010) Stochastic modeling and prediction for accrual in clinical trials. Stat Med 29:649–658

Part III
Case Studies

Chapter 17
A Case Study for Adaptive Trial Design Consideration and Implementation

Vladimir Dragalin and Michael Krams

Abstract The use of adaptive designs in dose ranging studies can increase the efficiency of drug development by improving our ability to efficiently learn about the dose–response and better determine whether to take a drug forward into confirmatory phase testing and at what dose. This approach can maximize the ability to test a larger number of doses in a single trial while simultaneously increasing the efficiency of the trial in terms of making better go–no-go decisions about continuing the trial and/or the development of the drug for a specific indication.

We show in a real case study of a dose ranging trial in patients with acute exacerbations of schizophrenia how such an adaptive design explicitly addresses multiple trial goals, adaptively allocates subjects according to ongoing information needs, and allows termination for both early success and futility.

Keywords Adaptive design • Adaptive dose ranging study • Allocation rule • Longitudinal modeling • Data monitoring committee • Normal dynamic linear model • Response-adaptive randomization • Stopping rule

17.1 Background

The development of drugs for psychiatric illnesses is complicated by limited knowledge of the pathophysiology underlying the illnesses. The reliance on a cluster of clinical signs and symptoms alone to make the diagnosis, assess severity of the

V. Dragalin (✉)
Aptiv Solutions, 4505 Emperor Blvd, Suite 400, Durham, NC 27703, USA
e-mail: Vladimir.Dragalin@aptivsolutions.com

M. Krams
Janssen Pharmaceutical Research and Development, 1400 McKean Rd,
Spring House, PA 19477, USA
e-mail: vdragali@its.jnj.com

W. He et al. (eds.), *Practical Considerations for Adaptive Trial Design
and Implementation*, Statistics for Biology and Health,
DOI 10.1007/978-1-4939-1100-4_17, © Springer Science+Business Media New York 2014

disease and judge improvement over time contributes substantially to the problems associated with clinical trials on investigational drugs. The inclusion of patients just on the basis of clinical signs and symptoms decreases the signal to noise ratio such that it is difficult to consistently observe a clinical efficacy signal especially in a limited number of patients. Patient selection may be compromised by including patients who respond to placebo and others who do not respond to approved marketed treatments. These problems may be further accentuated when trying to develop treatments that work by novel mechanisms of action, and are most pronounced in the earliest stages up to proof of concept as only limited information may be available on optimal dose and dosing regimen of the investigational drug.

This chapter focuses on how adaptive designs may improve the efficiency of drug development in psychiatric disease by improving our ability to efficiently learn about the dose–response in a Phase II dose ranging study.

Adaptive clinical trial designs allow the use of accumulating data in real time to decide how to modify aspects of the study as it continues maintaining its integrity and validity of final results (Dragalin 2006). Adaptations can include stopping early either for futility or success, expanding the sample size due to greater than expected data variability, or allocating patients preferentially to treatment regimens with a better therapeutic index. This ultimately can benefit patients within the trial and in the future (Gallo et al. 2006; Krams et al. 2009; Orloff et al. 2009). The efficiency of the adaptive design is dependent on time to information (the earlier, the better) and the recruitment speed relative to the readout of observations required to adapt. For a detailed discussion on planning and implementing adaptive dose-finding designs, see Fardipour et al. (2009a, b).

Bayesian modeling is used to estimate the dose–response relationship for the primary endpoint, multiply impute missing outcome values based on early measurements, and determine posterior probabilities. The proposed trial design uses response-adaptive randomization and Bayesian dose–response models to focus on identifying the minimally effective dose (MED) and the dose with maximum effect (MaxD). The trial may be terminated for futility at the end of stage 1 or during any of interim analyses occurring in stage 2.

17.2   Study Design

This was a randomized, double-blind, placebo-controlled, comparator-referenced, multicenter, parallel-group trial using an adaptive study design in the treatment of adult subjects with acute exacerbations of schizophrenia. Seven active treatment arms of Vabicaserin (50, 100, 150, 200, 300, 400, and 600 mg/day QD) may be tested over the course of the trial. Risperidone 4 mg/day was the active comparator used for assay sensitivity. Placebo was used as a control. The use of placebo as a control was necessary to provide reliable scientific evidence of safety, efficacy, and tolerability to ensure a reliable evaluation of the balance of benefits and risks. Subjects have an approximate 60 % chance of receiving an active dose of Vabicaserin, an approximate 20 % chance of receiving placebo, and an approximate 20 % chance of receiving Risperidone.

The adaptive study design consisted of multiple stages. In the first stage, subjects were equally randomized into 1 of 5 treatment arms: placebo, Risperidone, or 1 of 3 active doses of Vabicaserin. Interim analysis results were made available to an unblinded Data Monitoring Committee (DMC). The DMC evaluated the observed real-time data on the total Positive and Negative Syndrome Scale (PANSS) score between baseline and 4-weeks of treatment and other associated measurements. A statistical algorithm was applied to the data to adapt the treatment allocations of future subjects based on the response from previous subjects.

After the first interim analysis, enrollment to new dose groups of Vabicaserin was opened and weekly interim analyses were conducted and results provided to the DMC. The randomization scheme was modified at the end of each analysis until enrollment was complete. The goal of such a response-adaptive allocation of subjects was to find both the minimally effective dose that yields the desired effect (10-point difference in change (decrease) in the PANSS total score from baseline to day 28) and the dose with the maximum effect, and to estimate the dose–response curve as precisely as possible.

The primary efficacy endpoint was the change in the PANSS total score from baseline to the end of the double-blind treatment period (study day 28). The PANSS total score was also assessed at day 7, 14, 21, and a longitudinal model was used to incorporate these early measurements in the interim analyses to improve the precision of estimation of the primary endpoint. The PANSS score was assessed by the principal investigator and a central rater.

17.3 Data Monitoring Committee

Four sponsor employees, a psychiatrist, a neurologist, a biostatistician, and a programming expert who were neither part of the project team nor involved with the conduct of the trial constituted internal members of the core DMC. The core DMC received weekly estimates of the dose–response relationship, key efficacy and safety data, and updates of the probability of the trial warranting termination for lack of benefit or for success. The core DMC also reviewed the performance of the computer algorithm. The core DMC, enriched by five external experts, psychiatrists, and internists, constituted the full DMC, to evaluate potential safety issues.

The randomization of the 100th, 200th, 300th, and 400th subject was to be used as a trigger for meetings of the full DMC. The focus of these meetings was to primarily review safety, but available efficacy data on the total PANSS score and the Clinical Global Impression—Improvement scale (CGI-I) scores were also reviewed, so an adequate risk–benefit determination of the compound could be made. Full Interim Reports, as laid out in the interim Statistical Analysis Plan (SAP), using all currently available data were produced. During the conduct of the trial, it was the responsibility of the DMC to advise study personnel regarding the continuing safety of study subjects as well as the continuing validity and scientific merit of the trial. The scope of the DMC's responsibilities included endorsing or rejecting the weekly updates from the adaptive algorithm on the proportion of patients to be allocated to the different treatment arms, and recommending to the Executive Steering Committee (ESC) to stop treatment arms for safety or other reasons, or terminate the study for safety, lack of benefit or for success.

The ESC was composed by four senior executives of the sponsor appropriately removed from the conduct of the study. The ESC reviewed the DMC's recommendations, and either endorsed or amended them, and passed them on to the study team. For a more detailed description of trial committees for an adaptive clinical trial, see Fardipour et al. (2009a, b) and Antonijevic et al. (2013).

17.4   Overview of the Design

The primary efficacy endpoint was the change in the PANSS total score from baseline to the end of the double-blind treatment period (study day 28). This study has been designed to find the minimum dose that yields a 10-point difference in changes on the PANSS total score over and above placebo. A 10-point difference on the PANSS total score change was chosen because it was consistent with the magnitude of effect seen in the previous Phase 2 study with this compound and represented a clinically meaningful difference with a standard deviation of 19.4 units.

A maximum of 450 subjects was planned for this study. It was expected to randomize approximately 80 subjects to each of the placebo and Risperidone groups. The remaining 290 subjects were supposed to be allocated to various Vabicaserin dose groups based on the adaptive algorithm. Data from the previous phase II study indicated that 80 subjects per group should be able to detect a 10-point mean difference between placebo and either of Vabicaserin groups in changes of PANSS total score with 90 % power at the 0.05 level of significance assuming a common standard deviation of 19.4.

Subjects were randomized to different doses using an adaptive allocation rule. The adaptive allocation rule was based on two goals. The first goal was to find the minimum effective dose (MED), the smallest dose that achieves the clinically significant difference (CSD) of 10 points increase in the change in the total PANSS score over the placebo. The second goal was to find the dose with the greatest change (MaxD) in PANSS score. The details for randomization are given below in the *Allocation Rule* section. The trial stops when sufficient information is available, that is, when the drug has been shown to be sufficiently effective or that continuation is futile. The trial stops for sufficient success when the MaxD dose is likely to be better than the clinically significant difference of 10 units. The trial stops for futility when the likelihood that each dose achieves the CSD is small. The details for stopping are given in the *Stopping Rule* section below.

17.4.1   Dose–Response Modeling

The relationship between dose and the change in the PANSS total score from baseline at day 28 is not necessarily believed to be monotonic and it is modeled using a normal dynamic linear model (NDLM). The NDLM is a convenient model for describing the dose–response relationship of a drug and allows a great deal of flexibility in the shape and form of the response, assuming only that the response at each dose is normally distributed around a mean, and that the change in mean from one dose to another can be predicted using a simple linear model. The NDLM was originally developed for the analysis and forecasting of time series data by West and Harrison (1997) and applied later in modeling dose–response relationship in many adaptive dose ranging studies, see for example Berry et al. (2002), Smith et al. (2006), and Padmanabhan et al. (2012).

The label for the dose that subject i receives is d_i, where $d=1, \ldots, 8$. The respective amounts of active dose of Vabicaserin are 0 (placebo), 50, 100, 150, 200, 300, 400, and 600 mg QD, respectively. There is an active comparator (Risperidone), which is labeled dose 9. The posterior distribution of the comparator response is tracked separately from the dose–response modeling for Vabicaserin.

Let θ_d be the mean response for Y_i when $d_i=d$. The following error structure is assumed for Y:

$$Y_i \sim \theta_d + N\left(0, \sigma^2\right),$$

where

$$\theta_1 \sim N\left(0, \tau_0^2\right),$$

$$\theta_d \sim N\left(\theta_{d-1}, \tau^2\right), d = 2, \ldots, 8.$$

The "drift" parameter τ^2 represents the "borrowing" from one dose to the neighboring doses. This is the variance between responses at neighboring doses. The larger the value of τ^2, the less borrowing from neighboring doses. The prior distribution for the "drift" parameter and the error term in the NDLM are

$$\tau^2 \sim IG\left(0.001, 1,000\right),$$

$$\sigma^2 \sim IG\left(0.001, 1,000\right),$$

where IG is the inverse gamma distribution. These prior distributions carry little weight, allowing the data to identify the dose–response relationship. They are slightly informative, however, and were selected with the goal of preventing improbable dose–response curves from having large posterior probabilities early in the study. The priors were selected for this purpose—to guide the trial early, but have little effect later in the trial when the data are informative.

An important calculation is the posterior probability that each dose has the highest mean response for Y and the posterior probability that each dose is the MED. Likewise the posterior variance in the response at each dose plays a critical role in the allocation of subjects.

17.4.2 Longitudinal Modeling

The change in total PANSS score from baseline is measured not only at 28 days but after every week.

Let X_t be the change from baseline in total PANSS score at week t and Y be the final outcome at week 4. Let the dose group for the subject be d. We assume the following linear model:

$$Y = a_d + bX_t + \varepsilon$$

where ε are independent identically distributed normal random variables with a mean of 0 and a standard deviation of λ_d. In this modeling the a_d and λ_d are functions of dose d. The slope parameter b is assumed to be the same for each dose. So, for each time period there is a separate intercept for each dose and a separate standard deviation for the error. The slope is assumed to be constant across all dose values. Distinct models are fit for each time period—there is no borrowing across time periods. In the simulations study presented in the *Simulations* section, the prior distribution for b was $N(0.80, 0.25^2)$ and the prior distribution for each intercept was assumed to be $a_d \sim N(0, 10^2)$. The prior mean value for b was empirically established from data in the previous Phase 2a study, while the prior distribution for a_d was intentionally chosen to be vague.

In determining the posterior distribution of the dose–response curve, we incorporated incomplete data using this longitudinal model, resulting in a natural Bayesian imputation of the results for subjects having partial information. The Bayesian approach treats the missing values as random variables, with distributions that depend on all available data, including those values that are known for the subject in question. Calculating the posterior distribution of the dose–response curve required integrating over the distribution for each of the possible values for the missing observations but, using this Bayesian methodology, we were able to account for the uncertainty associated with the missing observations.

The goal of the longitudinal modeling was to find the posterior distribution of the dose–response model. While the distributions of the missing values were not intrinsically important, their effect on the uncertainty in the dose–response model was critical. The Markov chain Monte Carlo (MCMC) approach used to sample from the posterior of the dose–response curve, in the setting of missing values, proceeded as follows:

1. Using the current estimated dose–response model and the longitudinal model, values for each missing value were randomly imputed.

2. Using these imputed values to create a complete set of Y's, a single draw from the posterior of the dose–response curve was obtained.
3. Using the new dose–response curve and the longitudinal model, new values for missing data were then imputed, as in step 1.

Steps 2 and 3 were repeated to create a collection of dose–response curves that represented a sample from the posterior distribution. The known values of Y were held constant throughout this iterative simulation, but the missing values differed from one imputation to the next. This approach provided a posterior distribution for the dose–response curve that appropriately accounted for the uncertainty associated with the missing data, while taking into account the available information from every patient. The MCMC approach is standard, using Metropolis within Gibbs sampler.

17.4.3 Allocation Rule

The adaptive allocation rule was motivated by two goals. The first goal was to find the dose with the greatest change (MaxD) in PANSS score. The second goal was to find the minimum effective dose (MED), the smallest dose that achieves the clinically significant difference (CSD) of 10 points decrease in the change in total PANSS score over the placebo. Bayesian response-adaptive allocation rules (see for example Berry 2004) alter the allocation probabilities based on posterior probabilities $Pr(d=d^*)$ of each dose being the target dose d^* or based on the posterior probabilities weighted by the reduction in variance of the mean response θ_d expected from adding one more subject to that dose:

$$V(d) = Pr(d = d^*)\frac{Var(\theta_d)}{n_d + 1}$$

where n_d is the number of subjects at dose d at the interim analysis time. Thall and Wathen (2007) proposed a more flexible approach using V^c with $c \geq 0$. Clearly $c = 0$ corresponds to equal randomization and they recommend to use a dynamic value for $c = n/2N$, where n and N are the current and the total number of subjects planned in the study, respectively. We used a fixed $c = 1/2$ in this study.

For the goal of finding the MaxD the following vector of randomization probabilities is used:

$$q_{1d} = \frac{\sqrt{V_1(d)}}{\sum_{k=2}^{8}\sqrt{V_1(k)}}$$

where V_1 corresponds to V for $d^* = MaxD$. Similarly for the second goal of finding the $d^* = MED$ the randomization vector q_2 is created as follows:

$$q_{2d} = \frac{\sqrt{V_2(d)}}{\sum_{k=2}^{8}\sqrt{V_2(k)}}.$$

At each interim analysis the two vectors are calculated and they are combined (equally weighted) to form the updated randomization vector:

$$r_d = \begin{cases} 0.20, & d = 1 \\ (0.60)\dfrac{q_{1d}+q_{2d}}{\sum_{k=2}^{8}(q_{1k}+q_{2k})}, & d = 2,\ldots,8 \\ 0.20, & d = 9 \end{cases}$$

The probability for placebo is assumed constant at 0.20. The same allocation ratio 0.20 is assumed for the control arm. The remaining 0.60 proportion of subjects is allocated to the Vabicaserin doses.

17.4.4 Stopping Rule

The study continues accruing until at least 125 subjects have been enrolled and at least one of the following three conditions hold.

If the probability is at least $C_2=0.80$ that the most likely MaxD (d^*) improves over placebo by at least CSD=10 points and the probability that dose d^* is the MaxD is at least $C_1=0.60$ and the probability that the MED was identified is at least $C_3=0.60$, then the trial stops for success. Stop the trial for success if the following three conditions are satisfied:

$$\Pr(d = \text{MaxD}|\text{data}) > C_1 \text{ for some } d$$

$$\Pr(\theta_{d*} - \theta_1 > \text{CSD} \mid \text{data}) > C_2 \text{ for the MaxD}$$

$$\Pr(d = \text{MED} \mid \text{data}) > C_3 \text{ for some } d.$$

Stop for futility if all doses have at least five subjects and the probability that the dose achieves the CSD of 10 points is smaller than $C_4=0.01$, i.e.,

$$\Pr(\theta_d - \theta_1 > \text{CSD} \mid \text{data}) < C_4 \text{ for all } d = 2,\ldots,8.$$

If the sample size reaches the cap of 450 then the trial stops. In this case, the predictive probability that the MaxD dose can beat placebo in a new phase III clinical trial with 100 subjects per arm is calculated. If this predictive probability is greater than $C_5 = 0.80$, then we refer to this condition as Cap/Success, otherwise we call it Cap/Futility.

17.5 Simulations

An essential step in the development and fine-tuning of an adaptive study design is the simulation of the design across a range of potential dose–response pattern scenarios. The appropriateness of the actual design was confirmed through these simulations. In this section we provide additional details regarding the simulation methodology and describe some dose–response scenarios utilized in the fine-tuning the adaptive design of this trial. Then we present the observed operating characteristics of this design across these scenarios.

The fine-tuning design parameters are the cutoffs C_1–C_5. After many simulations with different values of these control parameters we determined that values

$$C_1 = 0.60, C_2 = 0.80, C_3 = 0.60, C_4 = 0.01, C_5 = 0.80$$

are the most appropriate for the purpose of this trial.

17.5.1 Simulation Scenarios

Simulations are created to summarize the operating characteristics of the proposed adaptive design. In order to simulate the design, assumptions have to be made about how the data are generated. These assumptions do not affect the design or the analysis, but they are necessary to simulate subject results. Subjects are accrued at a constant rate of 40 subjects over a period of 28 days. However, in order to model slower enrollment for the first 3 months in the study, we assume 10, 20, and 30 subjects per period for the first three periods, respectively. In the first stage, a total of approximately 50 subjects will be equally randomized into 1 of 5 treatment arms: placebo, Risperidone, or 1 of 3 active doses of Vabicaserin 50, 150, and 300 mg.

The following assumptions are made to simulate subject results. A first week change from baseline value for the total PANSS score is simulated as:

$$Y_1 \sim N\left(\theta_d, \sigma^2\right)$$

Because of the correlation through time the following weeks $(t=2,3,4)$ are simulated as follows:

$$Y_t \sim N\left(\theta_d + \rho\left(Y_{t-1} - \theta_d\right), \left(1 - \rho^2\right)\sigma^2\right),$$

Table 17.1 The mean changes from baseline for total PANSS score for each dose under different scenarios

Scenarios	Mean change in the total PANSS score							
	0	50	100	150	200	300	400	600
1	0.0	0.0	0.0	0.0	0.0	0.0	0.0	0.0
2	0.0	0.5	1.0	2.0	3.0	4.0	5.0	5.0
3	0.0	1.0	2.0	3.0	4.0	5.0	7.0	10.0
4	0.0	4.0	7.0	7.0	10.0	7.0	7.0	4.0
5	0.0	7.0	10.0	10.0	12.5	12.5	12.5	12.5
6	0.0	12.5	12.5	12.5	12.5	12.5	12.5	12.5
7	0.0	7.0	7.0	7.0	7.0	12.5	12.5	12.5
8	0.0	8.0	15.0	15.0	7.0	7.0	5.0	5.0
9	0.0	7.0	7.0	7.0	7.0	12.5	7.0	7.0
10	0.0	15.0	10.0	7.0	5.0	2.0	1.0	0.0

which implies that the following week is normally distributed with the same mean for the dose, θ_d, and is correlated to the previous week's value with correlation coefficient ρ. In each of the simulations runs in this simulation study, the values $\rho = 0.70$ and $\sigma = 20$ are used.

The parameters θ_d determine the efficacy of the different doses. By varying these parameters different scenarios are created. The following scenarios are used in the simulations (Table 17.1).

Scenario 1 is a null case, in which the treatment has no effect. The next scenario is also a futile case because even if there is a trend with increasing the dose the maximum magnitude is only half of the required CSD. The third scenario is the one with only the 600 mg dose achieving the CSD. Scenario 4 has dose 200 mg as the MED and a moderate difference from the neighboring doses. Scenario 6 has a strong difference from placebo across all doses. The next three scenarios are strong scenarios for the experimental drug. In each case there is a strong difference from placebo in total PANSS score and there is a strong difference between the doses. The last scenario has the smallest dose 50 mg as MaxD.

17.5.2 Design Operating Characteristics

In this section the operating characteristics of the design are presented. In each scenario 1,000 simulated trials are conducted and a summary of the operating characteristics are presented. The control arm was not considered in the simulation study. Therefore, the mean sample sizes are only for the placebo and Vabicaserin treatment arms. Because about 80 subjects are required for the final comparison of the control to placebo, the sample size cap in the simulation study was 370 subjects $(370 + 80 = 450$, the maximum sample size for the trial).

The operating characteristics are reported in Table 17.2. The probabilities the design stops early for success are reported in the second column. The probability the trial stops at the cap is reported in the "Cap/Total" column. The probability the

Table 17.2 The operating characteristics of the design for each of the ten scenarios

Sc #	Suc	Cap PIII	Cap Total	Fut	Mean SS		0	50	100	150	200	300	400	600
						Mean sample size								
						Probability selected MaxD								
						Probability selected MED								
1	0.017	0.002	0.151	0.832	229.8		48.098	33.662	25.334	26.564	22.224	24.823	22.334	26.712
							0	0.237	0.127	0.113	0.106	0.114	0.114	0.189
							0	0.309	0.143	0.106	0.099	0.099	0.105	0.139
2	0.046	0.076	0.587	0.367	305.6		63.063	33.470	26.703	31.347	32.084	38.016	37.830	43.061
							0	0.075	0.039	0.049	0.092	0.144	0.238	0.363
							0	0.127	0.051	0.077	0.124	0.147	0.242	0.232
3	0.081	0.401	0.817	0.102	337.4		69.706	32.837	27.564	31.600	32.461	38.932	45.247	59.098
							0	0.015	0.014	0.025	0.028	0.034	0.134	0.750
							0	0.072	0.034	0.034	0.064	0.085	0.217	0.494
4	0.127	0.369	0.786	0.087	325.8		67.090	40.018	39.908	41.285	43.463	35.458	29.932	28.600
							0	0.031	0.106	0.122	0.422	0.127	0.117	0.055
							0	0.180	0.232	0.160	0.307	0.057	0.046	0.018
5	0.251	0.688	0.743	0.006	313.2		64.560	37.505	35.236	36.566	36.051	37.326	31.840	34.138
							0	0.015	0.044	0.061	0.152	0.221	0.173	0.334
							0	0.389	0.252	0.117	0.137	0.045	0.036	0.024
6	0.472	0.509	0.528	0.000	263.2		54.780	39.141	30.810	32.042	26.162	29.244	24.550	26.516
							0	0.088	0.111	0.159	0.128	0.161	0.128	0.225
							0	0.863	0.075	0.031	0.013	0.010	0.005	0.003
7	0.235	0.703	0.760	0.005	317.0		65.506	38.619	30.227	31.588	30.208	42.873	38.481	39.520
							0	0.010	0.010	0.015	0.008	0.250	0.278	0.429
							0	0.400	0.062	0.054	0.044	0.293	0.108	0.039
8	0.677	0.296	0.317	0.006	236.8		49.546	36.295	40.997	39.303	19.311	21.068	14.255	16.038
							0	0.019	0.472	0.465	0.010	0.014	0.001	0.019
							0	0.441	0.497	0.062	0	0	0	0

(continued)

Table 17.2 (continued)

Sc #	Suc	Cap PIII	Cap Total	Fut	Mean SS	Mean sample size / Probability selected MaxD / Probability selected MED	0	50	100	150	200	300	400	600
9	0.216	0.533	0.758	0.026	315.6		65.376	42.551	34.728	35.561	32.880	46.218	28.361	29.880
							0	0.057	0.053	0.072	0.061	0.583	0.064	0.110
							0	0.414	0.114	0.075	0.068	0.293	0.018	0.018
10	0.828	0.145	0.164	0.008	195.3		41.177	47.639	27.140	24.396	15.474	16.395	10.775	12.337
							0	0.782	0.142	0.044	0.009	0.005	0.003	0.015
							0	0.988	0.006	0.004	0.001	0.001	0	0

trial stops at the cap but there is a dose with a 80 % chance of success in a phase III trial with significance level 0.05 and 100 subjects per arm is reported in the "Pr(Cap)/ PIII" column. The mean sample size is reported in the "Mean Sample Size" column. The allocation to different arms is shown in the top of the cell, the probability that the dose is selected as the MaxD is reported in the middle of the cell, and the probability that the dose is selected as the MED is reported at the bottom of the cell.

For Scenario 1, the probability of early stopping for futility or reaching the cap and failing to achieve a 0.8 probability of success in Phase III is 0.981. The mean sample size is only 229.8.

For Scenario 2, the probability of early stopping for futility is only 0.367, but still the probability of claiming success is small 0.122.

Scenarios 3 and 4 have a single dose with CSD, 600 and 200 mg, respectively. These doses receive maximum of subjects (about 59 subjects for Scenario 3 and about 43 for Scenario 4) and the probability of reaching the cap is 0.817 and 0.786, respectively.

For Scenario 5, the MED is dose 100 mg and the MaxD is dose 200 mg. The MED is correctly identified with probability 0.255, the dose 50 mg with the true response of 7 units was selected as MED with probability 0.389. The MaxD has been selected as one of the doses 200–600 mg with probabilities 0.15–0.33. Notice that all these doses have the total PANSS score 12.5 under this scenario.

For Scenario 6, the probability that the trial stops for early success is 0.472. The trial runs to the cap 52.8 % of the time and never stops for futility. 50.9 % of the trials ran to the cap, but a dose was found to be more than 80 % likely to beat placebo in a phase III study, the trial did not stop because it was not clear which dose was the MaxD. If we classify this outcome as a success along with the "Suc" outcomes, then the power of this study is greater than 98 %. The likelihood that the 50 mg dose is found as the MED is 86.3 %.

Scenario 7 is similar to Scenario 6 but only the three higher doses are efficient. Because two of these three doses are available only after the first stage, the mean sample size is much higher than for the previous scenario.

In Scenario 8, the trial is stopped for sufficient positive information in 67.7 % of the trials, with 31.7 % running to the cap and 30 % predicting success in Phase III. The probability of (correctly) finding the 100 mg dose as the MED is 0.497. Most of the subjects have been allocated to lower doses (up to 300 mg). Scenario 9 is a variation of Scenario 7 in which the top two doses have lower mean scores. The probability of (correctly) finding the 250 mg as the MaxD is increased to 0.583 as compared to only 0.25 for Scenario 7. Mean sample size for Scenario 10 is only 195.3 subjects. The MED is correctly identified in 99 % of the cases. Very few subjects are allocated to higher doses where the mean total PANSS score is small.

17.6   Trial Results

Detailed results of this study have been reported previously in Shen et al. (2011). Here we focus mainly on the process of implementing the response adaptive design during the actual trial. A total of 280 subjects were screened, and 202 subjects were randomized and treated between December 2007 and May 2008. Initially, subjects were equally randomized to placebo, Risperidone and three doses of Vabicaserin: 50, 150, and 300 mg. The first interim analysis took place on March 7, 2008. At that time, 69 subjects have been randomized and 29 of them completed the 28 days double-blind treatment. The adaptive design recommended to open enrollment to other doses of Vabicaserin. At weekly interim analyses thereafter, the adaptive design engine was run using the accumulating data on subjects that completed the treatment as well as on those with partial data (based on the longitudinal model) to determine treatment arm allocation probabilities for the next stage.

On April 24, 2008, the adaptive design algorithm first recommended to stop the study for futility because the posterior probability of achieving CSD over placebo on all Vabicaserin doses was smaller than 0.01. The primary driver for futility decision was high placebo response that was apparent from the start of the trial and persisted over subsequent interim analyses. Figure 17.1 shows the estimates of the dose–response as they were made available to the core DMC. The vertical axis describes the change from baseline to day 28 on the total PANSS. The horizontal axis lists the different treatment arms. The first number in [] behind the treatment arm indicates the total number of patients with some available data, as used by the model, while the second number indicates the number of patients with complete datasets. The modeled dose–response is shown in black (point estimate for mean response, including 95 % confidence interval), and the dose–response curve is interpolated across all doses with available data. The observed (not model based) data is shown in grey (point estimate for mean response, and 95 % confidence intervals), and the dose–response curve is interpolated across doses only if there is final data available on at least one patient. The NDLM model indicated a monotonic dose–response for Vabicaserin with the highest effect at the top dose 600 mg. However, the posterior probability of achieving CSD over placebo on all Vabicaserin doses was smaller than 0.01. Moreover, no separation between placebo and the active control Risperidone was observed. The posterior probability of Risperidone achieving at least 5 points difference over placebo at the end of the trial was estimated to be only 11 %. The DMC recommended to override the algorithm and to continue recruiting into the trial and proposed to review the study status with the EXC periodically thereafter. Interestingly, at the next interim analysis, the early stopping for futility was not satisfied because the posterior probability of achieving CSD over placebo on the 600 mg dose of Vabicaserin was 0.017. However, the stopping rule for futility was satisfied consequently at the following four weekly interim analyses.

On May 16, 2008, the DMC recommendation was endorsed by the ESC and recruitment into the study has been stopped for futility due to high placebo response. European centers would have been ready to include patients into the trial by July 2008.

Table 17.2 shows the results used by the DMC in their recommendation. Figure 17.2 shows the estimates of the dose–response at that interim analysis that has the same format as Fig. 17.1 and Table 17.3.

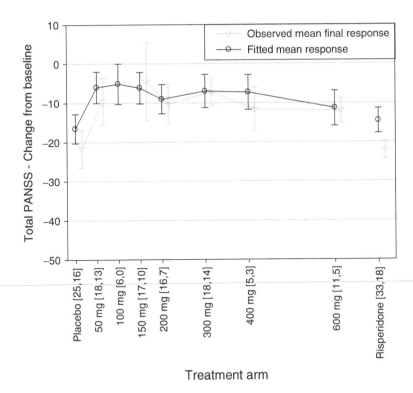

Fig. 17.1 Estimates of the dose–response based on the data available on April 25, 2008 when the adaptive design recommended for the first time to stop the study for futility

17.7 Discussion

In this study, real-time learning about the dose–response was deployed in a large, multicenter, international psychiatric study. The adaptive design allowed early determination of the failed nature of the study, i.e., the inability to separate the active control, Risperidone, from placebo. This led to significant conservation of research resources: a non-adaptive approach would have involved enrolling over twice the number of patients (i.e., 450 vs. 202); the enrollment in the European centers has not been even initiated. The adaptive approach exposed fewer patients to the unnecessary potential risk inherent in the study of an investigational compound. At the same time, the adaptive design allowed a more efficient learning about the dose–response of the investigational drug than would have been possible in a conventional fixed dose study, in particular, the use of the NDLM model in this study would have permitted the ability to assess for a potentially non-monotonic dose–response curve.

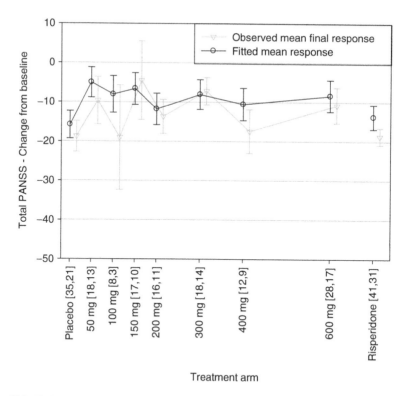

Fig. 17.2 Estimates of the dose–response based on the data available when the DMC made the recommendation to stop the trial for futility due to high response on placebo

A common misunderstanding is the concern that the confidence in the findings on a given dose in an adaptive trial design such as this one is compromised by the small number of patients on any 1 of the 7 doses of investigational drug tested in this study. However, the modeling approach of the adaptive design uses information from all doses in estimating the dose–response curve rather than simply doing pairwise comparisons between study drug dose arms and placebo.

Allocation to placebo and Risperidone was fixed to 20 % each, i.e., 40 % of all patients were used to generate reference points. Of note, the variability of the data on placebo was nearly twice as great as the data on Risperidone. For this reason, it might have been beneficial had the algorithm been enabled to increase the number of patients allocated to placebo or Risperidone beyond 20 %, conditioned on the emerging data, to better estimate the mean response for placebo treated patients. This should be considered in doing future studies employing this methodology.

Running a trial with nine different treatment arms (i.e., Risperidone, placebo, and seven doses of the investigational drug) was challenging, both conceptually and logistically. Population PK provided evidence for successful administration of the different doses across the dose range. For supply reasons, the study began with only

Table 17.3 The interim results at the time when the DMC made the recommendation to stop the trial for futility due to high response on placebo

Treatment group	Randomized Completed	Baseline mean (SD)	LS mean change to W4 (SE)	NDLM fitted mean (SE)
Placebo	35 21	94.74 (11.18)	−14.46 (3.11)	−15.81 (3.19)
50 mg	18 13	95.44 (9.64)	−6.40 (4.33)	−6.41 (3.52)
100 mg	8 3	97.25 (14.72)	−2.44 (6.50)	−8.73 (3.78)
150 mg	17 10	100.47 (12.83)	−2.70 (4.51)	−6.98 (3.72)
200 mg	16 11	93.06 (8.84)	−11.76 (4.60)	−9.66 (3.42)
300 mg	18 14	94.39 (8.73)	−5.44 (4.33)	−8.04 (3.15)
400 mg	12 9	92.83 (10.25)	−14.51 (5.31)	−9.58 (3.84)
600 mg	28 17	95.54 (12.46)	−6.38 (3.47)	−8.42 (3.33)
Risper	41 31	91.49 (10.96)	−14.23 (2.89)	−13.63 (3.18)

three doses of the investigational drug and the other four doses were added when they became available at week 12 in the trial. The study design allowed for subsequent subjects to be preferentially assigned to these other doses to test their effectiveness. Nevertheless, the recommendation for future studies would be to start with all of the doses at the beginning.

To avoid excessive wastage of study drug, only three dose strengths were produced. To ensure complete blinding each dose was prepared by using four bottles and taking one capsule out of each. Compliance was less of a concern, given that patients were hospitalized and medication was prepared for them by nursing staff. However, had this been an outpatient study, blistering study medication and preparing more dose strengths would have been beneficial.

The unanswered question with this study is: Why did it fail to separate the active comparator from placebo? No single prominent cause was identified, and a full discussion is beyond the scope of this paper. However, here are some considerations, with an emphasis on their impact on the adaptive design performance:

Adaptive designs assume exchangeability of patients, i.e., a patient entering the trial in one center early on should be exchangeable with another patient entering the trial in another center at a later stage. However, post hoc analyses revealed "study center" as a factor contributing to the placebo response observed in the trial reported here. Quality control is of paramount importance to reduce variability within and across study sites, at all times, starting with selecting the right study centers, providing appropriate education and monitoring study center work throughout the conduct of the trial to ensure that all aspects of the protocol are rigorously followed.

In response-adaptive-designs there is an "optimal" recruitment speed to learn about the research question, and very fast recruitment may be suboptimal. In the trial reported here, enrollment was more rapid than anticipated, such that 202 patients were recruited in less than 6 months, using 27 study sites in the USA. Recruitment was particularly rapid early during the winter season. This also begs the question whether some sites may already have had a pool of patients to enroll. In hindsight it would have been beneficial to run even more extensive upfront simulations to explore the impact of different scenarios for exchangeability of patients (or lack thereof) and recruitment speed onto the operating characteristics of the design.

Another issue is the assessment of the primary endpoint and associated rater variability: The adaptive algorithm and the initial decision whether a patient could be included in the trial used the PANSS total score as observed by investigators. Interestingly the PANSS total score ratings from the investigational sites were on average 10 points higher than the scores from the central rater, but the variability of the observations was comparable.

The problem of failed trials is not unique to the study reported here and has been observed in other randomized clinical trials conducted in acute schizophrenia patients in recent years. On the one hand the adaptive design was beneficial in establishing the failed nature of the trial early on. On the other hand this case study highlights that jointly with designing an innovative design methodology, there has to be an emphasis on getting the fundamentals of the clinical trial right: choosing a patient population and the endpoint with a goal to optimize the ability to detect a treatment effect, avoiding confounding factors such as uncontrolled concomitant medication and an urge to recruit quickly at all cost. This is particularly relevant in CNS indications where disease and outcome are clinically described through subjective endpoint measures.

Although the investigational drug failed to demonstrate efficacy in this trial, we feel that the design and analytic approach performed well. The NDLM modeling across dose groups, the longitudinal modeling, and the adaptive allocation to treatment all facilitated efficient learning about the dose–response curve. The emerging dose–response estimates, together with the various posterior probability estimates associated with the model and the end-of-study predictions, provided the information needed for decision-making.

In retrospect, we feel that the futility criterion was overly stringent. The motivation for the conservative rule was concern that one of the frequent interim looks would satisfy the futility criterion (even for an efficacious drug), thereby inflating the type II error rate. In actuality, the consistency of the results over many weeks (always indicating little chance of a meaningful advantage over placebo) made the DMC quite comfortable with the decision to terminate for futility. Further support of this decision was provided through pharmacokinetic analyses.

Pre-study simulation work is critical to fine-tuning the decision rules and optimizing the operating characteristics of an adaptive design. The futility criterion must be carefully assessed, recognizing that a less stringent rule increases the chance of a "quick kill" but at the risk of an increased type II error rate. To address the concern that multiple looks may lead to a spurious futility decision, we may wish to require that the futility criterion be satisfied more than once before stopping the trial (e.g., at three consecutive interim analyses). Extensive simulation work is necessary to assess the futility criterion and other design options, as we develop future applications of the present methodology that perform best across the range of potential response patterns.

References

Antonijevic Z, Gallo P, Chuang-Stein C, Dragalin V, Loewy J, Menon S, Miller E, Morgan CC, Sanchez M (2013) Views on emerging issues pertaining to data monitoring committees for adaptive trials. Drug Inf J 47:495–502

Berry D (2004) Bayesian statistics and the efficiency and ethics of clinical trials. Stat Sci 19:175–187

Berry D, Muller P, Grieve AP, Smith MK, Parke T, Blazek R, Mitchard N, Krams M (2002) Adaptive Bayesian designs for dose-ranging trials. In: Carlin B, Carriquiry A, Gatsonis C, Gelman A, Kass RE, Verdinelli I, West M (eds) Case studies in Bayesian statistics V. Springer, Berlin, pp 99–181

Dragalin V (2006) Adaptive designs: terminology and classification. Drug Inf J 40:425–435

Fardipour P, Littman G, Burns DD, Dragalin V, Padmanabhan SK, Parke T et al (2009a) Planning and executing response-adaptive learn-phase clinical trials: 1. The process. Drug Inf J 43: 713–723

Fardipour P, Littman G, Burns DD, Dragalin V, Padmanabhan SK, Parke T et al (2009b) Planning and executing response-adaptive learn-phase clinical trials: 2. Case studies. Drug Inf J 43: 725–734

Gallo P, Chuang-Stein C, Dragalin V, Gaydos B, Krams M, Pinheiro J et al (2006) Adaptive designs in clinical drug development – an executive summary of the PhRMA working Group. J Biopharm Stat 16(3):275–283, Discussion 285–291, 293–278, 311–272

Krams M, Sharma A, Dragalin V, Burns D, Fardipour P, Padmanabhan SK et al (2009) Adaptive approaches in drug development. Opportunities and challenges in design and implementation. Pharm Med 23:139–148

Orloff J, Douglas F, Pinheiro J, Levinson S, Branson M, Chaturvedi P, Ette E, Gallo P, Hirsch G, Mehta C, Patel N, Sabir S, Springs S, Stanski D, Golub H, Evers M, Fleming E, Singh N, Tramontin T (2009) The future of drug development: advancing clinical trial design. Nat Rev Drug Discov 8:1–9

Padmanabhan SK, Berry S, Dragalin V, Krams M (2012) A Bayesian dose-finding design adapting to efficacy and tolerability response. J Biopharm Stat 22:276–293

Shen J, Preskorn S, Dragalin V, Slomkowski M, Padmanabhan SK, Fardipour P, Sharma A, Krams M (2011) How adaptive trial designs can increase efficiency in psychiatric drug development: a case study. Innov Clin Neurosci 8(26):26–34

Smith M, Jones I, Morris M, Grieve A, Tan K (2006) Implementation of a Bayesian adaptive design in a proof of concept study. Pharm Stat 5:39–50

Thall PF, Wathen JK (2007) Practical Bayesian adaptive randomisation in clinical trials. Eur J Cancer 43:859–866

West M, Harrison J (1997) Bayesian forecasting and dynamic models, 2nd edn. Springer-Verlag, New York

Chapter 18
Case Study: Design Considerations for a Phase Ib Randomized, Placebo-Controlled, 4-Period Crossover Adaptive Dose-Finding Clinical Trial

James A. Bolognese and Yevgen Tymofyeyev

Abstract A new formulation of a test drug was to be studied in patients for the first time. Preclinical studies yielded a wide range of effective doses across species, so there was a desire to include at least 6 doses in the dose-finding trial. Adaptive design was chosen to focus the dose assignments on those that yielded at least 75 % of maximal response (ED75). A 4-period crossover in which each of 68 patients received 3 doses of test drug and placebo was chosen since it optimized performance characteristics. Frequent interim analyses were performed to optimally choose the 3 doses of test drug to maximize dose assignments to the doses estimated to be closest to ED75 based on analysis of study data accumulated up to each interim analysis time. The completed study yielded minimal assignment of doses away from ED75 and successfully identified, and focused dose assignment around, the target dose. The table below shows the numbers of assignments to each dose and the respective observed mean responses.

	Dose1(Pbo)	Dose2	Dose3	Dose4	Dose5	Dose6	Dose7
N	67	42	0	30	66	25	36
Mean	3	7	n/a	13	10	9	12

Keywords Frequent adaptation • Adaptive dose-finding cross-over • Isotonic regression

J.A. Bolognese (✉)
Cytel Inc., 675 Massachusetts Avenue, Cambridge, MA 02139, USA
e-mail: bolognese@cytel.com

Y. Tymofyeyev
J&J, One J&J Plaza, New Brunswick, NJ 08901, USA

264 Hampshire Drive, Plainsboro, NJ 98536, USA
e-mail: YTymofye@ITS.JNJ.com

W. He et al. (eds.), *Practical Considerations for Adaptive Trial Design and Implementation*, Statistics for Biology and Health,
DOI 10.1007/978-1-4939-1100-4_18, © Springer Science+Business Media New York 2014

18.1   Description of the Problem

An informed decision on doses of a new formulation of a commonly used drug was
needed for future studies to optimize chances of success of the drug development
program. Little was known about the dose–response shape and dose range for the
new formulation to guide dose selection. This information could not be obtained
from PK/PD studies due to nature of formulation. Based on previous experience
with the approved formulation, the dose–response curve was expected to be very
steep, that is, increasing from minimum to maximum across narrow dose range.
*Thus, it might be easy to miss the informative part of the dose range and encounter
study failure unless some preliminary learning about the dose–response relationship is accomplished in this trial.* Failure would be especially costly since later trials
might potentially include monotherapy and combination therapies, requiring rather
large studies. A very wide potential dose range and a large number of doses (about
6 or 7) needs to be studied in order to *properly* evaluate the dose-finding objectives
of the trial. Not enough preliminary information was available to narrow the dose
range to only 3 or 4 doses, and a limited budget was available. Thus, adaptive
designs were considered to permit study of more doses than the usual 3–4 of a more
traditional completely randomized design.

Study design logistics were favorable for adaptive design. In particular, the time
from randomization to observation of the key response was a week. Enrolment was
expected to occur over several months offering adequate time for interim analyses
for adaptation. Additionally, there was a limited number of centers, making implementation of adaptations logistically feasible.

At the protocol concept stage, the following design options were considered.
A 4-period crossover design with 44 subjects was the default option, i.e., the traditional non-adaptive design that would have been implemented if adaptive design
was found infeasible or with no advantage. This design would include 3 active treatment doses and placebo; hence, it would provide limited information about the
overall dose–response curve.

In order to increase the number of doses, an incomplete block design with 88
subjects was considered. It would include 6 doses of active treatment and placebo.
However, there still would be limited information about the dose–response curve
since estimation of treatment effects would be based on a combination of within-
and between-subject variability. Also, if balance were not achieved due to dropouts,
there would be confounding of dose–response effects with between-subject effects.

A seven-arm parallel design with 448 subjects was also considered. It would
include 6 doses and placebo to provide more complete information about the dose–
response curve than the 3-dose 4-period crossover design. However, it would be
much more costly due to the large number of subjects, and likely take longer to
complete.

A 2-stage adaptive 3-period crossover design in 88 subjects was considered.
Stage 1 in the first 44 subjects would include placebo, a mid-dose, and a high dose.
At the interim analysis, after Stage 1, 2 additional doses would be selected for

inclusion in Stage 2 along with placebo. The remaining 44 subjects would comprise Stage 2. However, since only 4 active doses could be included in this trial, it would provide incomplete information about the dose–response curve.

The penultimate design considered was a frequent-adaptation Bayesian dose–response modeling approach including 6 doses and placebo in 40 patients if crossover or 120 patients if parallel. This approach would provide information on the overall shape of the dose–response curve with emphasis on estimation of the dose with 75 % of maximal efficacy ("ED75"). The only drawback of this approach is complexity of implementation.

The chosen design was a frequent-adaptation fixed-algorithm-based 4-period crossover design in 64 subjects. Each subject was assigned 3 of 6 possible doses and placebo. This design, as did the Bayesian design, permitted evaluation of the widest range of doses and targeted estimation of ED75. It was much easier to implement, and easier to explain to clinicians; hence, it was chosen for implementation for the clinical trial. More detail on this design follows in the remaining sections of this chapter.

18.2   Methods/Key Aspects of the Chosen Design and/or Operational Features Considered

The frequent adaptation fixed algorithm 4-period crossover design was chosen. Although a formal interim analysis for the purpose of stopping the study early for futility or superior efficacy was not performed, there were multiple unblinded evaluations for the purpose of identifying the best doses for patient allocation. Unblinded data were evaluated by an unblinded statistician on a regular basis to determine patient-dose allocation. Study enrollment was going on at the time of these unblinded evaluations. Blinding to treatment assignment was maintained at all investigational sites. The results of unblinded evaluations were not shared with investigators or other SPONSOR personnel. Patient-level unblinding was restricted to an internal unblinded statistician performing the unblinded evaluations, who had no other responsibilities associated with the study.

The 3 initially selected doses (1, 4, and 6) were used at the start of the trial. At each adaptation time point, if the review of available responses suggested that using doses other than the 3 currently used doses would better identify the target dose yielding 75 % of maximal placebo-adjusted response (according to the specified algorithm), then a new combination of 3 doses was used for subsequent patients, until the next adaptation took place. A score function was used during the adaptive process to identify the best doses (closest to the target dose yielding 75 % of maximal placebo-adjusted efficacy). The score of a given combination of 3 active doses (i.e., a combination of 3 active doses that a given patient is randomized to receive during the study) was computed based on responses estimated at those 3 dose levels based on available data. A particular 3-dose combination was randomly selected from the set of three combinations with the highest scores. The performance and operating characteristics of the algorithm were evaluated by extensive simulations under different scenarios. The adaptation algorithm can be described as a data-driven allocation. No formal inference was done at the review points because sample sizes were not large enough to provide high confidence level statements.

Dose adaptation can be logically split into two parts:

- Estimation of the underlying dose–response relationship from observed data
- Selection of the best allocation scheme (based on the estimated dose–response) that best meets the adaptation objective.

At each time point of adaptation, the algorithm described here will update the allocation scheme in use at the time of adaptation. The updated scheme will then be used for subject randomization from that time forward until the next adaptation is performed. The first adaptation can be performed as soon as data are available from at least 21 responses as observed over at least 4 different dose levels. Adaptation can then be performed as often as the logistical constraints of data processing will permit; the planned frequency of adaptation is twice weekly.

18.2.1   Estimation of Dose–Response

The first adaptation takes place when data from at least 4 dose levels are available. The estimates are obtained by means of isotonic regression under the assumption that the underling true dose–response relation is a monotonically non-decreasing function. For this study, the Pool Adjacent Violators Algorithm (PAVA) will be used (Barlow et al. 1972).

- *Algorithm input*: Observed mean responses at the ordered dose level; available sample sizes are used to weight each dose level.
- *Algorithm output*: Least-squares error fit to the observed mean responses at each dose level, weighted by sample sizes (and subject to monotonicity constraint); response estimates for dose levels where data are not available are obtained by linear interpolation (Fig. 18.1).

18.2.2   Selection of the Optimal Dose Levels

Each subject is randomly assigned to one of four possible treatment sequences described in the protocol (sequence of 3 active dose strengths and placebo). Thus, the allocation scheme is completely defined by specification of the 3 active dose levels. There are a total of 20 different combinations that include 3 active dose levels out of 6 possible dose levels (Doses2 through 7, with placebo as Dose1), as listed in order in Table 18.1. Note that this translates into a total number of

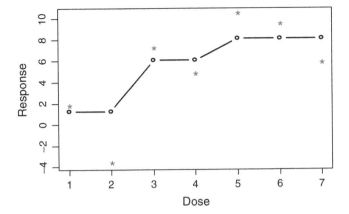

Fig. 18.1 Example of PAVA fit. *Red* stars are observed means

Table 18.1 Active dose combinations for crossover sequence assignments

Combination	1	2	3	4	5	6	7	8	9	10	11	12	13	14	15	16	17	18	19	20
Dose A	2	2	2	2	2	2	2	2	2	2	3	3	3	3	3	3	4	4	4	5
Dose B	3	3	3	3	4	4	4	5	5	6	4	4	4	5	5	6	5	5	6	6
Dose C	4	5	6	7	5	6	7	6	7	7	5	6	7	6	7	7	6	7	7	7

$20 \times 4 = 80$ different randomization sequences, but only 4 are used at a time once dose levels are selected.

Each combination of 3 dose levels will be assessed by computing its score. Then, one 3-dose combination is randomly selected from the set of three combinations having the highest scores. This 3-dose combination is then used (i.e., these 3 active doses) for each patient until the next evaluation (and possible dose adaptation) is performed.

The score of a 3-dose combination is computed based on estimated responses at the dose levels contained in that combination, and calculated in the following way:

The score function ranks dose-level combinations according to proximity of their 3 dose levels to the target dose ED 75. Let $r_1, r_2 \dots r_7$ be estimated responses via isotonic regression at placebo and 6 active dose levels, respectively. Compute $q_i = (r_i - r_1)/(r_7 - r_1)$ for $i = 2 \dots 7$, which reflect dose effectiveness relative to the maximum observed response adjusted for placebo. For each 3 dose combination, say $\{A, B, C\}$, the score is $S(q_A) + S(q_B) + S(q_C)$. The score function $S()$ is presented by the plot in Fig. 18.2. This score function was defined to yield maximum score for the target dose at ED75 and still yield high scores for doses near ED75, and decreasing away from ED75. Obviously many such score functions exist, and this one was chosen arbitrarily.

For example, suppose that the observed response means and estimated dose–response curve are as presented in Fig. 18.1. Then the scores for each of the 20 three-dose combinations are presented in Table 18.2.

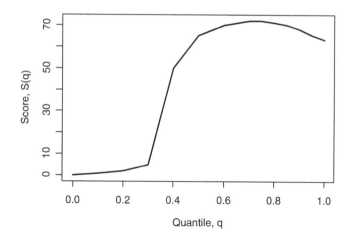

Fig. 18.2 Score function

Table 18.2 Score function values for active dose combinations

Combin.	1	2	3	4	5	6	7	8	9	10	11	12	13	14	15	16	17	18	19	20
Dose A	2	2	2	2	2	2	2	2	2	2	3	3	3	3	3	3	4	4	4	5
Dose B	3	3	3	4	4	4	5	5	6	4	4	4	5	5	6	5	5	6	6
Dose C	4	5	6	7	5	6	7	6	7	7	5	6	7	6	7	7	6	7	7	7
Score	144	135	135	135	135	135	135	126	126	126	207	207	207	198	198	198	198	198	198	189

The dose combination to be used (until next adaptation) is randomly selected from among the 3-dose combinations with the three highest scores, which in this example (Fig. 18.1 and Table 18.2) are {3,4,5}, {3,4,6}, and {3,4,7}. If there are several combinations that have the same score, then ties are broken by using the lower combination number listed in the first row of Table 18.1.

18.2.3   Simulation Setting

18.2.3.1   Evaluation of the Design

The algorithm performance was evaluated by means of extensive simulations. Figure 18.3 displays the true underlying dose–response profiles (scenarios) that were used.

The following entries were simulated for each trial:

- For each calendar day the number of subjects that enter the trial is a random number that follows Poisson distribution. The start time of each subject is recorded. For each subject, time to next treatment is 7 days.

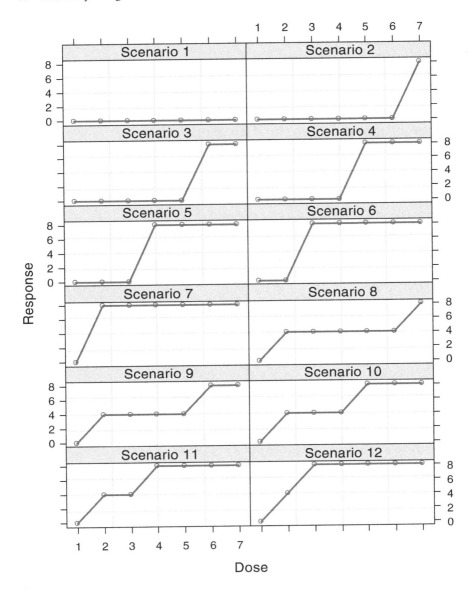

Fig. 18.3 Dose–response scenarios

- At each time point, there are four different treatment sequences with fixed 3 active dose levels and placebo. A subject is randomly assigned to one of the sequences.
- For each subject, the response is generated according to the underlying true dose–response at each dose level, imposing appropriate correlation structure regarding between- and within-subject variability. Only responses from the dose level corresponding to subject treatment sequence are used at the corresponding time points.

- Predefined proportions of subjects who did not complete all treatment periods. These subjects are selected at random. After that, a treatment period starting from which (inclusively) subject dropped from a trial is randomly picked from 2, 3, and 4 with equal probabilities.

18.2.4 Parameters Used in Trial Simulation

- Number of possible dose levels = 7 (placebo and 6 active dose)
  - Starting doses = 1 (Placebo), 2, 5, 7
- Number of subjects in each trial = 65 (adjusted for patient dropouts)
  - Dropout rate = 8 % (proportion of patients not completing all treatment periods)
- Standard Deviation (SD)
  - Within-subject SD = 13
  - Between-subject total SD = 18 (incorporates within-subject SD and subject random effect).
- Patient and data accrual
  - Poisson accrual with rate = 0.5 (Example of the resulting number of subject per week: 4 4 4 1 5 1 0 1 3 2 3 5 3 2 5 2 4 6 5 3)
  - Delay in response = 1 day
  - Time between treatment periods = 4–7 days
  - Timing to perform Adaptation = every 3, 4 days
- No early stopping rule.

18.2.5 Simulation Results

Simulation results are based on 5,000 simulations per dose–response scenario. Table 18.3 reports the proportion of the total sample size allocated to each dose level obtained by averaging across simulations. The actual allocation observed in the particular trial deviates from the presented value with a half interquantile range (0.5*IQR) equal to 3–7 %. Table 18.4 reports power for testing superiority of a dose level versus placebo (1-sided test at alpha level 2.5 %, without adjustment for multiplicity).

Figures 18.4 and 18.5 graphically present information from Table 18.3 and provide information from Table 18.4 in the title of each plot. Also, each title includes the true dose–response scenario for which information is presented.

Table 18.3 Proportion of total sample size allocated to each dose

Scenario	Dose1	Dose2	Dose3	Dose4	Dose5	Dose6	Dose7
1	0.25	0.17	0.05	0.07	0.17	0.08	0.21
2	0.25	0.14	0.06	0.07	0.13	0.11	0.23
3	0.25	0.11	0.06	0.07	0.11	0.18	0.23
4	0.25	0.10	0.04	0.07	0.21	0.16	0.17
5	0.25	0.07	0.04	0.15	0.18	0.14	0.17
6	0.25	0.07	0.11	0.15	0.17	0.12	0.14
7	0.25	0.19	0.11	0.09	0.17	0.07	0.13
8	0.25	0.14	0.08	0.09	0.15	0.11	0.17
9	0.25	0.13	0.08	0.09	0.15	0.13	0.17
10	0.25	0.13	0.08	0.09	0.18	0.12	0.14
11	0.25	0.11	0.08	0.13	0.17	0.11	0.14
12	0.25	0.11	0.11	0.13	0.16	0.10	0.13

Table 18.4 Power for comparison of each dose versus placebo

Scenario	Dose1	Dose2	Dose3	Dose4	Dose5	Dose6	Dose7
1	NA	0.022	0.021	0.022	0.026	0.020	0.020
2	NA	0.018	0.021	0.018	0.024	0.026	0.906
3	NA	0.021	0.025	0.024	0.017	0.841	0.913
4	NA	0.017	0.019	0.018	0.876	0.840	0.866
5	NA	0.016	0.014	0.728	0.869	0.806	0.849
6	NA	0.016	0.548	0.763	0.843	0.756	0.786
7	NA	0.748	0.612	0.559	0.853	0.495	0.793
8	NA	0.263	0.206	0.234	0.308	0.266	0.804
9	NA	0.258	0.221	0.233	0.314	0.716	0.834
10	NA	0.250	0.208	0.233	0.846	0.742	0.795
11	NA	0.229	0.204	0.686	0.852	0.720	0.791
12	NA	0.224	0.615	0.702	0.835	0.691	0.754

18.2.6   Conclusions from Simulations

On average, as it can be seen from Table 18.3 and Figs. 18.4 and 18.5, the algorithm allocates subject to the neighborhood of the effective and the highest sub-effective dose levels for the studied dose response scenarios. (Note that doses with the same level of response are assigned different proportions of patients; in particular, assignment peaks at the left side of the plateau since emphasis of the scoring system for adaptation is at ED75.) This translates to a high power to declare those dose levels superior to placebo, see Table 18.4. For reference, 43 subjects per treatment would be required for 80 % power to yield a statistically significant (alpha = 0.025, 1-sided) difference from placebo via pairwise comparison using a traditional crossover design. Type I error rate is controlled well: refer to Tables 18.3 and 18.4 to the row which corresponds to scenario 1.

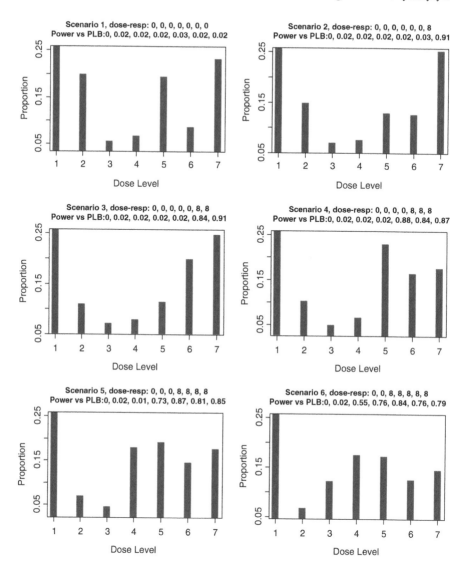

Fig. 18.4 Average proportion of the total sample size at each dose level (Scenarios 1–6)

18.3 Remarks on the Adaptive Study Design Chosen, in Comparison to Traditional Design Choices

The average number of subjects that completed all treatment is around 60. The adaptive design uses $60 \times 4 = 240$ total observations from 60 subjects. Depending on scenario the power of the adaptive design is around 80–91 %. A standard crossover

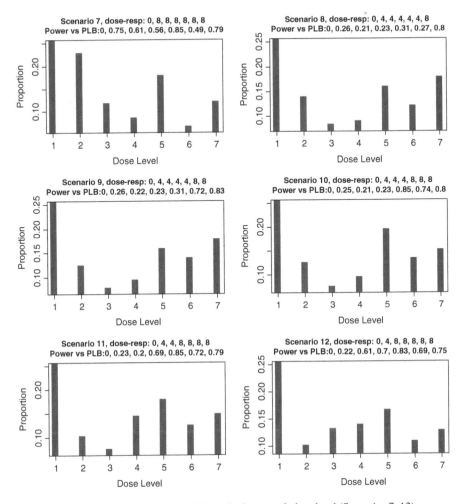

Fig. 18.5 Average proportion of the total sample size at each dose level (Scenarios 7–12)

design will require about 47 subjects to yield similar power for the same effect sizes. That 4-period crossover would have $47 \times 4 = 188$ observations but it explores only 3 dose-levels and placebo. So the adaptive design requires 28 % more observations than the traditional 3-dose, 4 period crossover because it explores $6 + 1$ dose levels. On the other hand, a crossover design that explores 6 doses and placebo (a 7-period crossover design, which would not be feasible for this study), would have $47 \times 7 = 329$ observations. So theoretically the adaptive design is $329/240 = 1.37$ more efficient than a standard 7-period crossover design. In addition, it provides a shorter study duration for each subject. At the end of the study, treatments are compared at each time point separately using a mixed effect model including terms for treatment, period, and baseline covariate. An unstructured variance/covariance matrix was utilized to capture the correlation between repeated measurements within a patient.

18.4   Results from the Actual Clinical Trial and Conclusions

The 4-period crossover design was carried out. The clinical portion was similar to the usual approach for a pharmacodynamic crossover study of traditional design except that results were frequently reported to the unblinded statistician for interim analysis and determination of next doses. Those dose-determinations were e-mailed to the unblinded pharmacists at the respective sites so that they could prepare the appropriate test medications for the next set of subjects.

The final study data was analyzed using a standard mixed effects model for a crossover study including fixed effects for periods and treatments and random effect for subjects. Figure 18.6 displays the resultant lease squares (LS) mean change from baseline in the primary efficacy response across the doses; Table 18.5 shows associated summary statistics. Note from these that the response appears to plateau at Dose4, and that Dose3 was not assigned since response at Dose2 was low and not much larger than that of placebo. Dose3 was never assigned since Dose4 was estimated to be on the plateau, and Dose2 was estimated well below ED75; note that the outcome is most similar to simulated Scenario 11, and even in the simulations, Dose3 was rarely assigned. The outcome of the clinical trial was a case where Dose3 was not assigned. This aspect of the adaptive design performance was as intended. Furthermore, the maximum number of observations was at Dose5, which

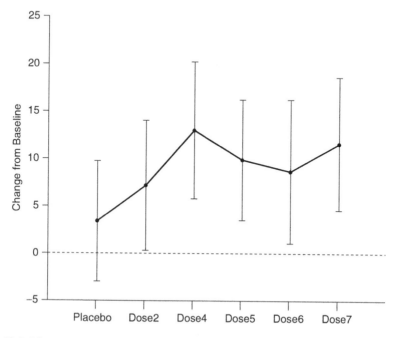

Fig. 18.6 LS mean response with 95 % CI. (Note: Dose3 was not assigned to any subject, so it does not appear)

Table 18.5 Summary statistics from analysis of primary endpoint responses from the completed trial

Treatment	N	Baseline Mean (SD)	Average over first 4 h Mean (SD)	Change from baseline Average over first 4 h Mean (SD)	LS Mean (95 % CI)[a]
Dose1(Placebo)	67	245 (64)	245 (66)	1 (25)	3 (−3, 10)
Dose2	42	239 (64)	247 (72)	8 (29)	7 (0, 14)
Dose4	30	255 (68)	267 (73)	12 (19)	13 (6, 20)
Dose5	66	246 (64)	255 (69)	10 (26)	10 (4, 16)
Dose6	25	256 (61)	266 (66)	9 (24)	9 (1, 16)
Dose7	36	238 (59)	251 (69)	13 (34)	12 (5, 19)

Pairwise comparison	Difference in LS Means (95 % CI)[a]	p-Value[a]
Dose2 vs. Placebo	4 (−1, 8)	0.096
Dose4 vs. Placebo	10 (4, 15)	0.001
Dose5 vs. Placebo	6 (2, 11)	0.002
Dose6 vs. Placebo	5 (−1, 11)	0.081
Dose7 vs. Placebo	8 (4, 13)	0.001

[a]Based on mixed-effects model with terms for treatment, period, and baseline covariate

approximates the ED75. However, since the maximum response was observed at Dose4, and the qualitative shape of the dose–response curve was non-monotonic, in hind sight it probably would have been better to have more observations on Dose4 to investigate if it provides maximal response. Since the design was built assuming monotonicity, its performance could be interpreted to be suboptimal for an observed non-monotonic situation.

18.5   Discussion (What Worked Well and What Did not Work Well)

18.5.1   Study Design

The consulting statisticians with special expertise in adaptive design contributed a lot to the design of the study. As at the time, very little was known about the dose–response for the new formulation; the goal was to obtain information on the shape of the DR-curve. The consulting statisticians guided the team in selecting the most appropriate design. They did many simulations and developed the algorithm for dose assignments. The collaboration between them and the project statistician worked really well and was essential in getting the protocol in place.

18.5.2   Planning for Study Execution

The design/protocol development stage took quite some time as the project statistician and clinical team were not familiar with this type of adaptive designs and had to go through a learning curve. Getting the logistics for the study in place (allocation schedules, drug supplies, etc.) was somewhat complex and required quite some discussion. It was important to take sufficient time during that stage to ensure everything was properly in place.

18.5.3   Study Execution

The study enrolled rather quickly and the team was using an internally developed spirometry system, not one by a vendor. The spirometry data was being constantly reviewed and any issues that were encountered were addressed with the site before data was uploaded to the database. There were issues with uploading to the database which were discovered after the study started. This is the reason that the unblinded statistician could not review the data in the database, but instead was reviewing in Excel format.

There were fewer interim looks than initially planned due to slower than expected data flow. The data flow from collection to the unblinded statistician was not fully set up before the first actual data transfer, and there were fewer subjects' data than expected at time of first interim analysis. Thus, it is recommended to set up and test the data flow mechanism prior to the actual data flow, and to more closely monitor the accumulation of subjects' data so the interim analyses occur with sufficient amounts of subjects' data as planned.

The study used an automated measurement device to obtain the primary endpoint readings from the subjects. It is possible that use of a vendor-developed system (to download information directly from the device to the database) may have alleviated some of the data issues, since the transfers would have been ironed out beforehand during UAT. For the internal data capture system, only the device was tested by users, not the data flow as a whole. There was no user testing environment to allow testing the upload from the data capture system to the database. If such user testing were possible, the data flow issues would have been discovered prior to study start and the unblinded statistician would have reviewed data in the database instead of in EXCEL spreadsheets.

Due to the limited amount of study drug and the fact that the doses might change, the team required the support of an unblinded Clinical Specialist (CS) and unblinded Clinical Research Associates (CRAs) to monitor the drug supply. The Allocation Numbers (ANs, with the treatment assignments) were sent to sites on an as needed basis. Initially, each site received 2 ANs, but subsequent numbers were sent only upon request and proof that they had patients in screening. This method permitted the team to be able to adapt the doses in near "real time." Once the blinded statistician analyzed the data, he updated the allocation schedule and communicated the schedule to the unblinded CS. The unblinded CS was then able to send out the updated ANs to sites upon request. Patients who were already on treatment did not have a change in dose, but completed the study with their original assignment. The CS sets up an "unblinded" restricted access eRoom for the unblinded team members since the information could not be placed on any share drives. This way the unblinded statistician and the unblinded CS could keep documents there and the information could be made available to anyone who would need to cover if needed. IVRS could have also helped with the execution of this part since it could turn arms on and off as needed by simply checking off the correct boxes for the treatments being used.

Given that the project team had really no idea where the dose–response curve would land, the data gave them useful information. The degree of "noise" in what was supposed to be the "flat" part of the dose–response did raise questions for some people looking at the data.

Reference

Barlow RE, Bartholomew DJ, Bremner JM, Brunk HD (1972) Statistical inference under order restriction. Wiley, New York

Chapter 19
Continual Reassessment Method for a First-in-Human Trial: From Design to Trial Implementation

Inna Perevozskaya, Lixin Han, and Kristen Pierce

Abstract We present a case study of a Phase 1 oncology dose-escalation trial utilizing modified Continual Reassessment Method (CRM). Learning about the dose–toxicity relationship and choosing the correct Maximum Tolerated Dose (MTD) to take forward into Phase II is one of the most challenging research questions in Phase 1 oncology trials. CRM is a Bayesian adaptive design targeting a specific Dose Limiting Toxicity (DLT) rate, e.g., 25 %. Similar to the traditional 3 + 3 designs used in oncology Phase 1 trials, learning about drug's toxicity profile with CRM occurs in real time. However, since CRM algorithm incorporates dose–toxicity modeling in the learning process, its ability to identify the correct Maximum Tolerated Dose is substantially improved, compared to the traditional 3 + 3 design. Such design also results in more patients being allocated to tolerable doses with therapeutic potential than would be the case in a more traditional 3 + 3 dose-escalation trial. This trial was designed and executed using a custom-developed and validated software package which helped to alleviate substantial increase in overhead cost typically associated with planning and implementation of such designs. We present the whole "story" of the trial from beginning to end, including selection of study design, assessment of its operating characteristics via simulations, execution, study results, and lessons learned.

I. Perevozskaya, Ph.D. (✉)
Statistical Research and Consulting Center, Pfizer, 500 Arcola Rd,
Collegeville, PA 19426, USA
e-mail: Inna.Perevozskaya@pfizer.com

L. Han, Ph.D.
Infinity Pharmaceuticals, 780 Memorial Drive, Cambridge, MA 02139, USA
e-mail: Lixin.Han@infi.com

K. Pierce, Ph.D.
Oncology Clinical Development, Pfizer, MS 8260-2132, Eastern Point Road,
Groton, CT 06340, USA
e-mail: Kristen.J.Pierce@pfizer.com

W. He et al. (eds.), *Practical Considerations for Adaptive Trial Design and Implementation*, Statistics for Biology and Health,
DOI 10.1007/978-1-4939-1100-4_19, © Springer Science+Business Media New York 2014

Keywords Continual-reassessment method • First-in-humans trials • Dose-limiting toxicity • Maximum tolerated dose

19.1   Introduction

Innovative statistical designs for Phase 1 dose-escalation studies have been gaining popularity in recent years as an alternative to the traditional 3 + 3 design. Original methodology development for many of these designs goes back to almost two decades ago (see, for example, a comprehensive review by Rosenberger and Haines 2002) but they remained largely unpopular among clinical trialists until recently due to additional complexity, lack of software, and need for more extensive statistical involvement. Perhaps one of the major catalysts of more general acceptance was FDA critical path initiative launched in 2004 and resulting surge in interest in Adaptive Trials in general Woodcock and Woosley (2008). As a result, considerable changes were seen in Phase 1 oncology practice with both industry and academia embracing innovative methods on a routine basis. This case study is one example of this more general acceptance within the industry: it was the first CRM-type study designed and executed within Pfizer.

There are many alternative design methods (to 3 + 3) available for designing Phase 1 oncology trials today (see, for example a review Tourneau et al. 2009). Most of these methods share a common goal: improving the efficiency of traditional 3 + 3 designs defined as increasing precision of Maximum Tolerated Dose (MTD) determination while maintaining trial sample size and exposure of patients to toxic doses as small as possible.

Continual Reassessment Method (CRM) is perhaps the oldest and most well-known method for oncology dose-escalation trials other than 3 + 3 design. Since the original manuscript by O'Quigly et al. (1990) was published, there were many follow-up developments including improvements of the original design to minimize toxic exposure and, exploring various working models (Goodman et al. 1995), incorporating efficacy endpoints (Braun 2002), extending method to Time-to-Event Endpoint (Cheung and Chappell 2000), and two-dimensional extensions (Yuan and Yin 2008) to name a few. Some good recent reviews of the CRM methodology with its multiple modifications and extension can be found in O'Quigly and Conaway (2010) and Cheung (2011). For our case study, we utilized a modified CRM procedure as described in Goodman et al. (1995) and Braun (2002). A brief overview of the procedure is given in Sect. 19.2. Other designs such as Up-and-Down (Gezmu and Flournoy 2006) and standard 3 + 3 design have been considered for this study as well, but CRM was chosen following careful evaluation of multiple methods.

Section 19.2 provides overview of study design including CRM methodology, Sect. 19.3 reviews simulation setup and key findings, and Sects. 19.4 and 19.5 present study results and discussion, respectively.

19.2   Study Design

This was a phase 1, open-label study of PF-05212384 administered once weekly as an IV infusion to subjects with solid tumors. The study was conducted in two parts: Part 1 was the MTD estimation phase, and was open to subjects with any solid tumor; Part 2 was the MTD confirmation phase, and was open to subjects with select tumor types that, based on preclinical considerations, were thought to be sensitive to the PI3K pathway, including breast, nonsmall cell lung, ovarian, endometrial, and colorectal cancer.

Part 1 of the study design utilized modified Continual Reassessment Method to determine the Maximum Tolerated Dose (MTD) of PF-05212384 to be taken further into confirmation part (Part 2). Target Dose Limiting Toxicity (DLT) rate was 25 %. The modified CRM algorithm utilized Bayesian methodology to consistently learn about dose–toxicity relationship after each cohort's DLT status became available. The algorithm operated on fine discrete dose grid consisting of 22 distinct doses: 10–319 mg in 20 % dose increments with two back-up doses of 6 and 8 mg in case of excessive toxicity at the starting 10 mg dose. The details of dose-escalation grid are given in Table 19.1. The algorithm was not allowed to skip more than three

Table 19.1 Dose grid utilized by CRM algorithm

Dose (mg)	Increment from prior dose (%) if the number of skipped doses is			
	0 (%)	1 (%)	2[a] (%)	3[a] (%)
10				
12	20			
14	20	44		
17	20	44	73	
21	20	44	73	107
25	20	44	73	107
30	20	44	73	107
36	20	44	73	107
43	20	44	73	107
52	20	44	73	107
62	20	44	73	107
74	20	44	73	107
89	20	44	73	107
107	20	44	73	107
128	20	44	73	107
154	20	44	73	107
185	20	44	73	107
222	20	44	73	107
266	20	44	73	107
319	20	44	73	107

[a]These dose escalations will not be allowed if two clinically significant grade 2 toxicities of the same type are seen in a cohort, or if one additional case of the same grade 2 toxicity or two other cases of clinically significant grade 2 toxicities of the same type are seen in the next cohort

doses in a single dose-escalation step which would roughly translate into no more than a doubling of the highest previously studied dose. Additional restrictions based on non-DLT toxicities are noted in footnotes of Table 19.1.

The relationship between the probability of DLT and dose was modeled using a binary endpoint ($Y = 1$: if DLT and $Y = 0$: if no DLT) and a one-parameter modified CRM model:

$$p_i = \Pr(Y = 1 \mid x_i; \beta) = f(x_i; \beta) = \left[\frac{1 + \tanh x_i}{2}\right]^{\beta}, i = 1, \ldots, 22 \qquad (19.1)$$

where the label for the dose that subject i receives is x_i, probability of DLT given that dose is p_i, and β is a parameter on which a prior distribution was placed at the beginning of the trial and later updated into a posterior distribution as the trial progressed. The actual amounts of active PF-05212384 doses corresponding to x_i's were 6, 8, 10, 12, ..., and 319 mg , respectively, as listed in Table 19.1. But the dosage strength in mg is not what was actually used in Eq. (19.1). In the latter, x_i refers to dose *labels*, i.e., the set of x_i, $i = 1, \ldots, 22$ obtained by solving (19.1) given $\beta = 1$ and user-supplied vector of p_i, $i = 1, \ldots, 22$ representing the "best guesses" of anticipated probabilities of DLT at each dose. Note: this approach is similar to the prior elicitation process of the original CRM method of Quigley et al. with the only difference that the function f in Eq. (19.1) was the power function (i.e., $p_i = x_i^{\beta}$) in the O'Quigly method. Since the user-supplied vector of $p_i, i = 1, \ldots 22$ "induces" the dose labels x_i, $i = 1 \ldots 22$ through the model (Eq. 19.1) relationship, this vector is often referred to as "skeleton" of the CRM reflecting that committing to it at the beginning of the trial is a fairly rigid assumption determining the shape of the model for the rest of trial, and consequently its performance.

The first cohort of patients was assigned to the starting dose of 10 mg. DLT assessment was performed after ~4 weeks of dosing. After the first cohort's DLT status update, the prior distribution of β was updated into a posterior distribution, defining a new set of toxicity probabilities p_i in model (19.1). The labels x_i, $i = 1, \ldots, 22$ in the model Eq. (19.1), once calculated at the beginning, remained the same throughout the trial. The current estimate of MTD would be the dose corresponding to $f^{-1}(0.25, \hat{\beta})$, given the posterior mean of β, and the next cohort dose assignment was chosen as the dose closest to this estimated MTD but not exceeding it. This process was iteratively continued until one of the stopping rules below was triggered:

1. Maximum sample size of 50 patients in Part 1 has been reached.
2. MTD has been identified with sufficient accuracy: 9 subjects have been accumulated on a dose that is currently estimated to be the MTD and there are at least 12 subjects overall enrolled in the trial.
3. Futility stop: all doses appear to be overly toxic (i.e., estimated Pr (DLT) > 25 % for the smallest dose) and the MTD cannot be determined in the current trial setting.

Starting from the second cohort and until the end of study, the above described modified CRM algorithm constantly incorporated additional information about dose–DLT relationship learned from the data via modeling and that was reflected on the projected MTD. By design, such dose allocation procedure was expected to cluster dose assignments around the dose that yielded approximately 25 % DLT rate.

Like any Bayesian method, the CRM might be sensitive to prior distribution placed on the model parameter β at the beginning of the study and the choice of "skeleton" $p_i, i = 1, \ldots, 22$. However, as the study progressed and the DLT data accumulated, it was expected to eventually overrule the prior information and the latter became less important. Furthermore, a non-informative prior distribution $\beta \sim \text{Unif}[0, 3]$ was used in this study. Through simulation, "skeleton" $p_i, i = 1, \ldots, 22$, representing a cautiously pessimistic DLT profile, was selected for this study to make the dose escalation more conservative. This profile assumed a 25 % DLT rate occurring at as low as 30 mg dose further increasing to 64 % at 154 mg dose.

Part 2 of this study was intended to confirm the safety and tolerability of the dose selected in Part 1, while assessing the antitumor activity of PF-05212384 in patients with solid tumors.

19.3   Overview of Simulation Setup and Results

Extensive simulations were performed to fine-tune the parameters of the modified CRM procedure and to study the operating characteristics of the chosen "best" CRM versus similar characteristics of the conventional 3 + 3 design. Those were summarized in detail in a study Simulation Report. Presenting all results and technical details here would not be feasible due to space limitation. We discuss only key setup features and findings.

The parameters explored to fine-tune the CRM included cohort size (2 or 3 subjects), CRM dose–toxicity model (power, 1-parameter logistic or *tanh*), maximum allowed dose increment between cohorts (3 or 4 doses), number of subjects on MTD to stop for success (6, 9, or 12 subjects), and prior information on toxicity (pessimistic vs. optimistic DLT profile).

Competing designs were evaluated against six different plausible scenarios of DLT profile varying in steepness of the dose–response curve and location of the true MTD within the dose range (Table 19.2). For each of the competing "variants" of CRM design, the key operating characteristics assessed were:

1. *Precision of MTD selection*: proportions of times when the dose selected as MTD had true DLT rate on-target, underestimated, overestimated, or NA were summarized. The four categories above were defined as follows:

   - On-Target MTD: selected dose produces 18–33 % true DLT rate.
   - Underestimated MTD: selected dose produces <18 % true DLT rate.
   - Overestimated MTD: selected dose produces >33 % true DLT rate.
   - N/A: trial stopped early for futility.

Note: the futility stop under the scenarios examined represents a false-negative decision because all six scenarios have at least one dose with $\Pr(\text{DLT}) \leq 0.25$.

Table 19.2 Dose–toxicity scenarios used in simulations and their respective target dose ranges

	Probability of DLT as a function of dose					
Dose	Sc. 1: MTD= 50 flat	Sc. 4: MTD= 40 steep	Sc. 2: MTD= 145 flat	Sc. 5: MTD= 135 steep	Sc. 3: MTD= 260 flat	Sc. 6: MTD= 210 steep
10 mg	0.15	0.14	0.00	0.01	0.00	0.00
12 mg	0.15	0.15	0.00	0.01	0.00	0.00
14 mg	0.16	0.15	0.00	0.01	0.00	0.00
17 mg	0.16	0.17	0.00	0.01	0.00	0.00
21 mg	0.17	**0.18**	0.00	0.01	0.00	0.00
25 mg	**0.19**	**0.20**	0.00	0.01	0.00	0.00
30 mg	**0.20**	**0.22**	0.00	0.01	0.00	0.00
36 mg	**0.22**	**0.26**	0.00	0.02	0.00	0.00
43 mg	**0.24**	**0.30**	0.00	0.02	0.01	0.01
52 mg	**0.27**	0.35	0.00	0.03	0.01	0.01
62 mg	**0.30**	0.42	0.00	0.04	0.01	0.01
74 mg	0.34	0.50	0.01	0.05	0.01	0.01
89 mg	0.40	0.60	0.02	0.08	0.01	0.02
107 mg	0.46	0.69	0.04	0.13	0.02	0.03
128 mg	0.52	0.78	0.10	**0.21**	0.03	0.04
154 mg	0.58	0.84	**0.26**	0.37	0.05	0.08
185 mg	0.63	0.87	0.47	0.57	0.09	0.15
222 mg	0.66	0.89	0.58	0.76	0.15	**0.31**
266 mg	0.68	0.90	0.61	0.86	**0.27**	0.55
319 mg	0.69	0.90	0.61	0.89	0.42	0.77

[a]Values in bold represent doses which deliver "acceptable" (18–33 %) DLT rates

[b]Scenarios are not named in consecutive order because initially only Scenarios 1–3 were considered. Their "steeper" version, i.e., Scenarios 4–6 were added later. For final results presentation it was chosen to group the dose–toxicity scenario by MTD location (low, middle, high) rather than number

2. *Design "cost"*: average trial duration (in weeks), average sample size, average number and proportion of subjects experiencing DLTs.

The two metrics of performance precision of MTD selection and design "cost" almost never pull the design choices in the same direction. More precision usually implies grater costs, so it is impossible to optimize the trial with respect to both. Conducting simulations and computing these metrics helped the team to quantify the trade-offs between precision of MTD selection and exposing more subjects to doses with higher toxicity levels, as well as trial duration. Competing variants of CRM design were chosen based on their performance with respect to the above operating characteristics under six scenarios in Table 19.2.

Among many design parameters examined, the stopping rule (number of subjects on MTD) had the most impact on the design's performance. As expected, increasing minimum number of subjects treated on MTD prior to stopping leads to a more precise MTD estimation; however this requirement would also lead to larger overall sample size, longer trial duration, and greater overall number of toxicities

Table 19.3 Operating characteristics of the CRM design versus conventional 3 + 3 design

| DLT sc. | Design | MTD dose selection decision (probability) | | | | Design "cost" | | | |
		Correct	Under	Over	NA[a]	Av. dur. (weeks)	Av. trial size	Num tox	Prop tox
1	3 + 3	0.330	0.393	0.089	0.187	23.0	17.3	3.7	0.25
	CRM	0.557	0.235	0.102	0.106	38.0	28.5	6.4	0.3
4	3 + 3	0.234	0.464	0.129	0.302	21.8	16.4	3.7	0.26
	CRM	0.643	0.185	0.082	0.089	38.7	29.0	7.0	0.3
2	3 + 3	0.352	0.601	0.048	0.000	48.9	36.7	3.8	0.10
	CRM	0.547	0.271	0.182	0.000	43.6	32.7	6.3	0.2
5	3 + 3	0.322	0.554	0.122	0.124	45.5	34.2	4.0	0.12
	CRM	0.468	0.289	0.244	0.000	44.4	33.3	6.4	0.2
3	3 + 3	0.257	0.692	0.000	0.050	55.9	41.9	2.9	0.07
	CRM	0.543	0.434	0.024	0.000	38.1	28.6	3.1	0.1
6	3 + 3	0.244	0.735	0.020	0.000	54.5	40.9	3.7	0.1
	CRM	0.349	0.588	0.063	0.000	40.6	30.4	4.8	0.2

[a]Trials with MTD not available (NA) were those where early "futility" stop was triggered (a false-negative conclusion) due to many toxicities observed at lower doses and trial not able to continue because all doses appeared to be overly toxic. This is more likely to occur in simulations due to high variability of binomial data with small samples rather than in real trial. In actual trial, the DLT data is collected rather than computer-generated; any extreme deviations from the expected values are examined on the basis of all safety information, so the trial is unlikely to be stopped based on DLT data alone

(but not necessarily the proportion of toxicities). Stopping rules with 6, 9, and 12 subjects on MTD were considered for this design and compared via simulations. Based on these results, it was decided that a stopping rule with nine subjects on the MTD provided the best trade-off between MTD precision and trial duration/toxicities. Other parameters chosen for the final "best" CRM design variant were cohort size 3, *tanh* toxicity model, and pessimistic DLT profile. This particular CRM variant was also compared to the traditional 3 + 3 design via simulations using the same metrics. The 3 + 3 design used in simulations was similar to the one described in Ji and Wang (2013) as 3 + 3^L design; the stopping rule of nine subjects on MTD was not implemented for the latter since the 3 + 3 design is not capable of accumulating that many subjects on any given dose by the way of its construction. Also, since the 3 + 3 design is not capable of skipping doses, the dose grid for 3 + 3 design was modified to resemble the modified Fibonacci sequence rather than fine grid of CRM. All dose–toxicity curves utilized in simulations were the same for both designs.

Based on these simulations, the selected "best" CRM variant provided, on average, a more accurate estimate of MTD than the 3 + 3 design, with comparable overall proportion of toxicities (<30 %). These results are presented in Table 19.3.

In all six scenarios, CRM identified MTD dose with target range of toxicity more frequently than the 3 + 3 design, with degree of "superiority" varying significantly depending on the scenario: best performance was 41 % advantage over 3 + 3 for Scenario 4 and the worst performance was for Scenario 6 with only 10 % advantage over 3 + 3 design. Other scenarios had 14–29 % advantage of CRM over 3 + 3 design in percentage of identifying the MTD correctly. Poor performance of Scenario 6 compared to Scenario 3 (both have similar profiles but one is steeper than the other) is probably due to the fact that the "true" MTD was at the end of the dose range and had toxicity rate 31 %: while still "acceptable" by the target range defined (i.e., 18–33 %), it was dangerously close to the unacceptable 33 % level resulting in more toxicities and possibly pushing the estimated MTD to the dose immediately below the true MTD. This is reflected by higher proportion of toxicities observed in CRM design under Scenario 6 (20 %) versus those observed under Scenario 3 (10 %) and higher number of times the MTD was underestimated under Scenario 6 as compared to Scenario 3 (58 vs. 43 %, respectively).

The number/proportions of toxicities observed in simulated trials were consistently slightly higher with CRM design (for all six scenarios) as compared to the 3 + 3 design, although still clinically acceptable. This observation is closely related to the higher percentages of MTD underestimated with 3 + 3 design because the latter frequently stops at lower than MTD doses.

With respect to the number of subjects (and resulting trial duration), the advantages of CRM became more prominent as the true MTD location moved from beginning of dose range to the end. For Scenarios 1 and 4 with "low" MTD location, the CRM design actually required more subjects than 3 + 3 (but that's the cost of added information). For Scenarios 2 and 5, the numbers of subjects were similar. Finally, for Scenarios 3 and 6 ("high" MTD location), the CRM design showed clear advantage over 3 + 3 design in average sample size to declare MTD. Scenarios 1 and 4 had many "competing" MTD doses and had to do more work differentiating between them while some of these doses were not available to the 3 + 3 design due to modified dose space mentioned earlier. These differences faded out for scenarios with mid- and high-MTD location (2 and 5, 3, and 6). These " competing doses" explain why CRM actually required more subjects than 3 + 3 in case of Scenarios 1 and 4 ("low" MTD).

To further take advantage of flexibility of the CRM design, cohort sizes of two and four patients were allowed in the actual trial. The maximum sample size of 50 was set for Part 1 of the study based on budgetary consideration as well as simulated average sample sizes from Table 19.3. The sample size of Part 2 was based on clinical considerations rather than statistical rationale.

19.3.1 Model Change Mid-trial

At some point during the trial, six cohorts had been assigned to doses up to and including 266 mg. The observed toxicity of PF-05212384 appeared to be lower than expected at the time of study design. Based on limited toxicity observed, it appeared quite likely that the algorithm would need to further escalate from 266 mg, raising a concern of potentially not having enough doses since 266 mg was already close to the maximum dose of 319 mg. To address this concern, the CRM model was updated to include dosing beyond 319 mg and the study protocol was amended.

The new model dropped the lower doses of 6 and 8 mg (there was no data on it, the lowest dose studied was 10 mg) and added four doses above 319 mg in 20 % increments: 383, 460, 552, and 662 mg, resulting in new dose range consisting of 24 doses: [10–662 mg]. The new model essentially assumed the same pessimistic DLT profile as the original model by utilizing the same "skeleton" of DLT probabilities $p_i, i = 1, \ldots, 22$ as the original model but shifted to the right. Specifically, the initial DLT rates for [6–319 mg] dose range in original model were shifted to become initial DLT rates for dose range [14–662 mg] in the new model. The remaining low doses 10 and 12 mg were assumed very low toxicity rates under the new model. Other aspects of the new model were the same as the original model. A new set of simulations was run to evaluate performance of the new model; the results were acceptable.

19.4 Study Results

A total of 78 patients were enrolled in the study and 77 received treatment with PF-05212384 (Part 1 and Part 2 combined). The MTD determination was based on 45 evaluable patients in Part 1 and concluded with 154 mg dose declared to be the MTD. This data was presented in Tabernero et al. (2011). At the conclusion of Part 1, additional 30 patients were enrolled in Part 2 to confirm tolerability and to perform preliminary efficacy assessment of the MTD found in Part 1 (i.e., 154 mg dose). We will refer to these additional 30 patients as a confirmation cohort. The size of confirmation cohort (30 patients) was driven not only by MTD confirmation objective, but also by a strong consideration for preliminary efficacy exploration. There were actually two cohorts in Part 2 for slightly different purposes: molecular selection cohort and tumor biopsy cohort; details of efficacy exploration are beyond the scope of this chapter. Twenty-eight out of 30 patients enrolled in confirmation cohort were evaluable for DLT at the end of Part 2. Because of the additional efficacy objective of Part 2 (evaluating preliminary antitumor activity in patients with specific cancers), the population of confirmation cohort (specific cancers) was slightly different from that of the Part 1 (all-comers). The main purpose of having a Part 2 was to confirm findings of Part 1 with respect to tolerability of PF-05212384 and not to further adjust or "refine" the MTD found in Part 1.

A summary of the Part 1 dose-escalation progress including number of evaluable patients and observed toxicities is given in Table 19.4 and Fig. 19.1. Table 19.4 also reports MTD candidate dose as estimated by CRM model, CRM-recommended dose assignment and the actual dose assigned to the next cohort following clinical review of all data. The first five cohorts were evaluated using the original CRM model; the remaining data (cohorts 6–12) was analyzed using the revised CRM model (see Sect. 19.3.1 for model change rationale).

Table 19.4 Part 1 dose recommendation and selection

Cohort	Dose (mg)	Evaluable patients	Patients with DLTs	CRM-estimated MTD (mg)	Next dose recommended by CRM (mg)	Next dose assigned (mg)
1	10	4	0	222	21	21
2	21	4	0	266	43	43
3	43	3	0	266	89	89
4	89	4	0	266	*185*	154[a]
5	154	4	0	266	266	266[b]
6	266	4	1	383	*383*	*319[c]*
7	319	4	2	266	266	266
8	266	4	2	222	222	222
9	222	2	1	222	222	222
10	*222*	*4*	*4*	*128*	*128*	*154[d]*
11	154	4	0	154	154	154
12	154	4	1	154	154	NA[e]

[a]Out of caution: 154 mg was maximum allowed at the time
[b]Model switch occurred after this cohort
[c]Other (non-DLT) AE's and investigators' input
[d]Based on cohort 5 (154 mg) safety results
[e]154 mg declared MTD, part 1 concluded

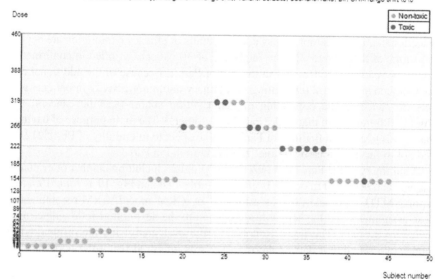

Fig. 19.1 Part 1 allocation and toxicity

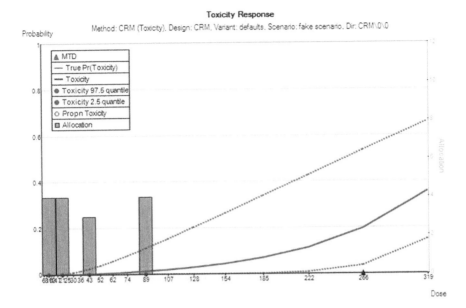

Fig. 19.2 Allocation and toxicity after cohort #4

19.4.1   Clean Versus Interim Data

The numbers of evaluable patients in Table 19.4 were based on communication with investigators at the time of review. After the study was completed and the data cleaned, the numbers of evaluable patients changed slightly. Specifically, the database reported that there were 3 (instead of 4) and 5 (instead of 4) evaluable patients in cohorts 1 and 10, respectively. The number of DLTs in the above cohorts remained unchanged from interim to final study data. These slight differences were not unexpected, as it happens with many interim decisions based on not "perfectly clean data." However, they did not affect the final MTD determination: additional sensitivity analysis comparing the two dose-escalating paths between interim data versus final study data was performed. That analysis demonstrated that 154 mg still remained the final estimate of MTD following 12 cohorts, based on the clean data used (results not shown). For simplicity, we present only the results based on interim data for Part 1, as it was done during the dose-escalation process. Cumulative study results (Part 1 and Part 2 combined) are based on the final clean study data.

19.4.2   CRM Progression Through Part 1

A detailed step-by-step illustration of how CRM model was performing dose assignments in Part 1 is given in Figs. 19.2, 19.3, 19.4, 19.5, 19.6, and 19.7. At each step, a Bayesian model described in Sect. 19.2 was fitted to all data available at that point

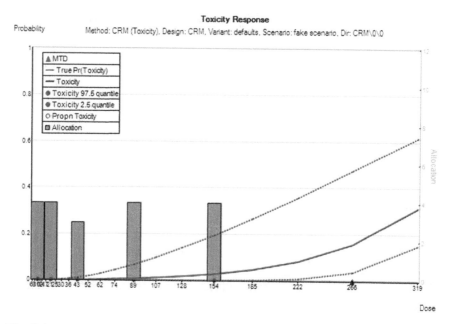

Fig. 19.3 Allocation and toxicity after cohort #5

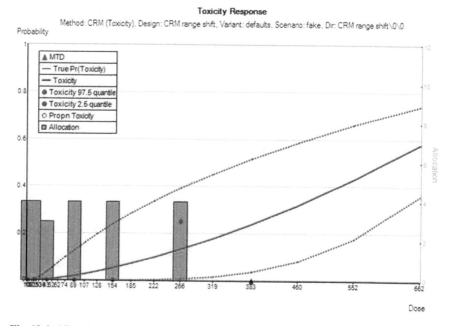

Fig. 19.4 Allocation and toxicity after cohort #6 (using new model)

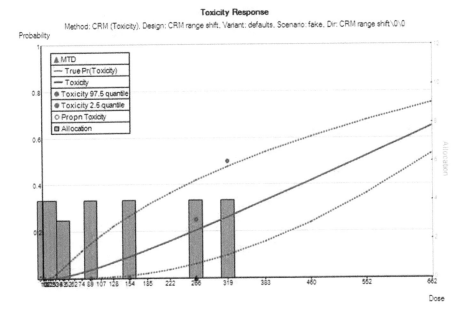

Fig. 19.5 Allocation and toxicity after cohort #7

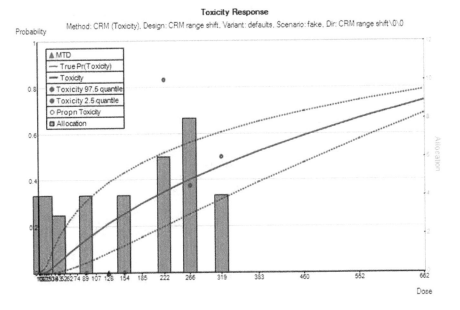

Fig. 19.6 Allocation and toxicity after cohort #10

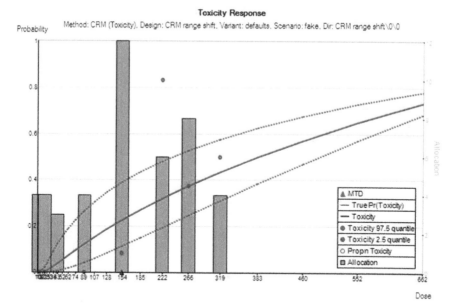

Fig. 19.7 Allocation and toxicity after cohort # 12 (end of part 1)

and the MTD was estimated according to that model. The next dose recommended was the one closest to the estimated MTD but below it. This is the dose reported in Table 19.4 as "CRM-estimated MTD." The "below-MTD" restriction makes the CRM algorithm more conservative in terms of safety (albeit less precise in some cases) than the one aiming at the dose simply "closest to MTD."

As can be seen from the early trial data (cohorts 1–5 in Table 19.4 and Figs. 19.2 and 19.3), the model-based MTD estimates could be quite misleading when no toxicities are observed. In our trial, the first five cohorts resulted in an estimated MTD substantially above its true value as well as the current dose being studied. This is a well-known concern associated with the classical CRM procedure (i.e., unrestricted dose escalation). In such cases, the "4 steps maximum" rule of the modified CRM procedure (described in Sect. 19.2) was activated resulting in the recommended dose being no more than a double of the previously studied dose. This rule explains substantial differences between "estimated MTD" and "recommended dose" columns of Table 19.4 for cohorts #1–5. In addition to the algorithm build-in "safety net" of maximum ~100 % dose increment mentioned above, the investigators and sponsor always had the option to override the CRM-recommended next dose suggestion based on aggregate data safety review. This situation had occurred three times during Part 1 of the trial, as can be seen from footnotes in Table 19.1. Brief descriptions of dose assignment "override" and underlying reasons are given below:

1. *After cohort #4 (89 mg dose)*, there were no toxicities observed in the trial and the CRM-recommended dose for the next cohort was 185 mg. However, a dose one step below it—the 154 mg dose—was chosen out of caution based on sponsor's

judgment and protocol criteria stating that 154 mg must be evaluated prior to assigning patients to higher doses. The 154 mg maximum dose restriction in the protocol was originally attributed to formulation impurity issue. The latter was cleared a long time before cohort #4 review was conducted, but the team felt that 154 mg was close enough to the recommended 185 mg dose and more cautious dose assignment would be best in that situation since 185 mg was already quite high compared to the starting dose of 10 mg.

2. *After cohort #6 (266 mg dose)* with one patient out of four experiencing DLT on the 266 mg dose, the CRM recommended the dose of 383 mg as the next cohort's assignment. However, there were some grade 2 toxicities seen in cohort #6, which influenced the sponsors and investigators decision to override the algorithm's recommendation and proceed with a lower dose of 319 mg for the next cohort.

3. *After cohort #10 (222 mg)*, with 4/4 DLTs experienced at the 222 mg dose, the CRM suggested 128 mg as the next dose assignment. This substantial dose reduction recommendation can be explained by high toxicity rates observed in the previous three cohorts, which reshaped the dose–toxicity model substantially, as can be seen from Fig. 19.6. Based on cumulative safety review, however, the sponsor and investigators felt that the dose 154 g would be more appropriate assignment than 128 mg since it was studied before with no DLTs observed and overall acceptable safety profile. This decision to implement a more aggressive dose escalation rather than the one suggested by CRM is rather unusual, especially in light of 100 % toxicity rate observed at the current dose (222 mg). At that point the trial was over 50 % of maximum planned enrollment (37 out of 50 patients enrolled) with no good MTD candidate available: every dose with acceptable DLT rate had no more than four patients on it while, per protocol, a nine patient minimum was needed to declare a dose to be an MTD. At that point, selecting 154 mg—a dose one step above the recommended 128 mg and having good safety profile based on earlier cohort's data—seemed a reasonable compromise between following CRM's recommendation and maximizing the trial's chance to find the MTD without exceeding the maximum number of patients.

Following data review from cohort #10, four more patients were assigned to the 154 mg dose in cohort #11; there were no DLTs observed at that dose leading to the next dose assignment (cohort #12) to be the 154 mg dose again. One out of four DLTs were observed in cohort #12. At that point, the 154 mg dose had 12 patients (three cohorts) assigned to it with model-based estimated toxicity probability of 0.225. This estimate was the closest to the target 0.25 but still below. The combination of toxicity estimate at 154 mg with three cohorts assigned to it had triggered a stopping rule described in Sect. 19.2 (at least nine subjects on dose estimated to be the MTD) and the CRM algorithm declared 154 mg as MTD. The total sample size at that point was 45 evaluable patients: just five patients short of the maximum planned trial size for Part 1. A decision was made to proceed with Part 2 of the trial.

At the end of Part 1, the raw proportion of toxicities observed at the MTD was only 0.083 (1/12 DLTs). The corresponding model-based estimate of DLT rate at MTD was 0.225 with 95 % Credible Interval of (0.112, 0.3892) (Fig. 19.7).

Table 19.5 Number of dose-limiting toxicities by dose level based on final study data (parts 1 and 2 combined)

Dose level (mg)	No. of patients	No. of DLT evaluable patients	No. of toxicities	Proportion of DLTs	Model-based probability of DLTs
10	4	3	0	0	0
21	4	4	0	0	0
43	4	3	0	0	0.010
89	4	4	0	0	0.054
154[a]	42	40	2	0.050	0.132
222	7	7	5	0.714	0.215
226	8	8	3	0.375	0.270
319	4	4	2	0.500	0.332

[a]The numbers presented for 154 mg dose are comprised of 1/12 DLTs observed in part 1 and 1/28 DLTs observed in part 2

The higher model-based estimates reflect toxicities observed at doses above the MTD therefore adjusting the estimate upward from the raw observed toxicity rate. As can be also seen from Fig. 19.7, the overall fit of one-parameter CRM model to Part 1 study data was quite poor, resulting in the credible interval at 154 mg not containing the empirical estimate. This property of 1-parameter CRM model is well known and not surprising, prompting a question of whether a richer model (e.g., a 2-parameter logistic model) should have been used. We will return to this discussion in Sect. 19.5.

19.4.3 Final Study Results (Part 1 and Part 2)

The toxicity data observed at 154 mg in Part 2 were generally consistent with the results of Part 1. There were 28 more patients treated at the MTD and evaluable for DLT in Part 2. One out of these patients experienced a DLT resulting in 0.036 estimated probability of DLT at 154 mg based on Part 2 data. Since safety profiles of 154 mg dose appeared generally consistent between Part 1 and Part 2 of the study, it was decided that it was appropriate to pool the Part 1 and confirmation cohort data to present the overall results.

The observed proportion of DLTs at 154 mg dose at the end of the trial was 0.050 (2/40) with 95 % Confidence Interval of (0.014, 0.165) based on Wilson method. Details of the estimated probability of toxicity by dose are given in Table 19.5. Slight differences between number of evaluable patients in Tables 19.4 and 19.5 are attributable to differences between interim and final study data. Both raw proportion of toxicity and model-based estimate of toxicity at the MTD consistently point out that the underlying true DLT rate at 154 mg dose is likely to be below the target rate of 18–33 %. However, the next higher studied dose (i.e., 222 mg) had an alarmingly high raw DLT rate of 71 %. Despite the model-based estimate of 21.5 % DLT rate at that dose which takes into account the effect of an outlier, it is hard to ignore the actual observed toxicity rate almost twice as high as the 18–33 % range that clinicians

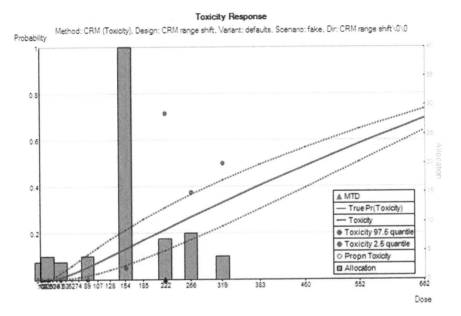

Fig. 19.8 Allocation and toxicity at the end of the study (part 1 and part 2 combined)

prespecified as "acceptable." Although it is possible that the observation of 5/7 DLTs on 222 mg was an overestimate of the actual true underlying DLT rate, it is hard to imagine that a dose with such toxicity profile would be selected as MTD even if model-based estimates suggest such a decision (Table 19.5). Model-based analysis was never prespecified in the protocol for final decision making; it was meant only to guide the dose-escalation decisions. In fact, it should be noted that the fit of one-parameter CRM model using the final study data is quite poor (Fig. 19.8), so any inferences based on that fit should be interpreted with caution. The poor fit issue is a well-known property of one-parameter CRM, so that finding is not surprising. These models are designed to "converge" to MTD, not to provide overall good description of dose–toxicity relationship. Based on all considerations above, no adjustment to MTD determination was made at the conclusion of Part 2 and 154 mg dose remained the final MTD estimate.

19.4.4 Sensitivity Analysis: Effects of Mid-trial CRM Model Adjustment

As was explained in Sect. 19.3.1, the CRM model had to be adjusted after cohort 5 to allow the possibility of including doses above 319 mg. Even though, in retrospect, such adjustment could have been avoided, at the time of cohort 5 data review, the

Table 19.6 Sensitivity analysis: dose-escalation decisions based on original vs. adjusted models

Cohort	Dose (mg)	Next dose recommended based on	
		Original CRM model[a]	Adjusted CRM model[b]
6	266	266	383
7	319	266	266
8	266	222	222
9	222	222	222
10	222	154	128
11	154	185	154
12	154	185	154

[a]Post hoc sensitivity analysis
[b]Actually used during trial

algorithm appeared to be escalating doses quite rapidly. The dose had been doubled four times already with no DLT observed, cohort 6 had been assigned 266 mg, and there was no way to accurately predict how high a dose needs to be pushed in order to get into MTD proximity range. If no DLTs were observed at 266 mg in cohort 6, further dose escalation would have put the next cohort at 319 mg. And if that were in fact a true MTD, the CRM algorithms were known from simulation experience to perform suboptimally in such scenarios because it was never "allowed to look" above the MTD to accurately estimate it. So, based on *partial* trial data (cohorts 1–5) available at that time, it seemed unavoidable that the MTD would be closer to 266–319 mg range than originally believed, thus necessitating the model change with dose expansion as a precaution. After the model change was implemented though (starting with cohort 6), the actual dose-escalation path never rose above 319 mg, prompting a natural question: what would have happened had we not adjusted the model?

Since the maximum dose studied in the trial was 319 mg, the trial data can still be fitted into the old CRM model as a sensitivity analysis. A comparison of dose-escalation paths between original versus adjusted models is given in Table 19.6. With a couple of exceptions, the impact of the new model on the dose-escalation path was minimal (as expected; the two models weren't very different after all). This statement has some limitation since the data was "retrofitted" into the old CRM model, i.e., its dose assignment recommendation was not followed because a different model was in place. Such comparison is furthermore confounded by presence of human oversight potentially overriding dose recommendations based on either model. So we may never know what would have truly happened had we not adjusted the model. We may only look at the final fit based on the two models and compare Part 1 MTD recommendations. This comparison is presented in Fig. 19.9 (original model—top, adjusted model—bottom); differences in available dose ranges reflect different dose spaces of each model. *Note: because CRM model is highly dependent on the initial "skeleton" of doses, it cannot be easily extrapolated beyond the originally selected dose range, thus resulting in a "truncated" graph on top. For the purpose of looking at both plots under the same scale, the dose range for both plots was chosen to be 10–662 mg (adjusted model) but the original model plot can be populated with data only up to 319 mg dose.*

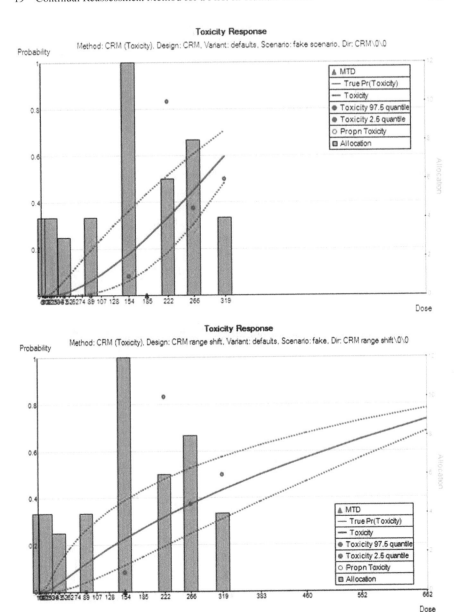

Fig. 19.9 Model sensitivity analysis: comparison of fitted toxicity at the end of part 1 using old model vs. new model. *Note*: *Top graph* represents old model (original dose range); bottom graph represents new model (expanded dose range)

As can be seen from Table 19.6 and Fig. 19.9, the final MTD recommendation at the end of Part 1 based on the original CRM model would have been 185 mg dose, not 154 mg dose. Perhaps having more data on 185 mg could provide additional insight into dose–DLT relationship and possibly yielded a MTD candidate dose with toxicity rate closer to 18–33 % target. But this was not pursued for a number of reasons.

At the time the MTD recommendation was made, the trial had reached nearly maximum sample size of 50 patients for Part 1. Considering a hypothetical scenario of overriding CRM's MTD recommendation after cohort 12 and continuing the trial, only five patients would have been left to enroll in Part 1 at 185 mg according to the study protocol. DLT data based on five patients at 185 mg would have provided only a "candidate" MTD dose at best. Since that dose had not been studied before, at least three additional cohorts would be required to achieve a minimum of nine patients on MTD—a criterion used by CRM algorithm to provide a reliable estimate. We use "reliable" here in a relative sense: compared to six patients necessary for the 3 + 3 design to declare MTD, nine patients provide more information, but it is by no means a "rule of thumb" or a guarantee of precision. Furthermore, in the light of extremely high toxicity rate observed at next higher dose (222 mg), more than nine patient data most likely would have been required to be collected at 185 mg dose in order to potentially recommend it for Phase 2, even under the ideal case scenario of the empirical DLT rate estimate being within the target 18–33 % range (e.g., 2 out of 9 DLTs or 22 % rate observed at 185 mg). Having additional cohorts enrolled to properly study 185 mg would require extending Part 1 trial size beyond the originally planned 50 patients and would have pushed back the study timelines significantly. Continuing the trial with only five additional patients would raise a risk of having an inconclusive Part 1.

The proximity of potential MTD candidate doses (184 mg is a 20 % increment from 154 mg) coupled with concern of not having convincing data on 185 mg weighted against tight study timelines has led the study team to the decision to accept CRM's recommendation for MTD after cohort #12 and to stop Part 1 of the study. This decision was consistent with study protocol (based on the adjusted model). This sensitivity analysis utilizing original model is presented here only as a post hoc assessment in order to gain more insight into how CRM worked. All trial conclusions are reported based on the adjusted model that was in place at the time the trial concluded.

19.5 Discussion

We have presented a story of an adaptive trial design and implementation for a first-in-human dose-escalation application in oncology. This study was the first of its kind designed and implemented within the company. As with every pilot project, there was no prior experience with such trials. Extensive planning was undertaken prior to implementation of the protocol in an attempt to foresee all likely hurdles. Despite very extensive planning, unexpected surprises still emerged. The biggest one was the need to adjust the CRM model mid-way through the trial. This was precisely the situation that the design team was trying to avoid: since CRM algorithm is known to be "inflexible" with respect to dose space changes, the very wide dose range of 10–319 mg was chosen for the original CRM model despite some internal critics saying that "it will never go as far as 319 mg." No one could predict at the design stage that a dose range increase would be necessary—otherwise the maximum dose would have been set higher. But in reality the DLT profile did not appear as planned. Even though, in retrospect, one could have stayed with the original model, the latter option appeared to be too risky at the time model adjustment decision was made. Another surprising part was the sharp increase in the probability of DLT with dose in the actual DLT profile observed. Small number of patients studied at each dose (except for MTD) allows little opportunity to guess whether that was an artifact of random variability or true DLT profile. In either case, this was not planned for in the simulations.

For dose–toxicity scenarios with sharp rise in toxicity like this one, a different type of model (e.g., 2-parameter logistic such as the one described in Neuenschwander et al. 2008) could have provided a better fit. The 2-parameter logistic model is more flexible and therefore capable of more realistic representation of the dose–toxicity relationship. It also allows for more accurate prediction of probability of overdose at the next dose assignment rather than relying on a purely empirical rule of restricting the number of steps that CRM can skip. With respect to overdosing, the method of Neuenschwander et al. (2008) is similar in spirit to Escalation with Overdose Control (EWOC) method of Babb et al (1998). They utilize a variation of Bayesian decision-theoretic approach (Whitehead and Brunier 1995; Haines et al. 2003) to target certain prespecified toxicity rate while the probability of overdosing is controlled. One common reason why one-parameter CRM models like the one we used is preferred over more flexible models is its parsimony: intuitively, estimating one parameter requires less data than estimating two parameters resulting in a smaller faster trials (one would hope). This trial actually can serve as an example that this is not always the case. With limited CRM case studies available in literature to date, it is hard to say whether 2-parameter models should be used routinely instead of the original CRM model. But they definitely should be considered when evaluating candidate designs for Phase 1 oncology trials. The trade-off between parsimony and precision can be evaluated on a case-by-case basis.

19.5.1 Algorithmic Decisions Versus Human Oversight

At all times during the trial a joint oversight committee consisting of sponsor clinicians and statisticians was in place to monitor the dose-escalation process. Study investigator's input was solicited on as-needed basis to support dose-escalation decisions. In three instances, the oversight committee had "overruled" the dose assigned by CRM to the next cohort. In 2 out of these 3 cases (cohort #4 and #6, i.e., relatively early in trial) the overrule decision was more conservative than CRM out of caution. In the third case of cohort #10, the "override" decision was rather unusual to implement a dose escalation slightly more aggressive than the one recommended by CRM algorithm. This was done because sufficient safety data had been accumulated at that point on the higher dose in question. All investigators supported that decision.

The need for such human oversight and the situations where it disagrees with a computer-recommended dose are reflection of the fact that CRM model has its limits on accurately predicting the MTD in all situations. CRM operates strictly based on binary data (DLT or no-DLT) and a rather restrictive one-parameter model. The latter is not well suited to describe all the complexities of dose–DLT relationships, not to mention more sophisticated dose–toxicity relationship incorporating multiple grades of adverse experiences, PK/PD information, etc. In other words, in all three situations of "deviation" described, the CRM method was essentially "blind" to additional safety info such as lower grade toxicities and PK/PD information. Without making the design's mathematical model overly complicated, that kind of information could only be incorporated in dose-escalation decisions by a human review performed *in conjunction* with CRM recommendations.

While human oversight is necessary, it can also be a limiting factor in interpreting final study results: the rules of oversight cannot be simulated and, since the actually implemented CRM-with-oversight procedure tends to be more conservative than the "optimal " CRM simulated, the advantages of CRM itself become less clear.

19.5.2   A Few Notes on Study logistics

A lot of research and planning were done prior to the protocol approval, contributing to approximately 2 months of additional development time. Most of that extra time was spent on designing the trial (including extensive simulations, fine-tuning the design through multiple iterations with team, and summarizing it all in the simulation report). Considerable time was spent on educating study investigators and their sites about new methodology in order to secure Investigational Review Board approvals. Following the protocol approval, most of the study logistics remained the same as for the 3 + 3 type of trials with perhaps the only overhead additional cost of custom-programming and User Acceptance Testing of the CRM allocation software (to perform actual dose assignments rather than simulations). Programming of the above software was contracted to the outside vendor (Tessella Inc). Tessella also co-developed Adaptive Design Explorer (ADE) software in collaboration with the sponsor. All simulations and graphs presented in this chapter were generated using ADE, which is an internal proprietary software within Pfizer. However, its core CRM algorithm (called BCRM (2005)) used for simulating this design is publicly available at MD Anderson Cancer center Software Download website: https://bio-statistics.mdanderson.org/SoftwareDownload/SingleSoftware.aspx?Software_Id=15.

It is estimated that availability of such powerful computational tool capable not only of simulating the CRM algorithm (which is not a very complicated task to program by itself) but also of organizing multiple scenarios, design variants, outputs, etc. had considerably reduced the trial planning timelines. The authors believe that planning and executing future adaptive trials similar to this one will take considerably shorter time because of the experience gained in this trial. This applies not just to design development but internal company review cycles: as the teams gain more experience with adaptive Phase 1 dose-escalation trials, such trials are viewed as less and less "daunting."

19.5.3 CRM Performance and Study Conclusions

At first glance, the final study results may look somewhat disappointing since the MTD appeared to be underestimated. When planning the very first adaptive trial it is only natural to hope for the outcome to be very much consistent with the "best case" scenario studied in simulations, i.e., deliver an MTD within 18–33 % range and possibly even close to 25 %. That's what this trial was designed to do, after all. At the end of the day, though, it is important to remember that the broader trial's objectives go beyond finding an MTD that delivers precisely 18–33 % DLT rate—the latter is simply an agreed-upon criterion we used to evaluate simulated performance. This trial was declared a success at the end because the MTD it found was very well tolerated and also showed some evidence of preliminary clinical activity. The PK/PD information (data not shown) was also supportive of 154 mg choice. By the time the confirmation cohort was completed, the MTD lower-than-targeted DLT rate became pretty evident. But because every dose above it had unacceptably high DLT rate (especially 222 mg—the next higher dose with 71 % observed DLT rate), there was really no choice other than to accept 154 mg as MTD or amend the protocol and continue the study beyond planned size to evaluate other intermediate doses. The latter was not considered to be a good option based on a trade-off of additional information/knowledge to be potentially gained versus additional resources invested.

The CRM algorithms seemed to do its job right, given the circumstances, but raised the question of whether the doses preplanned for the trial were right. In terms of the dose range, the answer to that question is probably "No," as evidenced by the need to change the model midway through trial. As for the dose grid, the 20 % increments seemed to be adequate: anything less than that would not generate a sufficiently different exposure from the PK/PD perspective. Looking at the final study data presented in Table 19.5, the most glaring difference in toxicity rates between two adjacent doses studied is between 154 and 222 mg (5 vs. 71.4 %, respectively). These two doses are separated by ~40 % increment. Had an intermediate dose of 185 mg been studied (185 mg is a 20 % increment from 154 mg), the toxicity "gap" probably would not be so huge and the dose grid based on 20 % increments would be adequate. The reason 185 mg was not studied is likely to be attributed to mid-trial shift in the CRM model, which altered estimated toxicity probabilities at each dose for cohorts #6 and beyond.

Another important point we would like to highlight is the difference between a single clinical trial experiment and the simulation experiment. While planning the trial, we simulated 5,000 trials for each of the six "hypothetical" scenarios we had to assume. The resulting choices of design parameters were based on the assumption that all six were equally likely. In reality we got a chance to run only one trial under the "true" scenario which may be different from what we hypothesized (we will never know for sure). One may hope that the results of this "one trial realization" of the simulation experiment will be consistent with "average "simulation performance, but unfortunately it is an unrealistic expectation.

Looking back to simulation results in Table 19.3 in Sect. 19.3, six dose–toxicity scenarios were considered in simulations for the original model. The actual observed toxicity profile was somewhat similar to Sc. 3 and Sc. 6. For both scenarios, the simulated chances of underestimating the MTD were pretty high: 43–59 % under the original model and 44–64 % under the new model. So what we are seeing in this trial is hardly a surprise considering the similarities between these scenarios and the observed data. In other words, the scenario observed was the least favorable for CRM among the six considered in a sense that CRM was least tailored to perform well in it.

Taking this into perspective, we would like to reiterate that when we perform simulations and evaluate their performance, we focus on a narrow set of criteria and rules to make the problem "manageable." However, in real life, the "performance" means a complex set of parameters, variables, etc. to assess benefit and risk, which goes beyond precision of MTD estimation. While this design did not deliver an MTD with range of toxicity of 18–33 % (which it was designed to do), it did deliver a well-tolerated dose. The PK/PD information observed (data not shown) was supportive of that choice as well. The overall proportion of toxicities in the trial was 24 % (11/45)—well in line with what clinicians consider acceptable and demonstrating that this "modified" version of the CRM is quite safe in protecting the patients from overly aggressive dose escalation. The precise dose–DLT relationship may never be known. The real measure of this trial's performance will be the overall development program success/failure (i.e., how well the selected dose will perform in Phase 2 trials and whether Phase 1 dose selection played a role in that).

Acknowledgements The authors sincerely thank Michael Krams for his pioneering work in making this adaptive trial happen; Vlad Dragalin and Amar Sharma for their instrumental help in designing this trial; Tom Parke for guidance with software; Charles Zacharchuk and Robert Millham for their leadership role in executing this trial; and Stephanie Green for careful review of the manuscript and insightful feedback.

References

Babb JS, Rogatko A, Zacks S (1998) Cancer phase I clinical trials: efficient dose escalation with overdose control. Stat Med 17:1103–1120

BCRM (2005) BCRM: bivariate continual reassessment method. Version 113. Department of Biostatistics, The University of Texas MD Anderson Cancer Center, Houston, TX

Braun TM (2002) The bivariate continual reassessment method: extending the CRM to phase I trials of two competing outcomes. Control Clin Trials 23:240–256

Cheung YK (2011) Dose finding by the continual reassessment method. Chapman and Hall, New York

Cheung YK, Chappell R (2000) Sequential designs for phase I clinical trials with late-onset toxicities. Biometrics 56:1177–1182

Gezmu M, Flournoy N (2006) Group up-and-down designs for dose-finding. J Stat Plan Inference 136:1749–1764

Goodman S, Zahurak ML, Piantadosi S (1995) Some practical improvements in the continual reassessment method for phase I studies. Stat Med 14:1149–1161

Haines LM, Perevozskaya I, Rosenberger WF (2003) Bayesian optimal designs for phase I clinical trials. Biometrics 59:591–600

Neuenschwander B, Branson M, Gsponer T (2008) Critical aspects of the Bayesian approach to phase I cancer trials. Stat Med 27:2420–2439

O'Quigly J, Pepe M, Fisher L (1990) Continual reassessment method: a practical design for phase I clinical trials in cancer. Biometrics 46:33–48

O'Quigly J, Conaway M (2010) Continual reassessment method and related dose-finding designs. Stat Sci 25:202–216

Rosenberger WF, Haines LM (2002) Competing designs for phase I clinical trials: a review. Stat Med 21:2757–2770

Tabernero J, Bell-McGuinn K, Spicer J, Bendell J, Molina J, Kwak E, Millham R, Houk B, Borzillo G, Shapiro G (2011) First-in-patient study of PF-05212384, a small molecule intravenous dual inhibitor of PI3K and mTOR in patients with advanced cancer: update on safety, efficacy, and pharmacology [abstract]. In: Proceedings of the AACR-NCI-EORTC international conference: molecular targets and cancer therapeutics 12–16 Nov 2011, San Francisco, CA. AACR, Philadelphia, PA. Mol Cancer Ther 10(11 Suppl):Abstract nr. A167

Tourneau C, Lee JJ, Siu LL (2009) Dose escalation methods in phase I cancer clinical trials. J Natl Cancer Inst 101(10):708–720

Whitehead J, Brunier H (1995) Bayesian decision procedures for dose determining experiments. Stat Med 14:885–893

Woodcock J, Woosley R (2008) The FDA critical path initiative and its influence on new drug development. Ann Rev Med 59, doi:0.1146/annurev.med.59.09056.155819

Ji Y, Wang SJ (2013) Modified toxicity probability interval design: a safer and more reliable method than the 3 + 3 design for practical phase I trials. J Clin Oncol 10:1785–1791

Yuan Y, Yin G (2008) Sequential continual reassessment method for two-dimensional dose finding. Stat Med 27:5664–5678

Chapter 20
Practical Considerations for a Two-Stage Confirmatory Adaptive Clinical Trial Design and Its Implementation: ADVENT Trial

Pravin R. Chaturvedi, Zoran Antonijevic, and Cyrus Mehta

Abstract In this chapter, we provide the details of an innovative two-stage, seamless adaptive clinical trial called ADVENT. This trial was conducted as a "final phase 3" clinical trial to establish the safety and efficacy of a first-in-class antidiarrheal agent, crofelemer, for the symptomatic relief of diarrhea in HIV patients receiving anti-retroviral therapy. Given that this was a trial with two-stage design that included a dose selection, it was necessary to demonstrate the strong control of Type 1 error. This was accomplished with a close testing procedure applied to combination tests that utilized the inverse normal combination function. We developed a one-sided significance testing procedure that ensures strong control of the Type 1 error at level 0.025. Using appropriate statistical methodology for combining the results from the two stages, a statistically significant outcome was obtained for the primary efficacy endpoint and crofelemer received marketing approval based on the ADVENT trial. While the authors acknowledge the importance of statistical methodology required to analyze the data from the ADVENT trial, this chapter also provides significant details on the clinical and regulatory challenges that were demanded for the conduct of this innovative, two-stage, adaptive clinical trial.

Keywords Two stage • Seamless • Adaptive design • HIV • Crofelemer • ADVENT • Antidiarrheal • Regulatory • Implementation

P.R. Chaturvedi (✉)
Napo Pharmaceuticals Inc., 185 Berry Street, Suite 1300, San Francisco, CA 94107, USA
e-mail: prchaturvedi@gmail.com

Z. Antonijevic • C. Mehta, Ph.D.
Cytel Inc., 675 Massachusetts Avenue, Cambridge, MA 02139, USA
e-mail: zoran.antonijevic@cytel.com; mehta@cytel.com

W. He et al. (eds.), *Practical Considerations for Adaptive Trial Design and Implementation*, Statistics for Biology and Health,
DOI 10.1007/978-1-4939-1100-4_20, © Springer Science+Business Media New York 2014

20.1 Introduction

Drug development is a time- and cost-intensive endeavor with the average cost of bringing a new drug to the market ranging between $800 million and $2 billion over a period of 15 years or longer from the initiation of research efforts in a given therapeutic area (DiMasi et al. 2003). It has been postulated that novel approaches to clinical trial design could improve the success rates of drug development programs through the adoption of a more integrated clinical development paradigm that efficiently uses the "knowledge" accumulated through the multiple years of drug development, rather than the traditional sequential, distinct, and discrete milestone-driven drug development phases. Innovative clinical trial approaches would thus need to be adaptive, parallel, and data driven, to allow regulatory submissions to be designated as "exploratory" and "confirmatory." An excellent review article on clinical trial design innovation was recently published that provides a broad overview of the innovative approaches in clinical trial design (Orloff et al. 2009).

One of the innovative clinical trial design approaches uses adaptive clinical trial designs in which interim data from a trial is used to modify and improve the study design in a pre-planned manner without undermining the validity and integrity of the study. If designed and executed appropriately, during the "exploratory" phase adaptive clinical trials can assign a larger portion of patients to the treatment groups that are performing well, reduce the number of treatment groups that perform poorly, and investigate a larger dose range to effectively select the optimal dose(s) for the "confirmatory" phase of the trial. As such, adaptive clinical trials would then allow judicious use of limited patient and capital resources as well as reduce unnecessary patient exposure to ineffective or poorly tolerated doses of drugs and lead to a "selection" of patient populations that are more likely to respond favorably to the treatment, leading to a maximized "benefit-to-risk" ratio. For example, Lawrence et a. (2014) described the INHANCE trial that was successfully included as a pivotal study in regulatory submissions for indacaterol, a once-daily maintenance bronchodilator treatment of airflow obstruction in adult patients with chronic obstructive pulmonary disease (COPD).

Central to the concept of adaptive (or flexible) clinical trial design is the use of accumulated data that can be used to modify various aspects of the clinical study, midstream, in a pre-planned manner without undermining the validity of the clinical study. Seamless adaptive designs improve the efficiency of clinical trials through the ability to combine objectives of clinical trials that were traditionally addressed through the conduct of separate phase 2 and phase 3 clinical studies. Possible advantages from conducting seamless adaptive clinical trials include the use of accumulated data to make beneficial changes such as sample size adjustment, allocation of patients to different treatment groups, addition or deletion of treatment groups, and adjustment of statistical hypothesis.

There are several requirements for the successful design and execution of seamless adaptive clinical trials. These include the ability to collect and analyze clinical response data in a timely (and preferably "real-time") basis and significant up-front statistical work to model the "expected" dose-response curves through simulations. Many simulations are required to determine the best combinations of sample sizes, randomization ratios between placebo and treatment dose levels, as well as the number of doses that can be included in the trial. Furthermore, several logistical and regulatory criteria must be fulfilled to avoid compromising the results from an adaptive clinical trial. Foremost amongst these is the pre-specification of the algorithm that determines the adaptation to implement the trial. This is accomplished through the establishment of an independent data monitoring committee (DMC) that is charged with the responsibility of performing unblinded interim analysis and communicating appropriately with the requisite members of the clinical team executing the trial. Furthermore, it is imperative that there be appropriate standard operating procedures (SOPs) to ensure the secrecy and confidentiality of such an algorithm to prevent any bias in the trial, either from the sponsor or the study investigators. The restricted knowledge of the interim results from seamless adaptive trials needs to be ensured to avoid any compromise in the interpretation of the results from such clinical trials.

An "inferentially" seamless adaptive clinical trial, such as the one used to determine the efficacy and safety of crofelemer in the ADVENT trial (described below), requires the use of data from both (exploratory and confirmatory) stages of the trial and requires absolute secrecy and integrity of the data from the first stage of the trial. On the other hand an "operationally" seamless adaptive clinical trial uses only the data from the second stage of the trial, after the dose selection has been made from the initial exploratory phase. Other important considerations for the conduct of adaptive clinical trials include the determination of the appropriate primary (and secondary) endpoints for the clinical trial. Modeling and simulations play a very important role in assessing the specific details of the seamless adaptive trial designs such as per-group sample sizes in the two stages of the clinical trial to maintain the robustness of the clinical trial. The final analysis plan must use statistical methodology that is appropriate for the clinical study design and "simple" comparisons of placebo vs. treatment groups are inappropriate from seamless adaptive trial designs.

In this chapter, we provide the details of an innovative two-stage, seamless adaptive clinical trial conducted as a "final phase 3" clinical trial to establish the safety and efficacy of a first-in-class antidiarrheal agent, crofelemer, for the symptomatic relief of diarrhea in HIV patients receiving anti-retroviral therapy. The details and results from this trial were recently presented (MacArthur et al. 2012). While the authors acknowledge the importance of statistical methodology required to analyze the data from the ADVENT trial, this chapter also provides significant details on the clinical and regulatory challenges that were demanded during the conduct of this innovative, two-stage, adaptive clinical trial design.

The ADVENT trial is to our knowledge the first phase 3 trial using this type of seamless adaptive clinical trial design that led to an FDA approval. Hence, in this chapter we describe all clinical, regulatory, strategic, methodological, and operational aspects that led to its approval. In Sect. 20.2 we provide clinical background on secretory diarrhea in HIV patients and on the study drug crofelemer, and rationale for the ADVENT confirmatory clinical study. In Sect. 20.3 we describe regulatory interactions, including the Special Protocol Assessment (SPA) process. Section 20.4 describes the details of the ADVENT clinical trial design and Sect. 20.5 describes design options and motivation for application of an adaptive design.

Section 20.6 provides details on the statistical methodology of the selected approach. Given that the initial design was rejected by the FDA, we will explain reasons why the original design was rejected and what made the revised design acceptable. Section 20.7 describes implementation of this trial. This section also describes the data monitoring process, including (a) membership, (b) rule for dose selection, and (c) how confidentiality on selected dose was maintained. Finally, Sect. 20.8 presents the final results and ultimate regulatory decision on the fate of crofelemer's marketing approval.

20.2   Clinical Background

20.2.1   Secretory Diarrhea: A Clinical Unmet Need Resulting from Various Etiologies

Diarrhea is a clinical symptom that is characterized by the passage of one or more watery or unformed stools. Secretory diarrhea occurs when the secretion of fluid and electrolytes in the intestinal lumen exceeds the absorption of water and electrolytes from the lumen. Secretory diarrhea is a significant global health issue and is a leading cause of morbidity and mortality worldwide (Murray and Lopez 1996). If not treated in a timely manner, secretory diarrhea can lead to severe dehydration, electrolyte abnormalities, acute renal failure, hypovolemic shock, and death. Treatment of secretory diarrhea is usually supportive and includes replacement of intestinal fluid losses with oral rehydration salts (ORS).

The majority of the secretory diarrheas result from bacterial infections such as *Vibrio cholerae* and *Escherichia coli* and from viral pathogens such as norovirus, rotavirus, and human immunodeficiency virus (HIV) (Malago 2010). For diarrhea resulting from infections, generally the enterotoxins from the pathogen bind to the mucosal cells and induce a dysfunction of the intestinal chloride channels such as cystic fibrosis transmembrane conductance regulator (CFTR) and/or calcium-activated chloride channels (CaCC), as a consequence of increased cAMP, cGMP, or 5-HT levels which enables the secretion of chloride and other ions accompanied by water into the gut lumen, resulting in diarrhea (Field 2003).

20.2.2   The Emergence of Noninfectious Diarrhea in HIV Patients Following Treatment with Highly Active Anti-retroviral Therapy (HAART)

The treatment of HIV patients with HAART has resulted in prolonged survival of HIV patients. Drugs such as HIV protease inhibitors, a major component of HAART, also produce secretory diarrhea by a variety of mechanisms, including increased calcium-dependent chloride conductance and cellular apoptosis, necrosis, and decreased proliferation of intestinal epithelial cells (Bode et al. 2005).

Protease inhibitors were also found to increase intestinal permeability suggesting a disrupted intestinal barrier function and/or altered small intestinal absorption, which would produce diarrhea (Braga Neto et al. 2010).

20.2.3   Treatment and Management of HIV-Associated Diarrhea Remains a Challenge

An excellent review of the etiology and pharmacological management of noninfectious diarrhea in HIV patients is provided by MacArthur and DuPont (2012). HIV patients receiving HAART therapy have noninfectious diarrhea as an adaptive response to drugs. As such no treatments are available for the management of secretory noninfectious diarrhea in HIV patients. Palliative therapies including the use of adsorbents such as attapulgite, bismuth subsalicylate, kaolin, and pectin and anti-motility agents such as diphenoxylate-atropine, loperamide, tincture of opium, and octreotide remain inadequate to treat secretory HIV diarrhea. Thus, there remains a large unmet clinical need for the treatment of secretory diarrhea to restore the physiological function of the intestinal ion channels that regulate fluid and electrolyte transport.

20.2.4   Crofelemer: A Novel Anti-secretory, Non-opiate, Non-antimicrobial Antidiarrheal Drug for the Treatment of Noninfectious Diarrhea in HIV Patients

Crofelemer (formerly known as SP-303, NP-303 or Provir), now marketed as Fulyzaq, is a novel drug that was recently approved by the US FDA for the treatment of watery diarrhea in HIV patients receiving anti-retroviral therapy. Crofelemer is extracted and purified from the latex of *Croton lechleri*, a plant distributed throughout Western South America. The details of the extraction, purification, and characterization of crofelemer have been described by Ubillas et al. (1994).

The anti-secretory mechanism of effect of crofelemer was first demonstrated in vitro in a cAMP-mediated chloride secretion model and in vivo in a cholera toxin (CT)-induced fluid secretion mouse model by Gabriel et al. (1999). In Ussing chamber studies, crofelemer had significant reductions on both basal current and forskolin-stimulated chloride current, coupled with increased resistance, suggesting an inhibitory effect on cAMP-mediated chloride ion and fluid secretion. In mice treated with cholera toxin (CT), crofelemer reduced the fluid accumulation induced by CT, with a half-maximal inhibitory dose of 10 mg/kg. These studies indicated that crofelemer has broad spectrum anti-secretory antidiarrheal effects.

Crofelemer inhibited the cystic fibrosis transmembrane conductance regulator (CFTR) chloride (Cl-) channel producing a voltage-independent block coupled with the closed state of the CFTR chloride channel. Crofelemer's effects on CFTR were prolonged and it was also found to strongly inhibit the intestinal calcium-activated chloride channel by a voltage-independent mechanism. The dual inhibitory effects of crofelemer on two structurally unrelated intestinal chloride channels are considered to account for the anti-secretory activity of crofelemer (Tradtrantip et al. 2010).

20.2.5 Crofelemer Has Demonstrated Excellent Antidiarrheal Effects in the Treatment of Secretory Diarrhea

Crofelemer is well tolerated and has demonstrated efficacy in the treatment of traveler's diarrhea as evidenced by the reduction in the duration of watery diarrhea (DiCesare et al. 2002). Crofelemer has also been well tolerated and shown excellent efficacy in adult patients with acute infectious diarrhea in combination with fluid and electrolyte replacement without the use of antibiotics (Sharma et al. 2008).

Crofelemer has also been effective in the treatment of severe acute infectious diarrhea in cholera patients when co-administered with fluid and electrolyte replacement as well as an antibiotic (azithromycin) (Bardhan et al. 2008).

Crofelemer has been evaluated in a multicenter, double-blind, placebo-controlled trial in adult men and women with diarrhea-predominant irritable bowel syndrome (d-IBS). Crofelemer was well tolerated and did not appear to have any significant effects on stool consistency or stool frequency in these patients following oral dosing for 3 months. Crofelemer showed significant improvements in the number of abdominal pain- and discomfort-free days following oral administration in female d-IBS patients (Mangel and Chaturvedi 2008). Further studies are needed to evaluate the use of crofelemer as a visceral analgesic.

Previous studies have been conducted with crofelemer in the treatment of diarrhea in HIV patients. A multicenter, randomized, double-blind, placebo-controlled study was conducted in HIV patients to evaluate the effects of 500 mg beads of crofelemer or placebo administered four times daily on stool weight and stool frequency following oral dosing for 4 days. Crofelemer was well tolerated and showed a significant reduction in stool weight and abnormal (watery) stool frequency following a daily measure analysis of these endpoints compared to placebo treatment (Holodniy et al. 1999). Primary analysis showed that there were larger decreases in stool weight from baseline to day 4 in the crofelemer group compared to placebo ($p=0.0354$ by generalized linear model). The crofelemer-treated group also experienced significantly greater improvements from baseline to day 4 in abnormal (i.e., soft or watery) stool frequency, a secondary endpoint ($p=0.0116$).

Crofelemer was evaluated in a double-blind, placebo-controlled phase 3 study in HIV patients for the treatment of diarrhea to evaluate its effects on stool weight and stool frequency following oral dosing for 7 days in an inpatient setting. This period was followed by an additional 21-day period of crofelemer dosing in patients that were considered responders by the clinical investigator (Shaman Pharmaceuticals Study 37554-210—unpublished results). Crofelemer was administered at dose regimens of 250 mg tablets, 500 mg tablets, or 500 mg beads four times daily compared to a matching placebo. In the primary endpoint, there were significantly larger decreases in stool weight from baseline to day 7 in the 500 mg tablet group compared with placebo (p=0.0107). Significantly greater decreases were also observed in the 500 mg tablet group compared to placebo in stool frequency (p=0.0254) and in a daily gastrointestinal (GI) symptom score which summed the mean scores for seven symptoms (nausea, vomiting, abdominal pain, gas, urgency, tenesmus, and incontinence) (p=0.0002).

The safety profile for crofelemer in these studies was consistent with the minimal systemic absorption of crofelemer. No significant differences were observed in the incidence of adverse events (AEs) between the crofelemer- and placebo-treated groups of patients. The results of these two studies showed that crofelemer was well tolerated and was effective in reducing stool weight and soft/watery stool frequency in HIV-associated diarrhea.

20.2.6 Rationale for the ADVENT Phase 3 Clinical Study for the Evaluation of Crofelemer for the Symptomatic Relief of Diarrhea in HIV Patients

The aforementioned discussion provided clear evidence that crofelemer is well tolerated and effective in the treatment of secretory diarrhea resulting from bacterial infections as well as in HIV patients receiving anti-retroviral therapy. However, these various studies evaluated different patient populations using different dose levels and dosing frequencies and different oral formulations of crofelemer. Consequently, the optimal dose regimen for crofelemer for the treatment diarrhea in HIV patients remained unclear from these studies. Furthermore, the regulatory requirements obligate the conduct of two adequate and well-controlled clinical studies to gain marketing approval for a new drug for the treatment of a disease or a condition. The design of the pivotal phase 3 study for crofelemer for the treatment of HIV-associated diarrhea was defined prospectively following discussions and agreement with the Food and Drug Administration (FDA) in accordance with a special protocol assessment (SPA). The SPA process included consultation with the Division of Gastrointestinal Products on key aspects of the study design, including, but not limited to, the criteria for selection and qualification of patients in the study, the choice of primary endpoint (i.e., clinical response), the appropriate methods for confirming efficacy, and the interim analysis process for dose selection.

20.3 Regulatory Background

20.3.1 Sponsor-Regulatory Interactions Determined the Nature of the Trial Design for This Phase 3 Study

The sponsor of crofelemer (Napo Pharmaceuticals) conducted an end-of-phase 2 (EOP2) meeting with the FDA to obtain the agreement from the FDA on the conduct of an additional proposed phase 3 study to support the regulatory submission of the New Drug Application (NDA) for crofelemer. The sponsor initially proposed conducting a multicenter, double-blind, placebo-controlled outpatient study for crofelemer in HIV patients at two different dosing regimens of crofelemer. The dosing period would include a placebo-controlled 4-week period and a placebo-free extension period of an additional 20 weeks (maintenance period) to provide long-term tolerability and durability of effectiveness data on crofelemer's effects in the symptomatic relief of diarrhea in HIV patients.

The previous studies were conducted on symptomatic endpoints of diarrhea such as stool weight and stool frequency in an in-patient (controlled) setting. The regulatory agency as well as the HIV patient community requested the outpatient study to provide clear evidence of safety and efficacy of crofelemer in HIV patients under their "daily routine" setting. Hence, the sponsor had to design a primary endpoint that would define a clinical response and identify the "responders" to crofelemer treatment. Since the definition of diarrhea (passage of watery stools) was unambiguous in the clinical setting (rather than defining normal bowel function), the sponsor worked with the clinical and regulatory opinion leaders to obtain consensus on the definition of a clinical response.

20.3.2   The Special Protocol Assessment (SPA) Process for the Design of an Acceptable Clinical Protocol

The FDA agreed with the sponsor's definition that a patient will be considered to have diarrhea if the patient has at least one watery stool per day (i.e., seven or more watery stools per week) at baseline. The FDA also agreed with the sponsor that a clinical response would be achieved when a patient has less than or equal to two (≤ 2) watery stools per week. The FDA recommended that additional endpoints such as frequency of bowel movements (watery and formed) and overall daily stool consistency needed to be assessed at baseline along with the use of prescription as well as over-the-counter (OTC) medications. Furthermore, there was agreement on a single-blind placebo-run-in period to ameliorate the high placebo response in the symptomatic relief of diarrhea in HIV patients.

Based on the guidance from the FDA, a new two-stage clinical study protocol was submitted by the sponsor to the FDA under SPA to evaluate the safety and efficacy of crofelemer in a randomized, double-blind, placebo-controlled study at dose levels of 125, 250, and 500 mg administered twice daily in HIV patients. The agency agreed with the sponsor's request to include patients that had at least one watery stool on 5 of the 7 days in the screening period and urgency on at least 1 of the 7 days during the screening period for this study. The agency did not agree with the overall design of the two-stage approach proposed initially by the sponsor or with their selection of a two-sided Type 1 error rate of 0.025. The initial suggestion from the FDA was to conduct two separate trials to better assess the dose-effect relationship for the three active doses proposed in the study. The FDA suggested doing a "responder analysis" and the use of Dunnett's procedure for multiple comparisons while accounting for the multiple comparisons. Furthermore, the regulatory authorities also suggested the Dunnett's approach as it would reduce the sample size requirements as compared to the use of Bonferroni adjustment for three possible pairwise comparisons between each active dose and placebo.

The FDA also had concerns about the decision making at the interim analysis for the initial two-stage design proposed by the sponsor. Specifically, the FDA wanted a confirmation that the interim analysis would only be used for selecting a dose that would be studied further and that the study would not be stopped for efficacy. Taking all the features of the trial design and in collaboration with the sponsor, the FDA recommended that the sponsor consider using an adaptive trial design methodology instead of the proposed two-stage design by the sponsor. The FDA provided guidance on several other key inclusion and exclusion criteria to be included in such a two-stage adaptive trial design and provided clear guidance on definitions of nonresponders including those patients that either switched their anti-retroviral therapy regimens or used antidiarrheal agents or opiates for more than 3 days in this study.

20.4 The ADVENT Clinical Trial

The ADVENT (*A*nti-*D*iarrhea therapy in HI*V* disease—*E*mergi*N*g *T*reatment concepts) trial was a randomized, double-blind, placebo-controlled two-stage adaptive clinical trial to assess the efficacy and safety of three doses of crofelemer (125, 250, 500 mg) taken orally twice daily. The trial consisted of three phases: a 10-day single-blind placebo *screening phase*, which enrolled the patients with a history of chronic diarrhea and were required to stop using antidiarrheal medications (ADM) upon entering the trial. This was followed by randomization into the trial which comprised a 31-day, double-blind, *placebo-controlled (PC) treatment phase* and concluded with a 20-week *placebo-free (PF) extension phase*. The 31-day double-blind phase consisted of a 3-day placebo-run-in period and a 28-day efficacy assessment period. In the extension phase, patients who were on placebo in the first 4 weeks were randomly assigned to one of the three crofelemer dose groups. The primary efficacy endpoint was evaluated at the end of the 4-week placebo-controlled phase. A subject who experienced two or less watery bowel movements per week during at least 2 of the 4 weeks of the efficacy assessment period was classified as a clinical responder. Details of the trial and its results have been recently presented elsewhere (MacArthur et al. 2012). Figure 20.1 displays the different phases of the ADVENT trial.

The trial was conducted in two stages, with one interim analysis between stages, in order to evaluate efficacy and safety and to make a dose selection. Stage I was activated in October 2007. During stage 1, subjects were randomized equally to the four arms of the trial. After enrolling a total of 194 evaluable subjects, enrollment

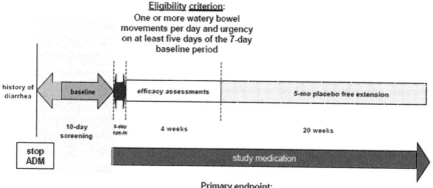

Fig. 20.1 Phases of ADVENT trial

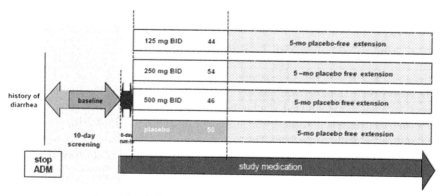

Stage 1 – 194 evaluable patients for Dose Selection

Fig. 20.2 Stage I of ADVENT trial

was temporarily halted in June 2009 and all enrolled subjects were followed in order to assess their 4-week efficacy outcomes. In August 2009, after complete 4-week efficacy data had been obtained from all stage I subjects, an independent Interim Analysis Committee (IAC) consisting of four physicians and a statistician reviewed the results and selected the 125 mg dose for further testing against placebo. Thereupon enrollment was re-opened for stage II of the trial. Between August 2009 and October 2010, 180 stage II patients were randomized between placebo and the crofelemer selected (125 mg) dose. Using appropriate statistical methodology for combining the results from the two stages, a statistically significant outcome (p = 0.0096) was obtained for the primary efficacy endpoint (MacArthur et al. 2012). The two stages of the trial are displayed separately in Figs. 20.2 and 20.3, respectively, and in Fig. 20.4 as one integrated trial.

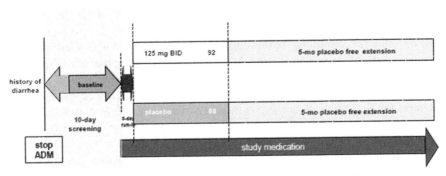

Stage 2 – 180 additional evaluable patients for Dose Assessment phase
(to be combined with Stage 1 patients for the placebo and 125 mg BID dose groups)

Fig. 20.3 Stage II of ADVENT trial

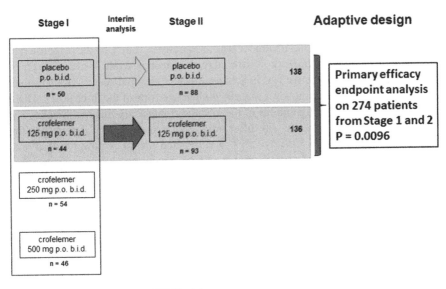

Fig. 20.4 Stages I and II of ADVENT trial

20.5   Design Considerations

While crofelemer had previously been administered as 250 and 500 mg tablets administered daily, the optimal dose of crofelemer remained unclear. Both doses were well tolerated and were associated with decreases in stool frequency compared to matching placebo. Since a lower dose might also be efficacious, it was decided to have three pairwise comparisons, of 125 mg, 250 mg, and 500 mg tablets, respectively, to matching placebo. For this purpose, three design options were considered. The first option was to design a four-arm study, perform three pairwise comparisons at the end of the trial, and use Dunnett's procedure to control for the multiple comparisons. The second option was to conduct two separate trials, one for learning and the other for confirming. In this option one would start out with a learning trial that included all four treatment arms. At the end of the learning trial one of the three doses would be selected for further study in a two-arm confirmatory trial vs. placebo. As the data from the two trials were kept completely separate, it was permissible to perform the final analysis of the confirmatory trial at the full level α without any adjustment for multiplicity. The third option was to conduct an adaptive two-stage trial with a learning phase and a confirming phase. This option bore some resemblance to option 2 in that the learning phase would start out with all four treatment arms and end with a dose selection. This would be followed by a two-arm confirming phase that only included the selected dose and placebo. In this option, however, the data from the learning and confirming phases could be combined. Special statistical methods would be required to control the Type 1 error which could potentially be inflated due to the dose selection at the end of the learning phase.

The primary endpoint was control of watery bowel movements over a 4-week period. A patient who had less than two watery bowel movements per week over a 4-week period was classified as a responder. Let $j=0, 1, 2, 3$ and denote the placebo, 125 mg, 250 mg, and 500 mg treatment arms, respectively. Let π_j be the response rate of treatment j and denote by $\theta_j = \pi_j - \pi_0$ the increase in response rate of treatment j over placebo. The design objective was to achieve 80 % power to detect a 20 % absolute improvement in response rate over placebo with at least one of the three doses. There are, of course, many configurations of the π_j values that satisfy this requirement and the sample size requirements will differ amongst them. Based on past results the configuration $\pi_0 = \pi_1 = \pi_2 = 35\%, \pi_3 = 55\%$ was targeted for 80 % power with a one-sided multiplicity adjusted error rate of $\alpha = 0.025$. Since the placebo response rate was expected to be much smaller than 35 %, this was a conservative assumption and diminished the risk of running an underpowered study. For each of the three options, sample sizes meeting the above power and Type 1 error goals were determined by simulation. These simulation results, along with the statistical methodology for guaranteeing strong control of Type 1 error at level $\alpha = 0.025$, are given below.

20.5.1 Single Four-Arm Trial

In this approach patients are randomized equally to the four treatment arms. There is no interim analysis. At the end of the trial one tests the three null hypotheses $H^{(j)}: \theta_j \leq 0$, for $j=1, 2, 3$, against one-sided alternatives of the form $\theta_j > 0$. Define the Wald statistic for the jth test as

$$Z_j = \frac{\hat{\pi}_j - \hat{\pi}_0}{\sqrt{\dfrac{\hat{\pi}_j\left(1 - \hat{\pi}_j\right)}{n_j} + \dfrac{\hat{\pi}_0\left(1 - \hat{\pi}_0\right)}{n_0}}}$$

where $\hat{\pi}_j$ is the estimate of π_j and n_j is the corresponding sample size for treatment j. Under the null hypothesis $H^{(j)}$ each Z_j converges to the standard normal distribution. For $j = 1, 2, 3$, Dunnett's test rejects $H^{(j)}$ if the corresponding $Z_j \geq 2.358$. This cutoff adjusts for the multiplicity induced by performing three hypothesis tests instead of one, and provides strong control of Type 1 error at the one-sided level $\alpha = 0.025$. In contrast, if only one hypothesis were to be tested the corresponding level 0.025 cutoff would be 1.96. Simulations under the configuration $\pi_0 = \pi_1 = \pi_2 = 35\%, \pi_3 = 55\%$ were used to establish that at least one null hypothesis is rejected with 80 % probability at the sample size $n_0 = n_1 = n_2 = n_3 = 125$. Thus a single four-arm trial achieves 80 % power at the specified configuration with a total sample size of 500 patients.

20.5.2 Two Independent Trials

This approach involves a four-arm learning trial followed by a two-arm confirming trial. The data from the learning trial are not combined with the data from the confirming trial. Therefore the hypothesis test to be performed at the end of the confirming trial can utilize the full level α without any Type 1 error inflation. The combined sample size over both trials that provides 80 % power to reject any $H^{(j)}$ under the configuration $\pi_0 = \pi_1 = \pi_2 = 35\%, \pi_3 = 55\%$ is obtained by simulation. Accordingly we simulated the two trials in succession. For the learning trial, 50 patients were randomized to each of the four treatment arms. The treatment arm with the highest observed response rate was selected, along with placebo, for the two-arm confirming trial. One hundred and eight subjects were randomized to each treatment arm for the two-arm confirming trial. Let $Z_s^{(2)}$ denote the Wald statistic for the selected dose vs. placebo utilizing only the data from the confirming trial. Then $H^{(s)}$ is rejected by a level 0.025 test if $Z_s^{(2)} \geq 1.96$. The simulations revealed that with 50 subjects per treatment arm for the learning trial and 108 subjects per arm for the confirming trial the combined process has 80 % power to reject at least one hypothesis. Thus a total of 416 patients are needed to achieve 80 % power at the specified power using two independent trials. This is a saving of 84 patients compared to the single four-arm trial based on Dunnett's test. In this design the confirming trial proceeds immediately upon completion of the learning trial but the data from the two trials are not combined for the final inference. Hence this design is termed "operationally seamless" and the schematic for the trial is shown in Fig. 20.5.

20.5.3 An Integrated Two-Stage Trial

This approach was eventually selected for the crofelemer trial. It involved a two-stage adaptive design where the objective of the first stage was to select the dose for the second stage, and the objective of the second stage was to confirm the efficacy of the selected dose. Stage 1 enrolled 50 subjects per group for the three dose groups (125, 250, 500 mg) plus placebo, while the stage 2 enrolled 75 additional subjects per group for the selected dose group and placebo group. Subjects from stage 1 were combined with stage 2 subjects for the final analysis of efficacy and safety. The final

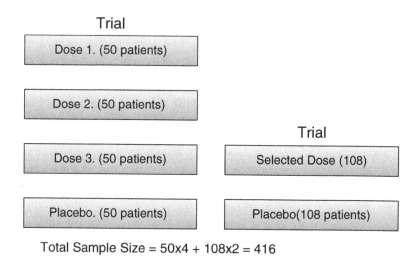

Fig. 20.5 Two separate trials (operationally seamless)

hypothesis test for the primary efficacy endpoint was based on comparing all 125 subjects enrolled in the placebo group with all 125 subjects enrolled in the group selected at the interim analysis.

After approximately 50 subjects were enrolled to each of the four treatment groups, the enrollment was *stopped* until all these subjects completed the placebo-controlled treatment period or terminated the study, and the interim analysis and decision for stage 2 were completed. Based upon an assessment of efficacy and safety, the sponsor selected one of the crofelemer doses to continue along with placebo into stage 2 (see Sect. 20.8.2.2 for details). The decision to perform an interim analysis after 50 subjects were assessed for the primary endpoint was based on clinical judgment, not a power calculation. This timing also permitted the majority of subjects analyzed for efficacy to be randomized during the second stage of the trial. Detailed statistical methodology of this approach is presented in the next section. This design is termed *inferentially seamless* because the data from both stages of the trial were combined for the final inference and a schematic of such a trial is shown in Fig. 20.6.

20.6 Methodology

20.6.1 Determination of Sample Size

Sample size and power calculations for the evaluation of efficacy during the placebo-controlled treatment phase utilized results from a previous phase 3 study (Protocol 37,554-210) in the HIV-positive patient population where a 20 % point improvement in response was observed for the treatment arm relative to placebo. With 125

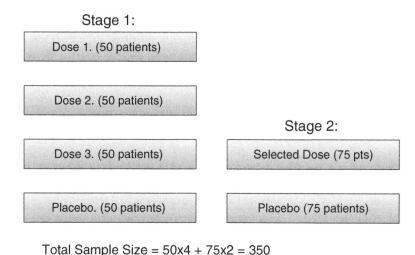

Total Sample Size = 50x4 + 75x2 = 350

Fig. 20.6 Integrated trial (inferentially seamless)

subjects randomized to both treatment groups (one crofelemer arm and placebo), the power of the study ranges from 71 % to over 91 % to detect a treatment difference at a one-sided alpha of 0.025 when the underlying response rate of one or more of the crofelemer dose groups exceeds placebo by 20 %. The analysis utilized the technique of Posch et al. (2005), based on the original work of Bauer and Kieser (1999), which controls the experiment-wise error rate for this two-stage adaptive design at a one-sided α of 0.025. The clinical response of 20 % is based on an estimated response rate of 55 % in crofelemer and 35 % in placebo during the 4-week efficacy assessment period. The size of the randomized population is described in Table 20.1.

Expecting that 33 % of subjects will fail screening, in order to obtain 350 randomized subjects, approximately 525 subjects must be screened. It is estimated that approximately 200 subjects will be randomized in stage 1 and 150 subjects in stage 2.

20.6.2   Strong Control of Type I Error

Given that this is a two-stage design that includes a dose selection, it is necessary to demonstrate the strong control of Type 1 error. This was accomplished with a close testing procedure applied to combination tests that utilized the inverse normal combination function. Details are given below.

Let $\pi j, j = 0, 1, 2, 3$ be the true response rates for the placebo and three treatment groups, respectively. Define $\theta j = \pi j - \pi 0, j = 1, 2, 3$. The global null hypothesis is $H(1,2,3)$: $\theta 1 = \theta 2 = \theta 3 = 0$. There are however other null hypothesis besides the global null, due to the presence of multiple treatment arms. Table 20.2 displays all possible null hypotheses and corresponding ways in which Type 1 error could arise.

Table 20.1 ITT sample size by treatment and stage (total randomized $n = 350$)

Stage	Placebo	Crofelemer 125 mg b.i.d.	Crofelemer 250 mg b.i.d.	Crofelemer 500 mg b.i.d.
I	50	50	50	50
II	75	0	75[a]	0
Total	125	50	125	50

[a]One of the three crofelemer doses will be selected for stage II; this table arbitrarily depicts the mid-dose as the one for stage II

Table 20.2 Null hypotheses and corresponding incorrect conclusions to be controlled at level $\alpha \leq 0.025$

Null hypotheses	[a]Type of incorrect conclusion
$H(1,2,3)$: $\theta 1 = \theta 2 = \theta 3 = 0$	The selected treatment is declared superior to placebo
$H(1,2)$: $\theta 1 = \theta 2 = 0$, $\theta 3 > 0$	Treatment 1 or 2 is selected and is declared superior to placebo
$H(1,3)$: $\theta 1 = \theta 3 = 0$, $\theta 2 > 0$	Treatment 1 or 3 is selected and is declared superior to placebo
$H(2,3)$: $\theta 2 = \theta 3 = 0$, $\theta 1 > 0$	Treatment 2 or 3 is selected and is declared superior to placebo
$H(1)$: $\theta 1 = 0$, $\theta 2 > 0$, $\theta 3 > 0$	Treatment 1 is selected and is declared superior to placebo
$H(2)$: $\theta 2 = 0$, $\theta 1 > 0$, $\theta 3 > 0$	Treatment 2 is selected and is declared superior to placebo
$H(3)$: $\theta 3 = 0$, $\theta 1 > 0$, $\theta 2 > 0$	Treatment 3 is selected and is declared superior to placebo

[a]Configurations with any $\theta j < 0$ will also control corresponding incorrect conclusions at level $\alpha \leq 0.025$

For a testing procedure to have strong control of Type 1 error at level $\alpha = 0.025$, it must be the case that under any configuration from Table 20.2, the probability of making one or more false statements must not exceed 0.025.

20.6.3 Hypothesis Testing Procedure

Based on the paper (Posch et al. 2005) we developed a one-sided significance testing procedure that ensures strong control of the Type 1 error at level 0.025. The method utilizes two principles:

1. Combine valid p-values from the two stages of the design with the inverse normal combination function. A valid p-value, p, under the null hypothesis H has the property that for any α

$$P_H\left(p \leq \alpha\right) \leq \alpha$$

Suppose p is a valid p-value from stage 1 and q is a valid p-value from stage 2. Let n_1 and n_2 be the sample sizes of the two stages. Then the inverse normal combination function, given by

$$C(p,q) = 1 - \Phi\left[\sqrt{\frac{n_1}{n_1 + n_2}}\Phi^{-1}\left(1 - p\right) + \sqrt{\frac{n_2}{n_1 + n_2}}\Phi^{-1}\left(1 - q\right)\right],$$

where $\Phi(.)$ is the left tail of the standard normal density, is a valid p-value for the combined data from the two stages.

2. Perform a closed test for the final analysis. To understand closed testing, suppose without loss of generality that dose 1 is selected at the interim analysis. To declare statistical significance for dose 1 with a closed test we must reject $H^{(1)}: \theta^{(1)} = 0$ with a level α test and in addition, we must reject every intersection hypothesis that contains $H^{(1)}$ with a level α test. To be specific:

- Must reject $H^{(1,2)}: \theta_1 = \theta_2 = 0$ at level α
- Must reject $H^{(1,3)}: \theta_1 = \theta_3 = 0$ at level α
- Must reject $H^{(1,2,3)}: \theta_1 = \theta_2 = \theta_3 = 0$ at level α

We will now apply these two principles to the ADVENT trial. Let $\hat{\pi}_{ij}$ be the estimated response rate for treatment j based only on the n_{ij} observations obtained from stage i for treatment j, i = 1, 2, j = 0, 1, 2, 3. Let

$$\bar{\pi}_{ij} = \frac{n_{ij} \hat{\pi}_{ij} + n_{i0} \hat{\pi}_{i0}}{n_{ij} + n_{i0}}$$

be the pooled estimate of response from the $(n_{ij} + n_{i0})$ subjects enrolled in treatments j and 0 at stage i and let $\bar{n}_{ij} = 0.5(n_{ij} + n_{i0})$ be the mean number of subjects enrolled in treatments j and 0 at stage i. At stage 1 we compute the Wald statistic:

$$z_{1j} = \frac{\hat{\pi}_{1j} - \hat{\pi}_{10}}{\sqrt{\bar{\pi}_{1j}(1 - \bar{\pi}_{1j})\left(\frac{1}{n_{1j}} + \frac{1}{n_{10}}\right)}}$$

and the corresponding one-sided p-value

$$p^{(j)} = 1 - \Phi(z_{1j})$$

for j = 1, 2, 3. Assume, without loss of generality, that $p^{(1)} \le p^{(2)} \le p^{(3)}$. Therefore treatment 1 is selected for stage 2. At stage 2 we compute the Wald statistic:

$$z_{21} = \frac{\hat{\pi}_{21} - \hat{\pi}_{20}}{\sqrt{\bar{\pi}_{21}(1 - \bar{\pi}_{21})\left(\frac{1}{n_{21}} + \frac{1}{n_{20}}\right)}}$$

and the corresponding one-sided p-value

$$q^{(1)} = 1 - \Phi(z_{21}).$$

Define the following p-values from the stage 1 data:

$p^{(1,2)} = \min(2p^{(1)}, p^{(2)})$

$p^{(1,3)} = \min(2p^{(1)}, p^{(3)})$

$p^{(1,2,3)} = \min(3p^{(1)}, 1.5p^{(2)}, p^{(3)})$

These p-values are based on Simes test (see Posch et al. 2005, Sect. 2.2.1). Since only treatment 1 is selected at the end of stage 1, set $q^{(1,2)} = q^{(1,3)} = q^{(1,2,3)} = q^{(1)}$. Now define the combination functions for the various intersection hypotheses as follows:

Reject $H^{(1)}$ if

$$C\left(p^{(1)}, q^{(1)}\right) = 1 - \Phi\left[\sqrt{\frac{\tilde{n}_1}{\tilde{n}_1 + \tilde{n}_2}} \Phi^{-1}\left(1 - p^{(1)}\right) + \sqrt{\frac{\tilde{n}_2}{\tilde{n}_1 + \tilde{n}_2}} \Phi^{-1}\left(1 - q^{(1)}\right)\right] \leq \alpha$$

Reject $H^{(1,2)}$ if

$$C\left(p^{(1,2)}, q^{(1,2)}\right) = 1 - \Phi\left[\sqrt{\frac{\tilde{n}_1}{\tilde{n}_1 + \tilde{n}_2}} \Phi^{-1}\left(1 - p^{(1,2)}\right) + \sqrt{\frac{\tilde{n}_2}{\tilde{n}_1 + \tilde{n}_2}} \Phi^{-1}\left(1 - q^{(1,2)}\right)\right] \leq \alpha$$

Reject $H^{(1,3)}$ if

$$C\left(p^{(1,3)}, q^{(1,3)}\right) = 1 - \Phi\left[\sqrt{\frac{\tilde{n}_1}{\tilde{n}_1 + \tilde{n}_2}} \Phi^{-1}\left(1 - p^{(1,3)}\right) + \sqrt{\frac{\tilde{n}_2}{\tilde{n}_1 + \tilde{n}_2}} \Phi^{-1}\left(1 - q^{(1,3)}\right)\right] \leq \alpha$$

Reject $H^{(1,2,3)}$ if

$$C\left(p^{(1,2,3)}, q^{(1,2,3)}\right) = 1 - \Phi\left[\sqrt{\frac{\tilde{n}_1}{\tilde{n}_1 + \tilde{n}_2}} \Phi^{-1}\left(1 - p^{(1,2,3)}\right) + \sqrt{\frac{\tilde{n}_2}{\tilde{n}_1 + \tilde{n}_2}} \Phi^{-1}\left(1 - q^{(1,2,3)}\right)\right] \leq \alpha$$

where $\tilde{n}_1 = 50$ and $\tilde{n}_2 = 75$ are the pre-specified sample sizes per treatment arm for the two stages. We will reject $H^{(1)}$ and conclude that dose group 1 is superior to placebo if

$$\max\{C(p^{(1)}, q^{(1)}), C(p^{(1,2)}, q^{(1)}), C(p^{(1,3)}, q^{(1)}), C(p^{(1,2,3)}, q^{(1)})\} \leq 0.025.$$

It is important to note that strong control of Type 1 error is maintained even when $\tilde{n}_i \neq n_{ij}$ as long as the values of $\tilde{n}_i$ have been pre-specified, or at least have been specified prior to any unblinding of the data. Indeed, it is even permissible to alter the stage 2 sample sizes after observing the stage 1 data as long as the weights that are used to combine the p-values from the two stages utilize $\tilde{n}_i$ values that have been selected prior to unblinding the data.

20.6.4   Analysis of the Primary Efficacy Endpoint

The primary efficacy analysis was conducted on the ITT population and was based on the data from the 4-week efficacy assessment period of the placebo-controlled treatment phase (MacArthur et al. 2012). The primary efficacy endpoint has a binary outcome, defined as two or less watery bowel movements per week during at least 2 of the 4 weeks.

Imputations for clinical response were handled as follows: A subject's data were evaluated for assessment of clinical response each week if at least five daily assessments per 7-day weekly period were available; that is, if 0, 1, or 2 days' data were missing, there was no imputation. If less than 5 days of data were available, then the subject could not be classified as a responder for that week. Subjects who discontinued prematurely (i.e., before scheduled visit 3) during the 4-week efficacy assessment period were classified as nonresponders.

Subjects who used an antidiarrheal medication (ADM) or opiate pain medication, including any combination of ADM or opiate pain medication, for greater than three consecutive or non-consecutive days during the 4-week efficacy assessment period were permitted to remain in the study, but were classified as nonresponders.

For the purpose of convention, if the screening phase was extended or contracted for any reason, visit 1 would still remain day 4 on the schedule of assessments. Therefore, the run-in period remained days -3 to -1, the first day of the efficacy assessment period remained day 1, and the last day of the efficacy assessment period remained day 28. The efficacy assessment period for the purposes of the primary and secondary efficacy variables remained days 1–28 regardless of the actual day on which visit 3 (days 28–34) occurs.

Patients in ADVENT trial were male or female of at least 18 years of age and presented with a history of diarrhea. Diarrhea was defined as either persistent loose stools despite regular use of antidiarrheal medications (ADM) or one or more watery stools per day without regular ADM use of at least 1-month duration, prior to the screening period. During the baseline period, which comprised a single-blind, placebo screening phase lasting for at least 10 days, the diarrhea symptoms were measured using patient diaries in an interactive voice response system (IVRS). If a subject had more than 7 days of baseline efficacy (IVRS) data, then the last 7 days were used. Patients who reported at least one watery bowel movement per day on at least 5 of the last 7 days of the baseline screening period and urgency on at least 1 of the last 7 days were eligible for randomization into the double-blind, placebo-controlled phase of the ADVENT trial.

20.7 Data Monitoring and Study Implementation

20.7.1 Data Monitoring Committee Membership

The Interim Analysis Committee (IAC) included three voting members, with medical experience in gastroenterology, HIV disease, and the conduct of clinical trials. Their primary responsibility was to implement the pre-specified dose selection criteria. Each of the three IAC members carried equal votes for dose selection. A quorum consisted of at least two of the three IAC members. In the case of a nonvoting member or tie, or an absent member, the Chairperson would cast the tie-breaking vote. The selected dose was revealed only to those personnel required to prepare and ship the study drug for stage 2.

The IAC was also responsible for ongoing safety monitoring by examination of unblinded AE and SAE data. If a significant safety signal emerged, it would be communicated to the medical monitor of the study.

This study also had a consulting statistician (CS) as a nonvoting member of the IAC. The CS played a dual role—preparing the data for presentation to the IAC members, and explaining the fine points of adaptive design.

20.7.2 Dose Selection Criteria

The IAC Charter stipulated that selection of the dose of crofelemer for stage 2 should be based on the following criteria:

1. The primary efficacy variable in the ITT population, concomitant with AE and SAE rates.
2. Assuming that there are no safety issues, the crofelemer dose selected for stage 2 is the one for which the primary efficacy variable in the ITT population is at least 2.0 % greater than the other crofelemer treatments. If there are safety issues, the decision as to dose selection is too complex to pre-specify.
3. If two or three treatment groups' percents are less than 2 % of each other, and there are no safety issues, the lowest of these doses will be selected for stage 2.

20.7.3 Interim Analysis

An interim analysis was to be performed when 50 subjects are randomized to each of the four treatment groups and completed the placebo-controlled treatment period or terminated the study (excluding the 14-day post-dosing telephone call). Enrollment was *stopped* at approximately 50 subjects per treatment group until the interim analysis and decision for stage 2 are completed. An analysis was conducted on the primary efficacy endpoint in the ITT population and various safety parameters. Based upon an assessment of efficacy and safety, sponsor selected one of the crofelemer doses to continue along with placebo into stage 2. The interim analysis was not used to adjust the sample size or to stop the study early due to positive efficacy treatment results.

20.7.4   Duration of Interim Analysis Period

There are two particularly interesting items related to the conduct of this trial. The first one is that the enrollment paused during the interim analysis period. The second is that there was an internal agreement by the sponsor to be blinded to the selected dose. The decision of dose selection at the end of stage 1 and the time needed for statistical analysis were kept to a minimum to avoid selection bias. Enrollment in stage 1 was temporarily halted when approximately 50 subjects had been randomized to each of the four treatment groups (approximately 194 subjects total). The time point at which the last of these subjects had completed the 28-day placebo-controlled treatment period or terminated the study marked the start of the interim analysis period. The CS received cleaned interim data from the CRO, compiled the necessary efficacy and safety tables and listings, prepared an electronic copy of the Interim Analysis Report, and convened a meeting of the IAC. Immediately upon termination of the IAC meeting the CS prepared four notification memoranda, one for the medical monitor, and three for the drug distribution vendors responsible, respectively, for quality assurance, clinical supply management, and IVRS. The medical monitor was only notified that a dose had been selected without identifying the dose. The three drug distribution vendors were given the identity of the selected dose. This marked the end of the interim analysis period. Enrollment was resumed to the selected dose and placebo. The duration of interim analysis period was not to be kept longer than 8 weeks.

20.7.5   Maintaining Confidentiality

Very strict procedures were applied to prevent from the interim results leakage that would bias the stage 2. All analyses were prepared by the CS and entered into the Interim Analysis Report. The CS was not a sponsor employee and had no direct relationship to the CRO handling the site monitoring and data management. The statistical software files used to prepare data tables and listings and electronic copy of the Interim Analysis Report were stored securely such that neither the sponsor nor the CRO could access them. The randomization code was stored on a computer that sponsor cannot access, and the selected dose was revealed only to those personnel required to prepare and ship the study drug for stage 2.

20.8   Results

20.8.1   Disposition, Demographics, and Efficacy

A total of 376 patients were randomized in the ADVENT trial with 238 patients in the crofelemer treatment groups and 138 patients in the placebo group. Of these 374 patients received drug (or placebo) and were included in the intent-to-treat (ITT) population for the primary efficacy endpoint (see Fig. 20.7). More than 85 % of the randomized patients completed the placebo-controlled (PC) treatment phase of the trial. Eighteen patients in the crofelemer group and nine patients in the placebo group discontinued during the placebo-controlled (PC) phase of ADVENT. In the placebo-free (PF) extension phase of the trial, 337 patients were treated with crofelemer at dose levels of 125 mg BID (n=220), 250 mg BID (n=67), or 500 mg BID (n=50). Of the 337 patients, 126 patients had received placebo during the PC phase of the trial.

Combined analysis of demographics indicated that most of the patients in the PC phase (84 %) in each treatment group were male with a mean age of 45 years. By race, Caucasians, African-Americans, and Hispanics constituted at least 98 % of the patients randomized in the trial. The baseline diarrhea characteristics and symptom scores were similar across crofelemer and placebo groups in the ITT population. The HIV characteristics were balanced across the groups and most patients in each group (78 %) had an HIV viral load <400 copies/mL at baseline and more than 96 % of the patients in each group reported the use of anti-retroviral therapy (ART).

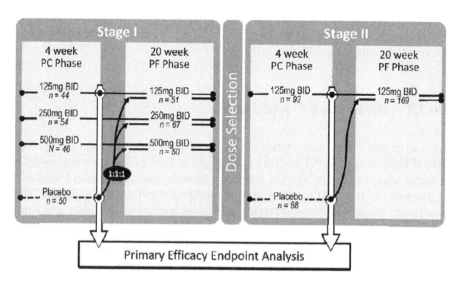

Fig. 20.7 Primary efficacy results by study stage in the ADVENT trial

Crofelemer demonstrated a statistically significant and clinically relevant treatment effect for the primary endpoint of proportion of patients achieving a clinical response. Clinical response was defined as reduction of number of watery stools per week of less than two (<2) for at least 2 out of the 4 weeks of the PC phase of the trial. The significance of crofelemer efficacy on the primary endpoint was further supported by the treatment effects of crofelemer on the secondary endpoints that evaluated various diarrheal symptoms such as daily watery bowel movements as a measure of watery stool frequency and stool consistency. The efficacy of crofelemer was also sustained and in fact improved, during the PF phase of the 20-week period, indicating the durability of the efficacy of crofelemer in the treatment of HIV-associated diarrhea.

A significantly larger proportion of patients treated with crofelemer at 125 mg BID group achieved clinical response compared to those treated with placebo (18 % vs. 8 %; one-sided p=0.0096, adjusted for dose selection and multiplicity by the Posch et al. (2005)) method in the ITT population. This result is statistically significant at the one-sided 0.025 level. Details of the computations resulting in this adjusted p-value of 0.0096 are given below.

Marginal Results for Each Stage

Dose	Stage 1 Results		Stage 2 Results	
	Response	P-value	Response	P-value
Placebo	1/50 (2%)	------	10/88 (11.4%)	------
125 mg	9/44 (20.5%)	0.0019	15/92 (16.3%)	0. 1690
250 mg	5/54 (9.3%)	0.0563	**The 125 mg dose was selected for Stage 2**	
500 mg	9/46 (19.6%)	0.0024		

The weights for combining the data from the two stages were computed from the total sample sizes of the 125 mg and placebo arms prior to unblinding the results. Thus the stage 1 and stage 2 weights are, respectively,

$$w_1 = \sqrt{\frac{(50+44)}{(50+44+88+92)}} = 0.5857 \text{ and } w_2 = \sqrt{\frac{(88+92)}{(50+44+88+92)}} = 0.8105.$$

Since $p_1=0.0019$, $p_2=0.0564$, and $p_3=0.0024$, the adjusted stage 1 p-values for the various intersection hypotheses are obtained by Simes method as follows:

$$p^{(12)} = \min\{2\min(p_1, p_2), \max(p_1, p_2)\} = 0.0038$$
$$p^{(13)} = \min\{2\min(p_1, p_3), \max(p_1, p_3)\} = 0.0024$$
$$p^{(123)} = \min\{3\min(p_1, p_2, p_3), 1.5\text{med}(p_1, p_2, p_3), \max(p_1, p_2, p_3)\} = 0.0036.$$

The corresponding Simes-adjusted stage 2 p-values are

$$q_1 = q^{(12)} = q^{(13)} = q^{(123)} = 0.1690.$$

Thereupon the combined p-values from both stages are

$$C(p_1, q_1) = 1 - \Phi\left[0.5857\Phi^{-1}(1 - p_1) + 0.8105\Phi^{-1}(1 - q_1)\right] = 0.0067$$

$$C\left(p^{(12)}, q^{(12)}\right) = 1 - \Phi\left[0.5857\Phi^{-1}\left(1 - p^{(12)}\right) + 0.8105\Phi^{-1}\left(1 - q^{(12)}\right)\right] = 0.0096$$

$$C\left(p^{(13)}, q^{(13)}\right) = 1 - \Phi\left[0.5857\Phi^{-1}\left(1 - p^{(13)}\right) + 0.8105\Phi^{-1}\left(1 - q^{(13)}\right)\right] = 0.0077$$

$$C\left(p^{(123)}, q^{(123)}\right) = 1 - \Phi\left[0.5857\Phi^{-1}\left(1 - p^{(123)}\right) + 0.8105\Phi^{-1}\left(1 - q^{(123)}\right)\right] = 0.0095$$

Since all these combined p-values are less than 0.025 we can claim, by the principle of closed testing, that the 125 mg crofelemer dose is statistically superior to placebo at the overall significance level of 0.025. The multiplicity-adjusted overall p-value is then

$$\max\left(0.0067, 0.0096, 0.0077, 0.0095\right) = 0.0096$$

The efficacy of crofelemer on the primary endpoint was further substantiated by sensitivity analyses controlling for the impact of protocol deviations on the outcome, using the per-protocol (PP) population and a Cochran-Mantel-Haenszel (CMH) test (18 % vs. 8 %, p=0.0181). Additional analysis controlling for geographic region also demonstrated a significant crofelemer treatment effect (18 % vs. 8 %, p=0.0127).

Subgroup analyses showed that crofelemer treatment effect was more pronounced in patients with a more clinically significant diarrhea at baseline and the clinical response endpoint was consistently correlated with other daily assessments of changes in diarrheal symptoms.

20.8.2   Review of Results

20.8.2.1   Stage 1

Crofelemer 125 mg BID and 500 mg BID dose levels performed similarly in stage 1 and one-sided treatment difference between crofelemer the placebo group was statistically significant for 125 mg BID (one-sided p=0.0019) and 500 mg BID (one-sided p=0.0024). A statistical trend in favor of crofelemer was also observed for the 250 mg BID dose group (one-sided p=0.0563) in the primary efficacy endpoint. A dose-response trend was observed in stage 1 responder analysis for the exploratory secondary endpoint of stool consistency (p=0.0039).

Monthly response rates observed at the interim analysis were 20.5 % (9 out of 44), 9.3 % (5 out of 54), and 19.6 % (9 out of 46) in 125 mg, 250 mg, and 500 mg crofelemer doses, respectively, compared to 2 % (1 out of 50) in placebo arm.

20.8.2.2   Interim Analysis

Based on the criteria for dose selection outlined in the Interim Analysis Charter (IAC), the lowest dose of 125 mg BID crofelemer was advanced by the independent analysis committee for stage 2.

20.8.2.3   Stage 2

The low dose (125 mg) was selected to advance to stage 2, based on these results and the pre-specified dose-selection criteria. Response rates in stage 2 were 16.3 % (15 out of 92) in crofelemer 125 mg arm, compared to 11.4 % (10 out of 88) in placebo arm. The proportion of responders in stage 2 did not result in a statistically significant treatment difference due to the higher proportion of responders in the placebo group (one-sided $p = 0.1690$). An analysis of baseline diarrhea in placebo patients between stages 1 and 2 showed a lower proportion of diarrhea in placebo patients in stage 2 (average daily watery bowel movements for stage 1 vs. stage 2 being 3.5 vs. 2.8, $p = 0.0443$).

Per the defined Statistical Analysis Plan (SAP), the results from stage 1 and stage 2 were combined to evaluate the efficacy of crofelemer treatment using the Posch and Bauer method (Posch et al. 2005). Following the combination of the results from the two stages, the clinical response rates were 17.6 % in crofelemer 125 mg arm, and 8.0 % in the placebo arm (one-sided p-value $= 0.0096$) (see Fig. 20.8).

20.8.3   Secondary Efficacy Endpoints (PC Phase)

Crofelemer produced a significant reduction in mean daily watery stool frequency from baseline to end of treatment ($p = 0.0424$). Similarly, crofelemer improved stool consistency compared to placebo ($p = 0.0166$). The secondary endpoints were exploratory and data for these two endpoints were combined from stage I and stage II portions for the placebo and crofelemer 125 mg dose groups only.

20.8.4   Long-Term Efficacy of Crofelemer (PF Phase)

Placebo crossover patients who received 125 mg BID crofelemer during the PF phase had significantly greater odds for achieving clinical response during each of the 5 months of the PF phase compared to their experience during the 1-month PC

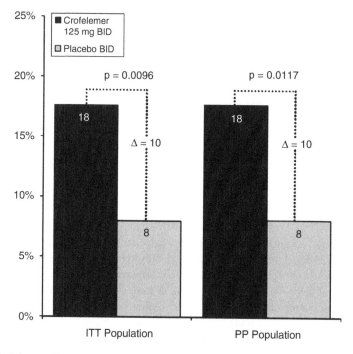

Fig. 20.8 Primary efficacy endpoint analysis from the ADVENT trial

phase (36 % vs. 9 %, odds ratio 5.85, p < 0.0001). The clinical response rates in this group of patients ranged between 36 and 55 % over the 5-month PF phase (p < 0.0001 for each month).

Weekly and monthly responder analyses in PF phase demonstrated the durability of crofelemer efficacy in HIV-associated diarrhea patients. The proportion of clinical responders during the 20-week PF phase was higher than during the 4-week PC phase when evaluated on a weekly or a monthly basis (see Fig. 20.9).

20.8.5 Crofelemer Safety

The safety profile of crofelemer in the ADVENT trial was comparable to that observed with placebo and consistent with an HIV-positive patient population. Crofelemer demonstrated a favorable safety profile for each dose group (125 mg BID, 250 mg BID, and 500 mg BID) during the double-blind, placebo-controlled (PC) phase and during the 5-month PF phase. Treatment emergent adverse effects (TEAEs) were observed in 27 % of crofelemer-treated patients compared to 33 % of placebo-treated patients during the 1-month PC phase. The incidence of severe

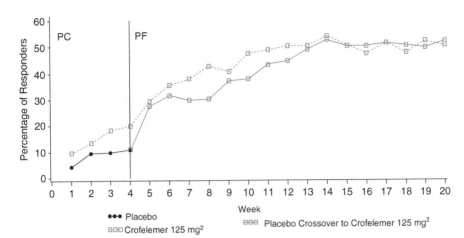

Fig. 20.9 Long-term efficacy of crofelemer in ADVENT trial

TEAEs was 1 % in the crofelemer-treated patients compared to 4 % in the placebo-treated group. Severe adverse effects (SAEs) were lower in crofelemer-treated group compared to placebo-treated group (1 % vs. 3 %) and TEAEs leading to drug discontinuation was 0 % in the crofelemer-treated group compared to 3 % in the placebo group.

Most frequently reported TEAEs were infections (10 % in crofelemer and 11 % in placebo groups) and gastrointestinal disorders (9 % in crofelemer- and 6 % in placebo-treated groups). During the long-term PF phase, the TEAEs were similar to the PC phase for crofelemer treatment. Most frequently reported TEAEs were upper respiratory tract infections (4 %), cough, nasopharyngitis, bronchitis, nausea and ALT elevation (3 % each) and AST increases, back pain, flatulence, gastroenteritis, and headache and sinusitis (2 % each). There were no ECG signals suggesting any cardiac safety risk with crofelemer treatment at any dose compared to placebo patients. Furthermore, crofelemer did not adversely affect the HIV status of the patients or the efficacy of ART in the ADVENT trial.

20.8.6 Pharmacokinetic Analysis

Population pharmacokinetic analysis using the sparse sampling technique showed that crofelemer absorption was negligible in all the treated patients. About 15 % of patients from the highest dose group of crofelemer (500 mg BID) in the PC phase had quantifiable crofelemer plasma concentrations exceeding 50 ng/mL. The dose selected for stage 2 (125 mg BID), less than 1 % of the plasma samples, had quantifiable crofelemer plasma concentrations.

20.8.7 Regulatory Recommendation

The NDA was submitted to FDA in December 2011 and crofelemer got approved for symptomatic treatment of HIV-related diarrhea on December 31, 2012. The drug is marketed as Fulyzaq.

References

DiMasi JA, Hansen RW, Grabowski HG (2003) The price of innovation: new estimates of drug development costs. J Health Econ 22:151–185

Orloff J, Douglas F, Pinheiro J, Levinson S, Branson M, Chaturvedi P, Ette E, Gallo P, Hirsch G, Mehta C, Patel N, Sabir S, Springs S, Stanski D, Evers M, Fleming E, Singh N, Tramontin T, Golub H (2009) The future of drug development: advancing clinical trial design. Nat Rev Drug Discov 8(11):949–957

Lawrence D, Bretz F, Pocock S (2014) INHANCE: An adaptive confirmatory study with dose selection at interim. In Trifilieff A (ed). Indacaterol – The first once-daily long-acting beta2 agonist for COPD, Springer, Basel, pp 77–92

MacArthur RD, Hawkins T, Brown SJ, LaMarca A, Chaturvedi P, Ernst J (2012) ADVENT trial: crofelemer for the treatment of secretory diarrhea in HIV+ individuals. Conference on retroviruses and opportunistic infections (CROI), Seattle, WA, March 2012, Poster O-117

Murray CJL, Lopez AD (1996) Global health statistics. World Health Organization, New York, pp 256–258

Malago JJ (2010) Diarrhea: causes, types and treatment. In: Wilson HM (ed) Diarrhea: causes, types and treatments. Nova, New York, NY, pp 1–41

Field M (2003) Intestinal ion transport and pathophysiology of diarrhea. J Clin Invest 111:931–943

Bode H, Lenzner L, Kraemer O et al (2005) The HIV protease inhibitors saquinavir, ritonavir and nelfinavir induce apoptosis and decrease barrier function in human intestinal epithelial cells. Antivir Ther 10:645–655

Braga Neto MB, Aguiar CV, Maciel JG et al (2010) Evaluation of HIV protease and nucleoside reverse transcriptase inhibitors on proliferation, necrosis, aproptosis in intestinal epithelial cells and electrolyte and water transport and epithelial barrier function in mice. BMC Gastroenterol 10:90

MacArthur RD, DuPont HL (2012) Etiology and pharmacologic management of noninfectious diarrhea in HIV-infected individuals in the highly active antiretroviral therapy era. Clin Inf Dis 55:860–867

Ubillas R, Jolad SD, Bruening RC, Kernan MR, King SR et al (1994) SP-303, an antiviral oligomeric proanthocyanadin from the latex of Croton lechleri (Sangre de Drago). Phytomedicine 1:77–106

Gabriel SE, Davenport SE, Steagall RJ, Vimal V, Carlson T and Rozhon EJ (1999) A novel plant-derived inhibitor of cAMP-mediated fluid and chloride secretion. Am J Physiol 276 (Gastrointest Liver Physiol 39):G58–G73

Tradtrantip L, Namkung W, Verkman AS (2010) Crofelemer, an antisecretory antidiarrheal proanthocyanadin oligomer extracted from Croton lechleri targets two distinct intestinal chloride channels. Mol Pharmacol 77:69–78

DiCesare D, DuPont HL, Mathewson JJ et al (2002) A double blind, placebo-controlled study of SP-303 (Provir) in the symptomatic treatment of acute diarrhea among travelers to Jamaica and Mexico. Am J Gastroenterol 97:2585–2588

Sharma A, Bolmal C, Dinakaran N, Rajadhyaksha G, Ernst J (2008) 48th Interscience conference on antimicrobial agents and chemotherapy (ICAAC), Abstract L-3595

Bardhan P, Khan WA, Ahmed S et al (2008) Evaluation of safety and efficacy of a novel anti-secretory anti-diarrheal agent crofelemer (NP-303) in combination with a single oral dose of azithromycin for the treatment of acute dehydrating diarrhea caused by Vibrio cholera. US-Japan Cooperative Medical Science Program. 43rd Conference on cholera and other bacterial enteric infections, Kyushu University, Fukuoka, Japan, Abstract

Mangel AW, Chaturvedi P (2008) Evaluation of crofelemer in the treatment of diarrhea-predominant irritable bowel syndrome patients. Digestion 78:180–186

Holodniy M, Koch H, Mistal M, Schmidt JM et al (1999) A double blind, randomized, placebo-controlled phase II study to assess the safety and efficacy of orally administered SP-303 for the symptomatic treatment of diarrhea in patients with AIDS. Am J Gastroenterol 94:3267–3273

Posch M, Koenig F, Branson M, Brannath W, Dunger-Baldauf C, Bauer P (2005) Testing and estimation in flexible group sequential designs with adaptive treatment selection. Stat Med 24:3697–3714

Bauer P, Kieser M (1999) Combining different phases in the development of medical treatments within a single trial. Stat Med 18:1833–1848

Index

CPSIA information can be obtained at www.ICGtesting.com
Printed in the USA
BVOW10*0333201014

371505BV00001B/13/P